# HIDDEN CAUSES OF INJURY, PREVENTION AND CORRECTION, FOR

## FOR

# RUNNING ATHLETES

## AND JOGGERS

## *John Jesse*

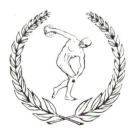

## *THE ATHLETIC PRESS*

Pasadena, California 91105

# HIDDEN CAUSES OF INJURY, PREVENTION AND CORRECTION, FOR RUNNING ATHLETES AND JOGGERS

Copyright © 1977 by John Jesse
All Rights Reserved

Published by The Athletic Press
A Division of Golden West Books
San Marino, California 91108 U.S.A.

Library of Congress Catalog Card No. 77-12214
I.S.B.N. No. 0-87095-065-7

**Library of Congress Cataloging in Publication Data**

Jesse, John, 1915–
    Hidden causes of injury, prevention and correction,
for running athletes and joggers.

    1.  Sports—Accidents and injuries.  2.  Running—
Accidents and injuries.  3.  Human mechanisms.
4.  Exercise therapy.  5.  Running—Training.  I.  Title.
RD97.J47 c.1          617'.L027          77-12214
ISBN 0-87095-065-7

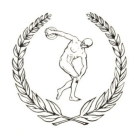

# THE ATHLETIC PRESS
P.O. Box 2314-D
Pasadena, California 91105

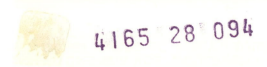

## DEDICATION

This book is dedicated to the following men who first brought to the attention of the athletic world, the predisposing causes of athletic injuries and overuse syndromes, and the hidden factors of muscular imbalance, postural faults, foot faults, and psychological conditions. They are Dr. Charles Lowman, Orthopedic Physician; Dr. W. E. Tucker, Orthopedic Physician; Dr. J. V. Cerney, Physical Medicine and Podiatrist; Dr. Bruce Ogilvie, Psychologist; Dr. Charles Tutko, Psychologist, and T. McClurg, Physiotherapist.

There is a dead medical literature and there is a live one. The dead is not all ancient, and the live is not all modern.

—Oliver Wendell Holmes*

*The Complete Works of Oliver Wendell Holmes (Boston: Houghton Mifflin Co., 1895).

# Preface

The first thing a coach, trainer, or orthopedic physician is likely to say on seeing a work like this is, "What? Another book on the injuries and disabilities of the athlete or physical fitness jogger?" I would understand his exasperation. This book, however, is entirely different from its predecessors; it deals with the prevention of athletic injuries and overuse syndromes through exercise. Fitness is the best prevention against injury.

For years, the writer has subscribed to more than 40 athletic and sports medicine journals from around the world. Rarely does an issue lack some type of article on the problems of treating athletic injuries. Both medical and athletic writers constantly comment on the tremendous increase in the total number of participants in competitive running and physical fitness jogging. These authors place emphasis on the need for year-round training, the results of running on hard surfaces and roadways, the total amount of mileage covered each week which results in an ever-increasing number of lower extremity minor strains, sprains, and overuse syndromes. Today, more and more medical practitioners and podiatrists are devoting their entire time to the diagnosis and treatment of such conditions.

The medical specialists who deal with athletic injuries have done an outstanding job in the rehabilitation process. They now recognize the importance of progressive resistance exercise as an essential part of rehabilitation. However, little has been written about the prevention of athletic injuries and overuse syndromes through use of specific exercises. Their have been only general admonitions that a high level of athletic fitness is the best prevention against injuries.

From the few books that do stress injury prevention, the reader can learn what to do; but their authors fail to explain how to prevent or correct the factors involving the athlete's body that predisposed him to athletic injury. This has been substantiated by many sports medicine specialists and coaches.

In 1969, Dr. Robert Kerlan, a prominent orthopedic sports medicine specialist, commenting on a knee injury incurred by Wilt Chamberlain, the star center for the Los Angeles Lakers basketball team, stated:

> Doctors have been making concentrated studies in the field of athletic injuries for about 20 years. They have made progress from the standpoint of taking care of minor injuries, but I don't know if any major progress has been made yet in the field where it is needed most. That is, in prevention.

In July 1974, Dr. James Garrick, speaking on football and skiing injuries, commented:

> Another aspect of this second problem, implementation, is the relative lack of attention paid to injury prevention. It is not uncommon to attend three- and four-day "sports medicine" conference/courses and hear not a word about injury prevention. We seem to be well-informed about the healthy athlete and how he functions and about the seriously injured athlete and how he might be repaired. We are not so well-informed about the task of keeping the healthy athlete from becoming an injured athlete.[1]

Starzynski, the Polish National Coach, in a speech before a National A.A.U. Track and Field Clinic in 1972, pointed out the necessity for a philosophy of prevention, stating:

> Prophylactics, the science of preventing injuries through specially conceived exercises, is becoming—due to the constantly increasing workloads and growing intensity of workouts—an absolute prerequisite in modern training. Again and again even the best athletes are prevented by injury from taking part in most important meets. The regenerating process, the chances for rehabilitation, as well as the growing scale and potential of the special, preventive exercises, are still only talked about—marginally at that.[4]

The author's interest in the subject of prevention of athletic injuries began three years ago with the realization that, despite a high level of strength, speed, endurance, or skill, the athlete is of no value to himself, his coach, or his teammates if he is unable to compete, or if his training is interrupted prior to a local, state, national, world, or Olympic competition.

This concept applies equally to the physical fitness jogger. How many joggers and runners have worked months to increase their oxygen intake capacity and reduce their pulse rate, then lost all of their gains in four to six weeks of forced inactivity due to a minor strain or sprain affecting their lower extremities or feet?

With few exceptions, little mention has been made in the sports literature relating to athletic injuries of the hidden factors of muscular imbalance, postural faults, foot faults, and psychological proneness to injury as predisposing causes of athletic injuries and overuse syndromes.

Lowman, the eminent American orthopedic specialist, in his writings directed to the medical, orthopedic, and physical education professions during the past 30 years, has been the lone proponent of the concept that postural faults are a major factor in athletic injuries. His talk before the American Medical Association on the "Effects of Postural Deviations on Athletic Performance" was a masterpiece. In summary, he stated:

> Any machine which on the whole or in any of its parts deviates from the true alignment cannot be expected to perform to the same potential as one which is properly aligned. Consequently, everyone having to do with physical training in athletics should recognize that: (1) The earlier the proper steps are taken to correct and/or ameliorate postural faults, the more proficiency there should be in later performance. (2) To coach an athlete to his maximum without attention to correctible details in his faulty body mechanics may contribute to later disturbances which will simply hasten the wear and tear that accelerates the aging process going on relentlessly in his musculoskeletal apparatus. . . . Junior coaches—in advising and coaching boys and girls—can lay a proper foundation for prevention of faults.[2]

In the late 1950's, Slocum, James, and Brubaker at the University of Oregon, and Klafs and Arnheim at Long Beach State followed in Lowman's footsteps, emphasizing the importance of postural faults in running efficiency and as a predisposing cause of athletic injuries and overuse syndromes.

W. E. Tucker, an English orthopedist, was, like Lowman, a man ahead of his time in emphasizing the importance of posture in the mechanics of athletic movement. He has consistently maintained over the past 30 years that postural faults represent one of the three major causes of athletic injuries.

T. McClurg Anderson, a Scottish physiotherapist, wrote one of the first books on kinesiology as applied to the athletic world. He, too, clearly pointed out that postural faults created poor body mechanics that led to injuries of the lower extremities.

Dr. J. V. Cerney, a podiatrist, was the pioneer in pointing out the importance of the foot in athletic performance and the contribution of foot faults to athletic injuries. He was followed by *Runner's World* magazine, the California School of Podiatric Medicine, and well-known podiatrists such as Barnes, Pagliano, Schuster, and Subotnick.

Dr. George Sheehan, a cardiologist and distance runner, has consistently advocated in his medical column in *Runner's World* that orthopedic physicians should pay greater attention to the foot in lower extremity injuries and overuse syndromes.

During the past few years, medical and sports literature has placed great emphasis on the troublesome "overuse" syndromes affecting runners and joggers. Various theories have been advanced as to the predisposing or actual causes of these syndromes, e.g., year-round running, total mileage covered each week, running on banked or hard surfaces, improper footwear, etc. However, in *Runner's World*, Sheehan, commenting on overuse syndromes among runners and joggers, stated:

> But evidence is accumulating that too many miles too fast is only part of the story. (Any number of perfectly healthy runners are handling the same distances/speeds.) Some biomechanical difficulty (malfunction in the running mechanism) has to be added to long mileage and high speed to cause disease. This biomechanical problem is most often in the foot.[3]

Three of the four hidden factors—muscular imbalance, postural faults, and foot faults—are so common among the general population that it is doubtful whether any young athlete enters the field of athletic competition without being affected to a lesser or greater degree by one or more of them.

The writer believes a more detailed and complete discussion of these factors and of the methods of correcting them or preventing their further development will enable the coach, trainer, and athlete to cope with them early in the young athlete's career. It will enable the athlete to reduce to a minimum the number of roadblocks and setbacks he suffers during training and in pursuit of his goals.

The information presented here should be of great value to the several million physical fitness joggers and runners in the population, because the book is aimed at providing understandable answers to all injuries that interrupt their progress toward attainment of an increased level of cardiovascular fitness, or that interfere with the psychological satisfactions obtained from engaging in such activities.

The human body supports itself against gravity, segment upon segment, relying on the muscles and ligaments that cross the joints, along with postural reflexes, to maintain an erect position and proper body alignment. Hence, there has to be a total or "holistic" approach to prevention and to correction of the hidden factors mentioned above. The reader must integrate his thinking to a total body concept.

If any body part deviates from its proper alignment, its weight must be counterbalanced by a deviation of another body part, above or below. Seldom is only one part of the body involved; usually, the entire body is out of alignment. It is, for example, of no value to correct foot faults without also correcting the compensating body faults in segments above the feet. The same holds true for correction of postural faults of the upper body; attention must also be given to correction of leg alignment and foot faults or foot positions in walking. The interrelationship of the different body segments and the interdependence of body faults in these segments will be emphasized as much as possible throughout this volume, although for learning and descriptive purposes the subject matter has been organized on a systematic segment-by-segment basis.

In stressing the importance of physical exercise as a preventive and corrective measure, the writer in no way intends to minimize the importance of surgery, casts, physical therapy, or orthotic appliances in the correction and rehabilitation of postural and foot defects that have altered the bone structure of the body or injuries that have seriously affected the body joints. The emphasis is on the importance and use of exercise in the prevention and correction of postural and foot faults which have not as yet altered the bone structure of the body. Neither is there any intention on the part of the writer to downgrade the importance of numerous factors given by authorities as causes of athletic injuries, e.g., inadequate warm-up or warm-down, improper footwear, hard and banked surfaces, changing from slow to fast running.

Finally, since this book is designed for distribution among professionals, specialists, coaches, trainers, athletes, and laymen, the dilemma of technical versus popular language presents itself. Some chapters, from the very nature of the subjects treated, require use of scientific terminology; but every effort has been made to keep technicalities down to their simpler terms. Wherever possible, anatomical terms and postural and foot fault terminology are explained by appropriate illustrations or explanations in parentheses, and a short glossary is included at the end of the book as an additional aid to the reader.

Hermosa Beach, California                                    John Jesse
April 1976

## REFERENCES

1. Garrick, James G., "Perspectives in Sports Medicine," *A.C.S.M. News,* July 1974.
2. Lowman, Charles L., "Effects of Postural Deviations on Athletic Performance," *A.M.A., Fourth National Conference on the Medical Aspects of Sports*, November 24, 1962.
3. Sheehan, George., "Look First at Your Feet," *Encyclopedia of Athletic Medicine, Runner's World Booklet No. 12*, June 1972.
4. Starzynski, Tadeuz., "Exercises to Prevent Injuries to Jumpers," *Track Technique*, No. 51, March 1973.

11

# Table of Contents

# Introductions

Fitness means different things to different people; it is not necessarily synonymous with health. The word "fit" nearly always implies fitness for some special activity. Jogging can create a state of preparedness for just about any sport. It can be combined with interval running, so important a part of training programme for the serious athlete. As well, a daily jog or run can keep the office-bound weekend sportsman's weight, circulation, heart and lungs in good order. Indeed it is also prescribed by many physicians, especially in the United States, as part of a rehabilitation programme for their post-heart attack patients.

This book goes much further than that. It covers the hidden causes of injury, not generally known, to sportsmen of all types. These are described in a clear and informative manner so that any sportsman (not only joggers and runners) can understand, and every medical man approve.

Faulty posture is frequently one of the causes of injury. It is a delight to me to see how well my conception of Active Alerted Posture is explained. Two laws govern movement: before motion starts the individual should be in the upright position so that the load, the force and the lever are one above the other. Then, when action takes place the activator muscles must be assisted by the synergic ones and they must work together on a firm prime-fixing base. When an accident or injury occurs it is usually one of these two laws—or both—that have been broken. So many sportsmen do not understand even the elementary principles of muscle action. The knowledge they can gain from this book will help prevent the accidents and injuries that so often take place during training and to avoid chronic postural strain.

John Jesse must be congratulated on producing such a well-balanced book with its wealth of knowledge so concisely and interestingly presented.

William E. Tucker, C.V.O., F.R.C.S.
Honorary Consultant Orthopedic Surgeon
Royal London Homeopathic Hospital

After carefully reviewing John Jesse's book, I can only say to all coaches, trainers, and anyone with an interest in helping athletes, to hurry out and buy the book. I also suggest that it become a part of the library of every high school and college.

John Jesse has done a remarkable job of explaining and diagramming significant therapy for problems that face all athletes sooner or later in their athletic career. He has done his homework well, researching the literature and has also come up with some original ideas, for which he deserves additional commendation. With the increased interest in jogging and running, and the vast number of people involved, this book should be a valuable aid.

Dr. Robert W. Barnes—Podiatrist
President, American College of Podiatric Sports Medicine
Fellow, American College of Foot Surgeons
Fellow, American College of Sports Medicine

Joggers and runners occur in a wide variety of ages, abilities, and body types. In common they have unbridled enthusiasm, an utter disregard for solitude, a hope of immortality, and numerous aches and pains.

John Jesse has sorted out the many factors influencing injury amongst these athletes in a most thorough and scientific manner. He is as painstaking in delineating exercises and training methods. This attention to detail comes as no surprise. I have known the author since our University days. He was then a fine athlete, and a diligent student of physical culture.

The years have added luster to his scholarly attributes. His enthusiasm is unquenchable, his writing is encyclopedic. He has organized and condensed in this volume an unbelievable mass of material.

Those who will study, not browse, through this book will be well informed; those who follow Jesse's method of training and exercise may well be rewarded with improved performance and fewer injuries.

J. Harold LaBriola, M.D.
Associate Professor, University of Southern California
Orthopaedic Consultant, Athletic Dept., University of Southern California
Director of Sports Medicine Clinic, Los Angeles Orthopaedic Hospital

By tradition physicians and podiatrists have looked upon sports related ailments with little or no concern. Only since the great sports participation explosion of the 1960's, have doctors found more and more of their patients coming to them with complaints that are specifically related to an athletic related injury. Most medical practitioners who have applied ordinary therapeutics to severely injured athletes find these do not necessarily work. Besides doctors are completely unaware of the cause or the preventative measures for such injuries unless they have engaged in sports medicine practices.

At long last we have finally bridged the gap between theory and prevention of injury in book form with John Jesse's new volume. His text deals with the hidden factors of muscular imbalance, postural and foot faults, leg alignment, and the psychological injury prone personality that are the predisposing factors in most athletic injuries and overuse syndromes.

A portion of this book deals with the role of exercise and manipulation in the prevention, correction and rehabilitation of the injured athlete. Jesse not only presents a clear and concise explanation of the various exercise regimes, but presents the theory behind their use and the role of strength and flexibility in injury prevention.

The prime theme running throughout this book is the concept of the body form as a total, rather than as separate, individual segments. He states that "the body supports itself against gravity, segment upon segment, relying on muscles and ligaments that cross the joints ... if any body part deviates from its proper alignment, its weight must be counterbalanced by a deviation of any body part.

17

It is seldom that one part of the body alone is involved ..." In just these few sentences, Jesse has presented the key to the prevention and cure of the athletic injury.

An extremely controversial concept brought out in this book is the hypothesis that muscular imbalance is a major predisposing and causitive factor that results in muscles and fascia strains, ligament sprains and other overuse syndrome complaints in the back, the legs, and the feet. A considerable amount of material is presented to support this theory. An interesting concept that Jesse points out is that most athletes develop one set of muscles, while failing to develop the antagonistic set. This he contends is the root of many athletic injuries.

This book is a "must" for all those in the medical profession concerned with athletic injuries. The athlete himself will find this book an invaluable tool in order to pinpoint his own physical faults and institute an injury prevention program.

Dr. John W. Pagliano—Podiatrist
Vice President, American Academy of Podiatric Sports Medicine
Associate, American College of Foot Surgeons
A.A.U. 50-Mile Champion (1972)
Staff Writer *Track Technique Magazine*
Member, American College of Sports Medicine

# Part One

## Background and Causes

# 1

# The Problem

During the past 30 years, sports participation has increased enormously. A parallel increase has been manifested both quantitatively and qualitatively in standards of performance and in the severity of training required to achieve success, particularly at the top levels of competition. In addition, there has been a tremendous increase in the number of relatively sedentary persons who have taken up jogging to improve their cardiovascular fitness. One result of these developments is a vast increase in the number of injuries to the lower extremities and the feet of those participating in the running sports. In particular, this increase in injuries has derived purely from the training process.

*Runner's World* magazine conducted a survey among 1600-plus runners to determine the extent of injuries suffered.[6] The report concluded that one runner in five had suffered knee or Achilles tendon damage. One in 10 had experienced shin splints, or forefoot breaks, bruises, and strains. The incidence of breakdowns among runners, many of whom had more than one injury, is reflected in the following chart:

| | | | | |
|---|---|---|---|---|
| 1. | Knee | 22.5% | 8. Calf | 6.8% |
| 2. | Achilles | 20.3% | 9. Hamstring | 4.6% |
| 3. | Shin | 9.9% | 10. Hip | 3.7% |
| 4. | Forefoot | 9.4% | 11. Back | 3.1% |
| 5. | Heel | 7.2% | 12. Groin | 1.8% |
| 6. | Ankles | 7.0% | 13. Thigh | 1.5% |
| 7. | Arch | 7.0% | 14. Stomach muscles | 0.2% |

Sperryn pointed out that most runners plant each foot over three million times each year, in addition to their normal daily activities.

He wrote:

> In modern track and field athletics rising standards of competition and training have imposed increasing strains on the limbs of athletes. Following Corrigan's (1968) classification into trauma and overuse injuries we find that in runners overuse injuries are becoming the biggest single barrier to the pursuit of a successful career. In a series of 150 consecutive sports injuries seen at King's College Hospital, 32 percent of all sports injuries were classified as overuse injuries but in track and field athletes these injuries accounted for no less than 64.3 percent of new attendances.[7]

He claimed that Eastern European statistics supported his studies of the high incidence of overuse injuries among runners.

Chapman classified the types of injuries occurring to 168 athletes.[2] The most common categories were strains (33%), stress fractures (16%), sprains (14%), tenosynovitis (12%), and miscellaneous (25%). The injuries were distributed by events as follows: sprinters (24%), middle distance (15%), distance (41%), joggers (3%), and undetermined (17%).

Strains of tendons and muscles (hamstring) were the most common. Stress fractures, mainly of tibia and metatarsals, made up the next injury group, followed by sprains, due primarily to irritation of tendon lining (ankle). Achilles tendon problems and a large percentage of various other types of injuries made up the rest.

Brubaker and James presented data on 109 cases of injuries to runners.[1] The most common categories of these were strains (33%), fractures (20%), sprains (14%), and tenosynovitis (12%). The injuries were distributed by event as follows: sprinters (24%), middle distance (15%), distance (41%), joggers (3%).

In 1949, Morehouse conducted a study on outer sole design of shoes to minimize landing shock among paratroopers.[5] He determined that the downward force at heel strike during walking was approximately 120 percent of body weight. It was pointed out that a 160-pound man, during a normal day's walking averaging 19,000 steps, would receive 3,705,000 pounds of repeated jolts to the musculoskeletal structure, and that in walking down an incline this force would be increased to 200 percent of body weight.

Though actual studies of such action have not been made, it is estimated that during running there is a downward foot strike on each foot of approximately 200 percent of body weight. Based on this estimate, a 140-pound runner striking the ground 5,000 times an hour would generate 1,400,000 pounds of repeated jolts each hour; a 150-pound man, 1,500,000 pounds; and a 160-pound man, 1,600,000 pounds.

From the above, it is readily understandable why there is such a tremendous increase in  injuries and overuse syndromes, particularly when the skeletal structure is biomechanically out of alignment due to muscular imbalance or minor postural and foot faults.

## REFERENCES

1. Brubaker, C. E. and James, S. L., "Incidence of Non-traumatic Injuries to Runners," *Abstracts of 20th Annual Meeting of American College of Sports Medicine*, May 7-9, 1973.
2. Chapman, Brian, "Running Injuries," *Modern Athlete and Coach*, January 1975.
3. Glick, James M. and Katch, Victor L., "Musculoskeletal Injuries in Jogging," *Archives of Physical Medicine and Rehabilitation*, March 1970.
4. Liljedahl, Sten-Otto, "Common Injuries in Connection with Conditioning Exercises," *Scandinavian Journal of Rehabilitative Medicine*, 3:1, 1971.
5. Morehouse, Laurence E., "Influence of Flexible Outsole on the Dynamics of the Walking Gait," *International Record of Medicine*, 170, No. 8, August 1957.
6. *Runner's World Booklet No. 25*, (World Publishing Co., July 1973). Reprinted by permission of the publisher.
7. Sperryn, P. N., "Runner's Heel," *British Journal of Sports Medicine*, July 1971.

# 2

## Neuromuscular Coordination and Body Movements

The two most important physical properties of muscle tissue in relation to the movement of the body or maintenance of an upright posture are: (1) contractibility—capacity to shorten and ability to develop tension (strength), and (2) irritability—ability to respond to a stimulus from the nervous system. Muscle contractions are of two types: phasic and tonic.

### PHASIC CONTRACTIONS

Phasic contractions of muscle tissue result in movements of the body. They may be either volitional or reflex in nature. They are volitional when the athlete intends to make a certain movement. They are reflex when they occur in reaction to a stimulus to the nervous system, such as a threat from the environment, e.g., a hot stove, a boxer's punch, etc. For this aspect of our discussion, we are more concerned with the volitional nature of phasic contractions.

When a muscle contracts, it actively develops tension (strength), shortens, and moves the bone to which it is attached. It may develop tension without shortening to maintain a held position or, when opposing a superior force, to resist lengthening of the muscle.

Skeletal muscles are almost completely dependent for their operation on the stimuli received from the central nervous system. Neuromuscular integration is the key to the capacity of the body to coordinate the action of the muscles of the body in the most efficient pattern to accomplish a specific movement or series of movements. It is a major factor in the development of a high level of speed and in the maximum expression of muscle strength against resistance.

24

1. Stimulation (contraction) of muscle tissue (fibers) is accomplished by volleys of nerve impulses from the central nervous system.

2. It is common knowledge that muscle contraction strength (tension) is adjusted to exert the amount of force required to carry out a muscular act. Muscles have the ability to contract strongly or weakly, or at any of a great number of graded intermediate levels. This mechanism of gradation is due to the ability of the central nervous system to send impulses to a greater or lesser number of motor units. The increase or decrease in the strength of a muscular contraction through gradation stems from the interaction of three factors: (A) the number of motor units stimulated; (B) frequency of the stimuli from the central nervous system; and (C) timing of the stimuli to the various motor units.

3. Three others factors have a strong influence on the amount of internal tension (strength) a muscle can develop when it contracts:

   (A) A muscle exerts its greatest tension when it functions at its greatest length. It can lift a greater load or produce a greater force the more it is pre-stretched from its natural length in the body prior to contraction.

   (C) As speed of muscle shortening increases, the amount of tension it can develop lessens. There is an optimum speed for a needed amount of force. Hill points out that optimum speeds for muscular efficiency and power are approximately similar in nature—20 to 30 percent of the maximum speed at which the muscle can shorten under zero load.[1]

4. The amount of tension which will stretch out a maximally contracted muscle to its original resting length is called the absolute muscle power.

5. A maximally contracted muscle is approximately 25 percent shorter than in the relaxed state. The greatest amount of passive stretching is 1.6 times its relaxed length. All motion by body joints must occur within these limits.

6. Whether or not a muscle shortens when it contracts and develops tension depends upon the type of resistance it encounters:

   (A) *Concentric contraction*—A muscle develops tension sufficient to overcome a resistance and produce work, so that the muscle visibly shortens and moves a body part despite the resistance.

   (B) *Eccentric contraction*—A specific resistance or load overcomes the muscle tension and the muscle actually lengthens. In this case, the muscle does negative work.

   (C) *Static or isometic contraction*—The muscle develops tension insufficient to move a body part against a given resistance and the length of the muscle remains unchanged.

*N.B.*: Both concentric and eccentric contractions are known as isotonic (dynamic) contractions.

## TONIC CONTRACTIONS

**The basic purpose** of tonic muscle tissue contractions is to maintain muscle tonus and control upright posture. Muscle tonus is the slight contraction of muscles in contrast to the very dynamic nature of phasic contractions. It provides the normal resistance to passive elongation or stretch of the muscles, and serves to prevent the full weight of body parts from falling on the ligaments binding the body joints together.

The impulses (stimuli) that bring about muscle tonus are derived from the sensory receptors (proprioceptors) in muscles and tendons. These stimuli result from changes in the tension of the muscle. The most important of them, in respect to muscle tonus and maintenance of posture, is the stretch reflex. When muscles are stretched, the sensory receptors in the muscles send impulses to the spinal cord which bring about a reflex contraction of the same muscle.

The extensor muscle (antigravity or postural) reflex stretch is well-developed in the antigravity muscles that maintain upright posture—the extensor muscles of the body joints, the supinator muscles of the foot, the abdominal and scapula adductors. Because of this fact, the muscle tonus in the antigravity muscles of the body theoretically should be greater than in the other muscles. In reality, however, the muscle tonus of the abdominal and scapula adductor muscles of the upper back in today's men and women is rarely developed to its greatest normal potential. This is manifested by the prevalence in industrialized societies of round upper backs and sagging abdomens.

## MOVEMENT

Muscles are classified by the roles they play in producing body movements. A mover or *agonist* muscle contracts and brings about movement at a body joint. A *prime mover* is a muscle primarily responsible for causing a specific joint action. An *antagonist* muscle contraction produces a joint movement directly opposite to a joint action caused by the contraction of an *agonist muscle*. A *fixator* or *stabilizer* muscle anchors, steadies, or supports a bone or body part so that an *agonist* or *antagonist* muscle has a firm base upon which to pull. A *neutralizer* muscle contracts to neutralize or counteract an undesired action of another contracting muscle. A *synergist* muscle assists a *prime mover* muscle in a supporting function to cause a joint movement.

26

Muscles are also classified by the action of a body joint or body part that results from their contraction. For the purpose of these classifications, the body is assumed to be in a standing upright position with arms hanging at the sides and palms of the hands facing forward.

*Flexor*        *A muscle that bends a limb at a joint.*

*Extensor*     *A muscle that straightens or extends a limb.*

*Abductor*    *A muscle that moves a limb away from the midline of the body.*

*Adductor*    *A muscle that moves a limb toward the midline of the body.*

*Rotator*      A muscle that brings about rotation at a joint. If a a rotation is inward toward the midline of the body, the muscle is an *inward rotator*. If rotation is outward from the midline, the muscle is an *outward rotator*.

1. Skeletal muscles seldom, if ever, act alone. Individual muscles are not represented in the nervous centers and pathways of the central nervous system, which thinks and acts in terms of movement, not in terms of single muscles.

2. When an athlete projects his body in movement, or acts against a resistance, his body acts as a whole. Most muscles have more than one joint action. The coordination of specific muscle actions in the most efficient manner to accomplish a specific movement is the result of a high degree of neuromuscular integration. *Agonist* muscles that are doing the work or bringing about a specific body movement have to contract; *antagonist* muscles must relax; *stabilizer* muscles have to contract and fix other body joints to provide a stable base and maintain balance.

3. An important aspect of neuromuscular integration in coordinating our muscle actions and movements is a neurological process known as reciprocal innervation or reciprocal inhibition of *antagonist* muscles. Sensory organs in the muscles and tendons are activated when muscles contract. They send impulses along nerve pathways to the cerebellum portion of the brain, which is the muscular coordinating system of the central nervous system. The cerebellum then sends impulses back to the opposite muscle groups, causing them to relax. This allows the *agonist* (mover) and *antagonist* muscles which control flexion and extension in a joint (knee of the runner) to contract and relax in an alternating synchronized manner, and permits the joint to move through its complete range of motion. The efficiency of the reciprocal innervation process is highly important to the development of maximum velocity or speed.

4. The athlete and jogger should be familiar with that aspect of muscular teamwork expressed in athletic movements as they relate

to running, hurdling, or jogging known as ballistic nature movement. Ballistic nature movement includes three phases: (A) an acceleration phase, characterized by contraction of *prime mover* muscles accompanied by relaxation of *antagonist* muscles; (B) a coasting phase, characterized by relaxation of both *prime movers* and *antagonists*; and (C) a deceleration phase, characterized by relaxation of *prime movers* and contraction of *antagonists*.

The limiting factors on body movement will be discussed in Chapter 24.

The movements of the principal body joints involved in running and jogging are shown in the illustrations below:

## MOVEMENTS OF SPINAL COLUMN

*Flexion*          *Extension*          *Lateral Flexion*          *Rotation*

## MOVEMENTS OF HIP JOINT

    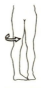

*Flexion*   *Extension*   *Abduction*   *Adduction*   *External Rotation*   *Internal Rotation*

## MOVEMENTS OF KNEE JOINT

*Flexion*          *Extension*

Muscular movements of the foot and ankle are illustrated in Chapter 17.

### REFERENCES

1. Hill, A. V., "The Design of Muscles," *British Medical Bulletin* No. 12 (1956), p. 165.

# 3

# Physical Properties of Soft Tissue Structures

Books on the physiology of exercise emphasize the importance of the muscle tissue properties of the human body, particularly the contractile property of muscle tissue that provides the power for moving the bony levers of the body. Little attention is given the connective tissues of the body which bind together the other body structures, other than mention that tendons are the attachment of the muscle tissue to bones or other muscle tissue and that ligaments bind the body joints together.

Books on injury prevention should stress all of the physical properties of both muscle and connective tissue. These are the body tissues that are subject to the strains, sprains, inflammations, and stress and overuse syndromes encountered by runners, hurdlers, and physical fitness joggers.

All soft body tissues are classified according to their predominant cell type. Muscle cells have been classified as striated, smooth, and cardiac tissue. Connective cells have been classified as collagenous, reticular, and elastic tissue.

The following discussion deals with the physical properties of striated muscle tissue and collagenous and elastic connective tissue only.

## MUSCLE TISSUE

Skeletal striated muscle tissue possesses four physiological properties: (1) Contractibility—capacity to shorten (contract) and ability to develop tension. (2) Extensibility—ability to stretch. (3) Elasticity—ability to regain its original size and length after being stretched. (4) Irritability—ability to respond to a stimulus.

## CONTRACTIBILITY

All movements involved in running, hurdling, and jogging result from contraction of skeletal muscles that provide the driving force for movement of the skeleton's bony levers. A muscle always pulls; it never pushes. Of the three types of muscle tissue found in the body, we are concerned here only with striated (skeletal) muscle tissue, which comprises about 40 to 45 percent or total body weight and is under the voluntary direction and control of the central nervous system (brain and spinal cord).

The basic component of skeletal muscle is the muscle fiber. Groups of 100 to 150 fibers are bound together with connective tissue to form a unit. This unit is bound together with others to form larger units and, ultimately, a whole muscle—itself covered by a connective tissue sheath. A single muscle will contain several thousand muscle fibers and units. The total muscle is attached to the bone by tendons.

The individual muscle fiber (a number of muscle cells) consists of a mass of sacroplasm in which are imbedded long filaments known as myofibrils, the contractile element of the fiber. Each fiber has a covering called the sacrolemma.

Two types of muscle fibers are found together in the individual muscle. White muscle fibers with a limited blood supply are designed for speech. They produce rapid powerful contractions of infrequent occurrence, but fatigue quite easily. They are preponderant in the flexor muscles. Red muscle fibers have three times as slow a contraction time as white muscle fibers. They produce slow frequent contractions and are better suited to endurance work because of a much greater blood supply, as they are not easily fatigued. They are prevalent in the postural extensor muscles.

Each bundle of muscle fibers is innervated by motor nerves consisting of numerous neurons (nerve cells) emanating from the central nervous system. A single motor nerve has from several dozen to several thousand branches. One motor neuron (nerve cell), its branches, and the group of muscle fibers it can stimulate to contraction make up a motor unit. A skeletal muscle may consist of several hundred motor units.

Skeletal muscles are also supplied with sensory nerve endings (receptors) located between groups of muscle fibers. The receptors are stimulated by changes in muscle tension (contraction, relaxation, and stretching) which send impulses to the central nervous system (CNS). These impulses play an important role in maintenance of muscle tone.

Muscular contraction involves the transformation of chemical energy into mechanical energy; chemical energy is derived from combustion processes (oxidation of carbohydrates, fats, and proteins). Each muscle receives oxygen and other nutrients required for its metabolic needs from the circulatory system. The arteries feeding the muscle divide up into an innumerable number of small capillaries that penetrate the outer covering of the muscle fiber. Their walls are extremely thin and allow an easy transfer of needed energy substances from the blood to the fiber.

## EXTENSIBILITY

The extensibility quality of muscle tissue permits the muscle to be stretched 1.6 times its original resting length before it ruptures. If the muscle is shortened due to other factors, the fibers will rupture before they reach their maximum extensibility range. Muscle tissue resistance to tear or rupture is much less than that of the tendon which attaches the muscle to the bone or another muscle.

## ELASTICITY

The elastic quality of the muscle tissue permits the fiber to return to its normal length after being stretched. Elasticity depends on the sacrolemma covering of the muscle cell and the connective tissue enveloping the muscle fiber. The elastic fibers take care of shortening when stretching ceases, and the collagenous fibers protect the muscle against overstretching. Elasticity is the passive structure of muscle tissue. The only stress to which it is subjected in this state is tension of an acute or continuous nature. The acute phase is due to sudden overstretching, while the continuous phase results when muscles are constantly under stretch due to body misalignment.

## IRRITABILITY

The irritability property of muscle tissue will be discussed in the following chapter.

## CONNECTIVE TISSUE

Connective tissue comprises a major portion of the total body mass. It binds together the muscle and skeletal structure of the body. It limits not only the range, but also the speed of movement. Many body components are entirely or largely composed of connective tissue. These include bones, cartilages, joints, aponeuroses (sheet-like tendons), muscle fascia, ligaments, and tendons, as well as the sacrolemma, endomysium, and periomysium that surround the units (cells and tissues) of the muscle tissue system.

The connective tissue of the body is subject not only to strains, ruptures, stress, and overuse syndromes, but—in addition—to sprains (knee and ankle ligaments) and deterioration of body joints, involving the articular cartilages, that lead to osteoarthritis of the joint.

Of the three types of connective tissue, only the collagenous (white) fibers and the elastic (yellow) fibers will be covered in this discussion.

Collagenous fibers, rich in protein, are essentially non-elastic and are found in the greatest proportion in tendons, ligaments, and fascia. Elastic fibers are the other important type of connective tissue fibers. They are characterized by the presence of the interstitial (between muscle cells) protein elastin. These fibers may be stretched, and when tension is relaxed will shorten again. They occur frequently mixed in with the more numerous collagenous fibers, but in certain locations of the body, such as in the posterior ligaments of the spinal column, rather large amounts of almost pure elastic fibers are found.

As a person grows older, the quality of elasticity in connective tissue tends to disappear. This tendency is greatly speeded up by inactivity, postural malalignment, and muscular imbalance.

## FASCIA

The connective tissue which forms enveloping sheaths around muscle is known as fascia. It consists principally of collagenous fibers, although the amount of elastic fibers varies with the functional activity of the muscle. Continuously active muscles have an abundance of elastic tissue, whereas the larger extremity muscles have a rather limited amount. Fascia resistance to tension stresses is very high. They can withstand momentary stresses during body movement up to their safety limits without rupturing. Protracted stress, however, results in a permanent elongation. Fascia also has a strong tendency to contract due to age, chilling, poor posture, and muscular imbalance. Contraction reduces the range of movement in body joints.

## LIGAMENTS

Most ligaments are almost pure collagenous tissue. There are pliant and flexible, but at the same time strong and inextensible. The exceptions to this are the ligaments of the spine and the spring ligament (Chapter 17, Figure 23) of the foot, which are made up almost entirely of elastin fibers and are quite elastic.

All ligaments can be permanently elongated if subjected to protracted stress from postural faults, bad leg alignment, or repetitive overstretching beyond their maximum safety limits. The term "sprain" refers to strained, torn, or ruptured ligaments.

# TENDONS

Tendons are generally composed of heavy collagenous fibers. Most tendons form narrow bands or rounded cords, with the exception of aponeuroses, which is a flat sheet and classified by some writers as fascia. Tendons have great strength and are practically inelastic.

As a rule, the tendon is stronger than the muscle to which it is attached. A normal tendon will not rupture. Tensions or loads large enough to tear tendon fibers or rupture the tendon will first rupture the muscle belly, separate the musculo-tendinous junction, cause the muscle origins to pull out, or fracture the bones to which they are attached.

Tendons undergo early degenerative changes since the central artery feeding blood to the tendon can disappear as early as the third decade of life. The tendon must then become dependent on circulation from the blood vessels in the area around itself. Tendon degeneration can also result from disease, stresses connected with postural faults, or extended overuse.

Rupture of the belly of the tendon is always preceded by degeneration. These spontaneous ruptures are most often seen in Achilles tendons of older runners. In the young athlete with normal tendons, an excessive load on the tendon severe enough to rupture the belly of it will instead result in avulsion (tearing away) of the tendon itself or parts of the bone to which it is attached.

# CARTILAGE

Cartilage is a rigid substance similar to the gristle in meat. Fibrous cartilage consists primarily of very thick collagenous fibers. These are found in the attachments of ligaments and tendons to the bone and in the inter-vertebral disks of the spinal column. In contrast, hyaline cartilage, which covers the articular surfaces of body joints, combines about 65 percent elastic fibers with 35 percent collagenous fibers. This provides it with a higher degree of flexibility combined with rigidity than that found in fibrocartilage.

1. The primary function of joint (hyaline) cartilage is to provide for the joint a smooth surface throughout its full range of motion. In carrying out this function, it is continuously subjected to stresses through the action of gravity on weight-bearing joints in lower extremities and to stresses produced by the tension of muscle in all joints.

2. In the normal joint under normal conditions, hyaline cartilage is highly extensible and compressible. This means that the cartilage can adapt itself to weight stress or loads by compressing, but will usually spring back into its original state after the stress or load is removed.

3. Two factors play an important part with respect to hyaline

joint cartilage—the amount of the load and the duration of the load. The latter factor is of particular importance. The longer the load continues, the less complete is the rebound of the hyaline cartilage after compression to its original state. Loads of short duration, within limits, show no deformation (compression), while similar loads repeated many times over or prolonged for a long period of time may cause permanent deformation and eventual degeneration of the hyaline cartilage.

4. The deformation of cartilage by compression is required if the greatest possible contact is to be achieved by the two bones composing the joint. It increases not only the contact area, but also the range of motion.

5. The stresses to which joint articulations are exposed must be met by relatively small areas of cartilage. The mechanical problems involved in body movement require that the fibers be arranged in such a manner that a sufficient number will always be at right angles to the imposed stress.

6. Hyaline cartilage may soften due to trauma or disease, or to abnormal joint mechanics resulting from postural faults, foot faults, muscle imbalance, and acquired or congenital malalignment of the legs. This is particularly so in the weight-bearing surface of lower body joints.

7. Deterioration of cartilage is the predisposing factor leading to osteo-arthritis (chronic degeneration) of body joints. Chondro-malacia patella—which is common among runners, particularly women—involves the degeneration and softening of the cartilage lining the posterior (under) side of the kneecap (patella). The predisposing factors are . poor leg alignment (knock-knees), also common among women, and foot faults. Repetitive stresses imposed by running lead to deterioration of the patella cartilage. Permanent deformation and eventual deterioration of the fibrous inter-vertebral disks of the spine are primarily due to poor posture.

8. During exercise, articular cartilage in body joints increases in thickness. During a rest period following exercise, the thickness diminishes approximately 10 percent.

9. Assuming that there is no malalignment of the legs due to congenital or acquired cases, that the legs are not excessively rotated inwards or outwards at the hip joint, and that the feet are pointed relatively straight ahead in walking and running, articular cartilage of lower body joints can be thickened. Rather than being worn down by excessive activity in weight bearing, the articular cartilage actually thickens and becomes healthier under the increased use and stress of exercise. The cartilaginous surfaces of the joint hypertrophy and the rate of repair of the cartilaginous friction loss is accelerated under these conditions of increased demand.

# GROWTH CARTILAGE AND THE TEEN-AGE RUNNER

Among specialists dealing with the histology of muscle and joint structures, it is well-known that fast-growing cells and tissues of youth, particularly during adolescence, are most vulnerable to damage or injury. Joint structures and epiphyseal growth cartilages are especially susceptible at this time.

Both static and dynamic stresses of the everyday activities of standing, walking, running, etc., to which the modern stress of training for runners is added, tend to increase the wear and tear on all joint surfaces, i.e., synovial lining of the joint, cartilages, and ligaments. If nutritional imbalances such as overweight or under-weight, postural malalignments, or glandular imbalance are present, the stresses are magnified. Imbalance of the glandular structure may cause a disturbance in growth and ossification of growth cartilages. This disturbed relationship between body height, weight, and skeletal ossification becomes a potential for injury, whether from sudden direct trauma, chronic postural stress, or repetitive stresses applied many times over during training.

Bone growth takes place at certain centers of ossification. In the long bones of the body, these centers are located near the ends of the bone. The bone shaft is called the diaphysis; the ends (tuberosities) which form the joint, the epiphysis. Between them is a layer of cartilage cells which forms the growth plate or epiphyseal line. Since growth takes place in it, this line is highly vulnerable to injury and the effects of stress or overuse syndromes.

Osteo-chondritis is inflammation of the growth cartilage. When inflammation is produced in bone, absorption of calcium takes place. Consequently, a softening or osteoporosis (reduction in density or weight) occurs even when the inflammation is too slight to produce pain. Under the stresses of weight-bearing and training activities, the inflammation becomes chronic. Actual injury followed by deformity or disability may result from the mashing down or dis-integration of the cartilage.

Among running athletes, osteo-chrondritis is most often found in the tibial tubercle (upper end of tibia). This is generally due to the great strain placed on the cartilage between the diaphysis and epiphysis, during the thousands of repetitive strikes of foot contact on the ground, by the patellar ligament. Such constant repetitive stress creates an irregularity in the ossification of the tibial tubercle which has been termed Osgood-Schlatter's disease.

# 4

## Definitions, Types of Injury, and Causes of Injury

The various body locations of strains, sprains, and the multiple types of overuse of stress syndromes that at one time or another affect the lower extremities and feet of the great majority of competitive runners in all events, as well as physical fitness joggers, are illustrated in Figures 1 and 2. Before proceeding further, however, the athlete in particular should have some understanding of the terminology used in the medical literature to identify the syndromes and injuries.

### DEFINITIONS

*Strains* apply to the muscles, their internal structure (fibers and connective tissue), and the fascia that encloses them. Strains also apply to the tendons that attach muscle to muscle or muscle to bone. Strains are classified into three degrees of severity: (1) a mildly pulled muscle or tendon; (2) a mild tearing of muscle fibers, connective tissue, or fascia, or tendon fibers; (3) a complete tearing or rupture of the muscle or tendon, within the muscle itself or through separation of one muscle from another, a muscle from its tendon, or a tendon from its attachment to a bone.

*Sprains* relate to the ligaments that bind the body joints together. They are divided into three degrees of severity: (1) a mild pull of ligament fibers; (2) a partial tearing of the ligament; (3) a complete tear or rupture of a ligament.

- Every grade of strain or sprain reflects varying degrees of pain and inflammation.
- An acute strain of a muscle or tendon results from a single violent contraction or overstretching beyond the capacity of the

36

muscle. An acute sprain of a ligament results from a single act of overstretching when a body joint is extended beyond its limit of movement or when the ligament is extended beyond its own range of extensibility. Loose ligaments can stretch further than tight ligaments before incurring a sprain.

- Acute strains or sprains may become chronic in nature if the pain, inflammation, and tissue damage is not completely healed through rest, physical therapy, or surgery, and the tissues restored to their original state prior to the resumption of training or competitive activities.

*Stress syndrome* and *overuse syndrome* are terms that have been used interchangeably in athletic literature. However, there is a feature that distinguishes the two terms in respect to their effect on athletes:

*Stress* involves a continuous factor that impacts upon the athlete both in his athletic activities and in his non-athletic activities.

*Overuse* involves repetitive stresses imposed on the body structure only in the athletic and occupational worlds.

Both syndromes involve the transmission of force to body tissue and body skeletal structure. The effect of this force depends on two basic factors: magnitude and duration.

*Stress syndromes* have as their underlying cause the application of continuous tension to the musculo-skeletal structure of the body. This continuous tension may result from: (1) physical tension in an occupational setting that keeps certain groups of muscle in a relatively sustained muscle contraction for a prolonged period of time; (2) emotional or psychological tension that through its somatic muscular component imposes equal muscular tension, in addition to the sustained contraction of physical work; (3) postural and foot faults and defects that distort the bony alignment of the body; and (4) muscular imbalance.

It should be noted that in the causes of stress syndromes are four factors which the writer maintains are "hidden" factors in predisposition to injury.

*Overuse syndromes* are due to intermittent stress imposed on the musculo-skeletal structure over long periods of time. An overuse syndrome can be the result of the stress of one sustained period of activity or of accumulated periods in the course of training.

The repetitive stresses affect the musculo-skeletal structure in two ways: (1) stresses imposed on the underlying predisposing factors of posture faults, foot faults, or muscle imbalance; and (2) overuse of soft tissue structures that are not prepared by training to withstand the stresses of training or a single competitive effort of sustained activity over a long period of time.

From the above, it can be seen that while stress syndromes are related to static, passive, and dynamic activities, overuse syndromes are directly related to dynamic activity only.

There are two other causes which, though rather uncommon, should also be considered in any discussion of overuse syndromes in runners and joggers:

1. Forcing a joint into an extreme range of motion so that actual contact is effected by the bones compressing the joint creates a condition of inflammation and irritation which will eventually activate the formation of new bone (extoses). This builds up to where an impingement is created when the joint is forced into a range where bones will contact each other. In runners and joggers, this condition can occur among those who do a great deal of hill running. Extreme dorsiflexion of the foot, when the foot is at the end of the support phase of running prior to the take-off, may cause extoses to form on the front edge of the tibia and the top of the astragalus (talus).

2. In runners and joggers, pathological changes in the joints, particularly the knee, may result from repeated microtrauma (minute injuries) or overtraining of the articular (joint) apparatus. In microtrauma, the joint is not always damaged directly. Lesions of soft tissues around joints involve muscles, cartilages, capsules, and ligaments. The repeated microtrauma disturbs tissue nutrition— which results in pathological changes of the entire joint. These usually begin when a runner or jogger suffers a very minor strain or sprain of the structures surrounding the knee or ankle and tries to "run it off," instead of restoring the slightly injured tissues to their original state.

In all stress and overuse syndromes, there are varying degrees of inflammation associated with the soft tissue structures of the body, or irritation and progressive degeneration of the bony structures of the body. In the medical literature, with rare exceptions, inflammations and irritations are identified by adding the suffix "itis" to the word describing the body part affected.

Figures 1 and 2 at the end of this chapter contain examples of syndromes affecting body structure many of which are not otherwise diagrammed in this work, e.g., bursitis, capsulitis, etc. Specific illustrations of each can be found in anatomy textbooks. For those who are interested, however, semantic descriptions are presented in the Glossary.

## TYPES OF INJURY

Not all of the injuries and syndromes depicted in Figures 1 and 2 are apt to occur to all runners, hurdlers, or joggers. This is particularly true with respect to runners and hurdlers in competitive activities. For this reason, the ensuing discussion is divided into three basic areas: (1) sprints up to 440 yards, including the hurdle races; (2) distance runs from 880 yards to the marathon

38

cross country runs and steeple chases; and (3) physical fitness jogging.

## SPRINTS

Sprinters are susceptible to hamstring, calf, and iliotibial muscle strains. Hurdlers are subject to hamstring, low back, and thigh adductor muscle strains. Rhoden, a former Olympic gold medalist in the longer sprints and now a podiatrist, pointed out that sprints impose most of the stresses on the forefoot.[16] He found that sprinters suffer from overuse or stress syndromes that cause stress fractures of the tibia, fibula, and the metatarsals, as well as anterior tibial syndromes, shin splints, Achilles tendon bursitis, and periosteal inflammation (heel spurs). Bould pointed out that sprinters are subject to inflammation of the lateral ligaments of the knee, while hurdlers are also subject to tendonitis of the peroneal muscle group.[4]

## MIDDLE AND LONG DISTANCES

A thorough study of Australia's 34 top middle and distance runners was made by Woodriff.[21] On the average, these athletes had been running seriously for six years, two months. Only serious injuries were tabulated for the average running years, while both serious and minor injuries were tabulated for a period of one year (1973).

| *Serious Injuries*<br>Area of Injury | Number of Injuries |
|---|---|
| Muscle and Tendon | |
| Achilles | 13 |
| Hamstring | 12 |
| Calves | 6 |
| Quadriceps | 5 |
| Back | 5 |
| Abdomen | 2 |
| Joint and Bone | |
| Foot | 17 |
| Knee | 13 |
| Ankle | 8 |
| Lower Leg | 6 |
| Hip | 2 |
| Other | 3 |

*Frequency of Serious Injuries*

| Form | Number of Injuries |
|------|--------------------|
| Muscle Strain | 31 |
| Joint Sprain | 21 |
| Achilles Tendonitis | 13 |
| Stress Fracture | 5 |
| Bruise | 3 |
| Dislocation | 1 |
| Other | 17 |

*Serious and Minor Injuries*

| Area of Injury | |
|------|------|
| Muscle and Tendon | |
| Calves | 55 |
| Hamstring | 19 |
| Achilles | 17 |
| Back | 9 |
| Quadriceps | 2 |
| Abdomen | 0 |
| Joint and Bone | |
| Ankle | 9 |
| Knee | 8 |
| Foot | 8 |
| Lower Leg | 5 |
| Hip | 1 |
| Other | 10 |

*Frequency of Serious and Minor Injuries*

| Form | |
|------|------|
| Muscle Strain | 86 |
| Joint Sprain | 22 |
| Achilles Tendonitis | 17 |
| Bruise | 3 |
| Stress Fracture | 2 |
| Dislocation | 0 |
| Other | 8 |

The average time lost in training for each serious injury sustained over a six-year period was two months, four days. Five athletes sustained no injuries at all during the period.

The average time completely lost per athlete for serious and minor injuries over the one-year period was found to be three weeks, six days. The average rate of injury (serious or minor) was slightly greater than four. The majority of the athletes received less than the average rate, but only six athletes sustained no injury, minor or serious, during the year. At the other extreme, seven of the athletes received 45 percent of all injuries. The interesting point about these figures is that five and six athletes sustained no injuries at all during either period.

With regard to women in track and field activities, Sharon Kosek, in a five-year study, found the most common injuries to be sprains, muscle strains, tendonitis, contusion, and patellar (knee) problems.[13] She commented that there was a greater tendency toward subluxation (partial dislocation) or dislocation of the kneecap because women, having a wider pelvis than men, tend to be knock-kneed. There was also a greater tendency for women to suffer from chondromalacia of the knee (degeneration of under surface of patella).

## JOGGING

Corrigan and Fitch have done an outstanding job in classifying by anatomical areas the types of injuries and overuse syndromes sustained by physical fitness joggers:[10]

1. *Foot*—tenosynovitis of calf muscle tendons; traumatic arthritis of second and third metatarsals; strain of arches; stress fractures of metatarsals; plantar fascitis; and heel spurs.

2. *Ankle*—Achilles tendonitis, bursitis, and rupture; talo-tibial exostosis; tenosynovitis of calf muscles; and subluxation of peroneal tendons.

3. *Leg*—tears of calf muscles; shin splints; anterior-tibial syndrome; and stress fractures of the fibula and tibia.

4. *Knee*—synovitis; bursitis; tendonitis; and chondromalacia of the patella.

5. *Hip*—tendonitis; bursitis; teno-periostitis.

They pointed out that degenerative joint disease (osteo-arthritis) is a common disability among people in "the jogging age group." The most likely locations of the disorder are the hip, knee, and foot. They also stated that a normal joint that is used normally should never be the site of osteo-arthritis, even if the jogger undertakes a high weekly mileage. A joint with some abnormality due to previous injury, disease, or incongruous joint surfaces from any cause (postural faults), is a likely site of osteo-arthritis, and the greater the use, the greater the prospect of developing this condition. They also noted that abnormal use of a normal joint, such as jogging with a short leg, may precipitate osteo-arthritis.

Allman, in commenting on adult exercise programs, maintained that foot problems are among the most frequent problems encountered therein.[1] The most common of these are: (1) plantar fascia strain; (2) medial longitudinal arch strain; (3) stress and fatigue fractures of the metatarsals and lower leg bones; (4) shin splints; and (5) knee problems.

Harris, Bowerman, *et al.* reported on a 12-week program of jogging involving 363 joggers.[11] There were 98 dropouts, 34 of them from sore legs or backs. These aches and pains were the most serious problems encountered in the early weeks of jogging and were a major cause of discouragement.

Blazina added one overuse syndrome to the list provided above.[3] He stated: "A most interesting problem in the knee developing in people over 30 is the horizontal cleavage lesion of the medial meniscus (cartilage)." He pointed out that this is not due to a single episode, as occurs in the young age group or in football players, but is the result of progressive degenerative changes within the cartilage over a period of time.

Clancy, maintaining that both the jogger and the competitive runner suffer similar injuries with the same predisposing factors, reported on his experience in treating 310 runners and joggers over a two-year period who had sustained a total of 316 injuries.[9] Approximately 10 percent of the patients were joggers; 30 percent were national and international caliber runners; and the remaining percent were high school runners. The important factors to be noted in his findings are the large number of syndromes affecting the lower back and the knee. The results of his study revealed the following injuries: 21 shin splints; 19 stress fractures; 6 cases of plantar fasciitis; 24 cases of tendonitis; 6 avulsion fractures; 42 muscle strains; 110 other injuries; 17 instances of iliac crest apophysitis (inflammation of upper edge of hip bones); 8 cases of infra-patellar tendonitis (knee); and 57 cases of chondromalacia patella (degeneration of the kneecap).

## CAUSES OF INJURY

In the traffic safety field, it has been well established over the last 50 years that 99 percent of so-called accidents are "caused occurrences." Further, if preventive or corrective action is to be taken to reduce the fatality and injury figures, the causes of such accidents must first be ascertained, so that future efforts will not be wasted—in terms of money and time—on the wrong objectives. The same approach should be made to reducing the ever-increasing number of injuries and overuse syndromes in the athletic world.

Armstrong broke down the causes of athletic injuries into three categories: (1) injuries from an outside agency; (2) self-produced injuries; and (3) injuries due to long-continued stress.[2] Williams classified athletic injuries as falling into two basic categories and several sub-categories.[20] The basic categories are: (1) consequential—directly due to athletic activity; and (2) non-consequential— directly due to athletic activity; and (2) non-consequential—not due to sports activity, but interfering with sports activity or training.

This volume favors the "holistic" or multi-factor approach to the problems of training and injury prevention and also the philosophy of caused occurrences. In all caused occurrences, someone is responsible for the occurrence. In the classification of the innumerable causes that have been advanced by various authorities on the prevention and treatment of athletic injuries, this fact should be kept in mind.

The writer's classification of causes is broken down into four broad areas: (1) intrinsic causes—within the athlete; (2) causes within the control of the athlete; (3) causes arising from outside influences—coach or trainer or, in cases of injury, the attending physician; (4) causes arising from outside agencies.

### INTRINSIC CAUSES

These are the causes that the writer classes as "hidden" factors, some of which are given relatively little attention in print, and of whose existence, in most cases, there is little or no awareness on the part of coach, trainer, or athlete.

1. Postural faults and defects.
2. Foot faults and defects.
3. Chronic postural stress due to faulty body alignment.
4. Congenital or hereditary bone anomalies and defects.
5. Lack of mobility due to faulty body alignment.
6. Muscle imbalance.
7. Nutritional deficiencies that lead to mental apathy, as well as poor body function.
8. Emotional stress, psychological factors, and proneness to injury.
9. Growth factors. Klein, in an article entitled "Flexibility—Strength and Balance," cited Dr. Don O'Donaghue's statement, "There is an amazing amount of lateral motion in the knee of the 14-, 15-, and 16-year-old youngster."[12] At this age level, the ligaments of the knee have not tightened up as much as in subsequent years. This is particularly true of the overgrown 14-, 15-, and 16-year-old boy, six feet tall, who has the physique of an adult, but the wobbly knee of a junior teen-ager. In the same article, Klein noted Dr. Milton Thomas' belief that this evidence of looseness of ligaments may well be due to serological changes that take place during puberty. The looseness of ligaments in this age group is of particular importance to the high school cross country runner who does a great amount of his running on hilly and uneven terrain, and who steps in a small hole on level terrain. This looseness of the collateral ligaments of the knee among adolescent runners is a strong contributing factor in the development of chondromalacia of the knee, evidenced by the high number of these cases cited in

Clancy's study of 310 runners mentioned earlier in this chapter. The second growth factor that should be considered in respect to young teen-age runners is the incomplete closure or separation of epiphyseal centers (ends of long bones) and incomplete ossification of bones. The most common failure or separation of epiphyseal centers in young runners occurs in the upper end of the tibia and is called Osgood-Schlatter's disease. The major causal factor here is the repetitive stress resulting from excess mileage in training for the longer distance runs.

## CAUSES WITHIN THE CONTROL OF THE ATHLETE

A. Earlier in this chapter, the injuries sustained by Australia's top middle and long distance runners were presented. In response to questionnaires, they submitted comments as to why they incurred these injuries. These comments are reflected below. The figure on the right represents the number of responses who suggested that specific reason.

| | |
|---|---|
| Unsuitable shoes | 9 |
| Running on rough surfaces | 7 |
| Training too hard, too soon | 6 |
| Change in type of training from winter to summer | 6 |
| Steeplechasing, i.e., stressful landing from steeple | 6 |
| Change from training in flat shoes to training in spikes | 5 |
| Training when not warmed up enough | 5 |
| Running on hard surfaces | 3 |
| Training while leg muscles are sore or tight | 3 |
| Lack of flexibility | 2 |
| Overtraining in track season | 1 |
| Too many hard races during track season | 1 |

B. *Improper Warm-up*: Some athletes have a tendency to spend too much time in warming up. If not in excellent condition, they may create a condition of mild fatigue prior to an intensive training session. The most common type of improper warm-up, however, is the use of uncontrolled ballistic type stretching movements that can easily result in minute muscle tears. These tears can be a predisposing factor to later injury, which may occur during a race involving maximum effort. This is particularly true with respect to the two-joint muscles, such as the hamstrings. The "Hurdle" exercise, where momentum is used to carry the head and trunk down to the knee in a bouncing movement that exerts tremendous strain on cold hamstring muscles, is an uncontrolled ballistic type stretching movement. The purpose of warming up is to raise the internal temperature and reduce the viscosity in the muscles. It should be noted that the Russians have found that including preliminary power (strength) exercises for the hamstring muscles in warm-ups prevents rupture of muscle fibers. Volkov and Mironova carried out studies of the temperature of the femoral (thigh) muscles and observed a decrease in the temperature of these muscles during common warming up exercises.[19] After inclusion of power exercises for the hamstrings at the beginning of the warm-up, an increase of 1.6 to 2.6 degrees (centigrade) was noted in their internal temperature.

C. *No Warm-up*

D. *Poor Mechanics of Walking and Running:* These include splay foot (toed outwards) running, use of a scissor gait in running (one or both legs crossing the midline of the body at the conclusion of a stride), and leaning too far forward while running.

E. *Fatigue*: Lactic acid is a by-product of muscular activity. Under normal circumstances, it is removed via the bloodstream. When lactic acid collects, the blood's alkaline reserve decreases. Although a part of this lactic acid is resynthesized to glycogen (sugar), it may be stored in the muscle. The result is fatigue—and fatigue, as the direct result of inadequate conditioning, contributes to injury. Most strains and sprains, outside of those due to body contact or falls, begin when fatigue sets in. Brewer commented on fatigue, stating:

> A tired muscle loses some of its ability to relax. The endurance of a muscle is characterized not only by its ability to produce power over a prolonged period of time, but also by the ability to maintain elasticity at the same time. In fatigue, a stiffening of the muscle, as well as slowed reaction time contributes to the hazards of athletic endeavor.[5]

F. *Momentary Incoordination:* This involves a breakdown in neuromuscular integration and the process of reciprocal innervation or reciprocal inhibitions of antagonist muscles to relax while prime mover muscles move a body joint through its complete range of movement. This failure is primarily due to fatigue or to cold and tight muscles that have not been properly warmed up. Sprinters and hurdlers are more apt to be affected by this than are other types of runners and joggers. Hamstring strains and ruptures are the direct result of momentary incoordination. However, the longer distance runners are more apt to be affected by the failure of the shin muscles to relax as the powerful calf muscles propel the body in forward movement. Travers commented on this saying:

> Thus the calf muscles have first to overcome the contraction of their antagonists before they can produce any propulsion effort at all. Efficiency is reduced, economy goes by the board, and an additional strain is thrown on the calf muscles, which may be enough to cause damage to the muscle or Achilles tendon. Another result is that since the full range of ankle movement is not used, the ankle joint

eventually becomes stiff and limits the work that the calf muscles can do even more.[18]

G. *Errors in Technique:* LaCava pointed out that technical errors, such as occur in hurdling and steeplechasing, are the most frequent cause of muscular lesions. [14] He maintained that constant repetition of a correct technique tends to create automatisms. The gradual adaptation of neuromuscular systems contributes to formation of muscular coordination.

H. *Lack of Balanced Strength or Flexibility:* James Nicholas showed a direct relationship between injury to body joints, strength, and flexibility.[15] Tight-jointed athletes were found to be more susceptible to muscle strains and tears, nerve pinch syndromes, and tendonitis; while loose-jointed athletes more readily suffer dislocations, subluxations, and ligament sprains. These findings, as they apply to runners, hurdlers, and joggers, emphasize the importance of developing an optimum balanced level of strength around the knee and ankle joints. The importance of muscular balance and muscular imbalance as major predisposing factors in athletic injuries and overuse syndromes will be discussed thoroughly in Chapter 6.

I. *Improper Conditioning:* Among competitive runners, there is a tendency to overemphasize the development of cardiovascular (aerobic and anaerobic) endurance, and in hurdlers the development of flexibility, at the expense of the strength factor.

J. *Overuse or Overexertion:* In the writer's opinion, this factor is overemphasized as a contributor to injuries. A well-conditioned athlete with good body alignment, no hidden postural or foot defects, no emotional or psychological problems, and good hygienic habits (adequate sleep, rest, etc.) should have no trouble in adapting to the training stresses of modern-day running athletes. Racing presents the exception to this statement. Participation in competitive racing generally involves a great amount of nervous tension or emotional stress, both of which are strong contributing factors to fatigue. A combined indoor and outdoor competitive racing season, added to training stresses, can easily lead to injuries and overuse syndromes.

## CAUSES ARISING FROM OUTSIDE INFLUENCES

A. *Coach and Trainer:* Though the track athlete is perhaps the best-informed of all athletes as to the physiology and techniques of training, he is still subject to the influence of a coach or trainer. This is particularly true in the case of young high school athletes. The coach or trainer can be a major contributing cause of injuries in many ways:

(1) Incorrect organization of training lessons and sports competitions.

(2) Failure to notice or correct poor mechanics of walking and running.[7]

(3) Neglect of minor soft tissue and joint sprains.[6] In too many cases, a coach or trainer will advise an athlete to "run out" a slight or moderate muscle strain or joint sprain. Smith pointed out that the term "strain," which is a nonspecific one, implies inflammation, and inflammation leads to exudation (inflammatory fluid) or, in the case of a joint, to effusion (flowing out of liquid).[17] He went on to state that ignoring so-called minor injuries can lead to early osteoarthritis, particularly in the knee joint. Cross country runners, joggers, and hurdlers are more prone to suffer minor knee strains. Smith stated there is no such injury to knee as a minor one; because of the effusion factor, all injuries to the knee are serious. Cerney pointed out that a once-pulled thigh muscle is susceptile to the same injury in the future, no matter how good a "healing job" has been done.[8]

B. *The Doctor:* Burry, in an article on the late effects of neglected soft tissue injury wrote:

Neglect of an injury may be the responsibility of the patient or of the doctor. On the one hand, the player may regard his symptoms as trivial in the early stages, as he often does with lesions of the adductor origin (groin), or he may in his anxiety to return to training before his hard-won fitness is lost, disregarding his doctor's advice. On the other hand, the advice he receives may be poor, ill-informed, unenthusiastic or, not uncommonly, both.... It is the view of many doctors that injuries to athletes are trivialities, that athletes are very lucky to be so fit, and that they should accept a prolonged period of rest without any other treatment and not waste the doctor's time. Such a view is not only damaging to the medical profession, but totally irresponsible.[6]

## CAUSES ARISING FROM OUTSIDE AGENCIES

A. *Cold Weather.*

B. *Uneven Terrain (holes in ground, rocks on ground, etc.) and Hard Pavement:* Cross country runners and joggers and long distance runners who use hill running as a training device are subject to the effects of uneven terrain.

C. *Poorly Fitting or Well-worn Shoes: Runner's World* magazine has published comprehensive articles and also two booklets on the importance of shoes in running. Poorly designed shoes have always been considered one of the major predisposing factors in the foot problems of the general population.

D. *Banked Roads:* Physical fitness joggers in particular have suffered the consequences of running on only one side of a banked road. Banked road running is a predisposing cause of knee pains and chondromalacia of the patella.

## COMMON INJURIES AND OVERUSE SYNDROMES AFFECTING RUNNING SPORTS

### Strains-Sprains-Inflamation and Internal Joint Degeneration

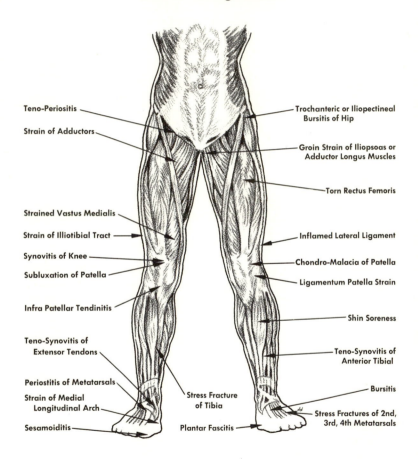

*Figure 1*

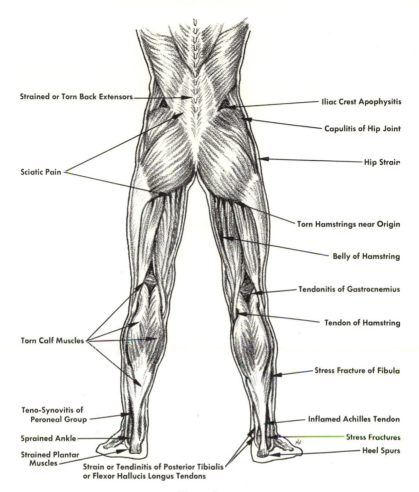

**Figure 2**

## REFERENCES

1. Allman, Fred L., "The Prevention and Treatment of Orthopedic Problems Related to an Adult Exercise Program," *Journal of Occupational Medicine,* Vol. 13, No. 12, 1971.
2. Armstrong, J. R. and Tucker, W. E., "Mechanism of Production of Injury," *Injury in Sport* (London: Staples Press, 1964).
3. Blazina, Martin E., "Orthopedic Problems Seen in Exercise Programs," *Nebraska Medical Journal,* December 1972.
4. Bould, C., *Hints on Athletic Injuries* (London: British Amateur Athletic Association).

5. Brewer, Bruce J., "Athletic Injuries: Musculo-tendinous Unit," *Clinical Orthopedics,* November 23, 1962.

6. Burry, Hugh C., "Late Effects of Neglected Soft Tissue Injury," *Proceedings of the Royal Society of Medicine,* Vol. LXII, September 1969.

7. Burt, H. A., "Effects of Faulty Posture," *Proceedings of the Royal Society of Medicine,* Vol. XLIII.

8. Cerney, J. V., *Athletic Injuries* (Springfield, Illinois: Charles C. Thomas, 1963).

9. Clancy, William G., "Lower Extremity Injuries in the Jogger and Distance Runners," *The Physician and Sports Medicine,* June 1974.

10. Corrigan, A. B. and Fitch, K. D., "Complications of Jogging," *The Medical Journal of Australia,* August 12, 1972.

11. Harris, W. E.; Bowerman, William; McFadden, Bruce; and Kerns, Thomas; "Jogging," *Journal of the American Medical Association,* Vol. 201, No. 10, September 4, 1967.

12. Klein, Karl K., "Flexibility—Strength and Balance," *Journal of N.A.T.A.,* Summer 1971.

13. Kosek, Sharon, "Nature and Incidence of Traumatic Injury to Women in Sports," *Current Sports Medicine Issues* (American Association of Physical Health, Education, and Rehabilitation, 1974).

14. LaCava, G., "The Prevention of Accidents Caused by Sports," *Journal of Sports Medicine and Physical Fitness,* December 1964.

15. Nicholas, James, "Injuries to Knee Ligaments," *Journal of the American Medical Association,* June 29, 1970.

16. Rhoden, George, "Overuse Syndrome of the Foot and Leg as Related to Short Distance Runners," *Second Annual Sports Medicine Seminar, California School of Podiatry, April 27 and 28, 1974.*

17. Smith, D. S., "The Late Effects of Injury to the Knee," *British Journal of Sports Medicine,* Vol. 4, No. 3, August 1969.

18. Travers, P. R., "Injuries Due to Faulty Style," *Track Technique,* No. 11, March 1963.

19. Volkov, M. V. and Mironova, Z. S., "Prophylaxis and Basic Principles of the Treatment of Trauma in Sportsmen," *"Proceedings of International Congress of Sports Sciences* (Tokyo: Japanese Union of Sports Sciences, 1966).

20. Williams, J. G. P., "Aetological Classification of Injuries in Sportsmen," *British Journal of Sports Medicine,* Vol. 5, No. 4, July 1971.

21. Woodriff, Jim, "Injuries to Australian Distance Runners," *Modern Athlete and Coach,* July 1974.

# 5

## The Mechanics of Correct Running Form

In determining how postural and foot faults, muscle imbalance, lateral asymmetry, and poor leg alignment specifically affect the performance of the runner, hurdler, or jogger, and how they predispose to soft tissue injuries and overuse syndromes, we must first determine what is considered by experts to be the correct mechanical form for the most efficient and energy-saving type of running and jogging.

Slocum and James, orthopedic surgeons at the University of Oregon, and Bill Bowerman, America's premier authority on middle and long distance running and physical fitness jogging, have done pioneering research on the biomechanics of the most efficient and correct form of running. They have presented their findings in several articles which have appeared primarily in medical journals. Slocum and Bowerman have outlined the biomechanical principles involved in establishing correct running form from the standpoint of postural balance.[1]

1. The smoothness and efficiency of the stride are the result of minimal body displacement in the sagittal (front to back) plane, of maximal forward displacement at take-off, and minimal deceleration by the leading leg at foot strike. The forward displacement of the upper body that is associated with the upright erect position in middle and long distance running or jogging should not be confused with the forward lean of the sprinter or middle distance runner at the start of a race.

2. The position of the pelvis is the key to postural control in running. The forward or backward rotation of the pelvis controls the motion of the lumbar spine, the degree of flexion relative to the ground, and the degree of outward rotation of the hip.

3. The leg plus the pelvis and low back from the lumbar joint complex downward provide the length, motive power, and motion necessary for running.

4. The normal working rate of motion of the lumbar spine in running is about 40 degrees; the full range of motion in the runner, from forced flexion to forced extension, usually exceeds this by 20 to 25 degrees.

5. The greatest functional range of extension of the lumbar spine is present when it is in the flat-backed flexed position at the foot strike and moves to the sway-backed, lordotic, extended position as the trailing leg leaves the ground. The flat-backed position facilitates spinal rotation, as well. In running, the spine undergoes a twisting motion, the lower spine rotates backwards with the extension of the trailing leg while, at the same time, the upper spine rotates forward synchronously with the arm to maintain equilibrium. Such action is carried out more easily and more efficiently about a relatively straight rod than a curved one. The flatbacked position effects a straighter axis and affords a slightly greater degree of rotation in the lumbar spine, which, in the extended lordotic position, is restricted by the vertebral articular (joint) facets that act as anatomic doorstops in motion.

6. The correct running in the sagittal plane involves two fundamental factors: (A) The entire leg must be moving strongly backwards at the time of the foot strike, in order to lessen resistance at impact and avoid deceleration; (B) The position of the trunk should be erect, as this favors the flat-backed position of the lumbar spine in midstance preparatory to take-off, requires less effort in maintaining postural equilibrium, and provides good respiratory position and free movement of the scapula (shoulder blades) over the rib cage.

7. The principal causes of forward shift of the center of gravity in the trunk are fatigue, technique, and faulty posture. With a forward lean, the full working range of the lumbar spine is not utilized to assist in extending the leg to the rear, and flexion of the hip is relatively decreased because of the forward pelvic tilt that accompanies forward lean.

8. In the frontal plane (looking at the runner from the front), side-by-side sway should be reduced to a minimum to lessen the burden borne by the postural muscles in maintaining balance and to sustain the trunk in a position of the greatest working efficiency. The gravitational line of weight must fall through the supporting foot, and the upward projection of the line must divide the body weight into two equal halves, if the runner or jogger is to maintain lateral balance. This balance is best achieved when the weight-bearing foot falls in the line of progression and the head is carried directly above this line.

9. The less the vertical (upwards) displacement of the body, the greater the efficiency of the runner. Energy is not wasted in raising the body upwards with each step, but is primarily used to project the body forward into the "float" phase of the stride.

## REFERENCES

1. Slocum and Bowerman, "Biomechanics of Running," *Clinical Orthopedics,* No. 23, 1962. Reprinted with permission of publisher, J. B. Lippincott Co.

# Part Two

## Hidden Factors and Their Effects

# 6

# Muscular Imbalance

Muscular imbalance has finally been recognized as a major predisposing cause of athletic injuries by the various disciplines concerned with the cause and treatment of such injuries. The purpose of this chapter is to emphasize the importance of preventing muscular imbalance through adequate testing and properly designed athletic conditioning programs.

An evaluation of studies relating to the testing of muscular strength in human beings can be of assistance to those concerned with the training of athletes in determing the body areas to which specific attention should be given in conditioning programs to prevent or correct muscular imbalances. In any proper evaluation of these studies, several points should be kept in mind:

1. Absolute strength of body musculature cannot be measured.
2. There is no location in the body, with the possible exception of the extraocular (eye) muscles, where agonists and antagonists are exactly equal to each other in strength due to their anatomical size and length.
3. Dynamic body movements generally are not involved in testing muscular strength. The persons tested are in most cases lying supine, prone, or on their sides, or sitting up, or lying supine or prone with legs hanging over the edge of the testing table.

4. Testing has been carried out in age groups ranging from 2 to 81 years of age, generally with normal untrained persons of both sexes.
5. It is impossible to test the strength of a specific individual muscle in a living subject because muscles work in groups of two or more to create movement of body joints. Research tech-

nicians, however, make every effort to isolate agonist (prime mover group) muscles being tested to minimize the contribution of synergist (assisting muscle group) during testing.

Knapp reported very accurate tensiometer muscular strength tests conducted by Beasley in 1956 on 386 children, aged 10 to 12, that reflected: (1) neck extensors 2-½ times stronger than flexors; (2) elbow flexors 1-1/5 times stronger than extensors; (3) wrist flexors 1-2/5 times stronger than extensors; (4) hip extensors 1-⅔ times stronger than flexors; (5) knee extensors 2 times as strong as flexors; and (6) plantar flexors 5-¼ times stronger than dorsal flexors.[15]

In studies to show the relationship between knee extension and knee flexion strength, Klein commented that the strengths of muscles around the knee and other body joints are not necessarily equal and that they vary at different age levels.[14] His studies reflected the percentage of strength in flexors as compared to extensors to be 76 percent at 9 years, 72 percent at 13 years, 57 percent at 15 years, 53 percent for high school seniors and college freshmen, and 60 percent for college football players.

Korobcov pointed out that researchers in Russia conducted extensive static strength tests of various groups of muscles (flexors and extensors of finger, hand, forearm, arm, neck, body, hip, shin, and foot) on 15 age groups from 2 to 81 years of age and older.[16] Studies of strength reflected it was first registered at 4 to 5 years of age. Development of strength is disproportional for various groups of muscles. Strength of the antigravitation muscles—calf, back muscles, front surface of hip, neck, and masticatory muscles—develops best of all.

Between 1916 and 1920, Martin and his associates, using a spring balance testing device, conducted numerous studies on muscular strength and symmetry in children and adults.[18] In the first study, 240 children and adolescents (128 males and 112 females) 4 to 18 years of age were tested; second study, 65 male adults tested; third study, 50 female adults tested. The results as tabulated by Martin are reflected in the following table on the page opposite.

Using a cable tensiometer, Clarke conducted tests of several groups of muscles on 64 Springfield College students.[3] In a seated position, the mean average of trunk flexion was 126.68 pounds and extension 234.66 pounds (ratio 1 to 1.85); in a supine lying position with legs straight, trunk flexion was 226.21 pounds and extension 271.20 pounds (ratio 1 to 1.2).

Hutchins tested 92 undergraduate women at the University of Oregon to determine the relationship between muscle balance and antereo-posterior posture.[10] Her tests reflected a mean average for trunk flexion of 34.88 pounds and for extension, 55.83 pounds (ratio 1 to 1.6). She maintains, along with other research investigators

## AVERAGE PERCENTAGE DISTRIBUTION OF STRENGTH AMONG THE MUSCLES

| Muscle Group | Age | | | | |
|---|---|---|---|---|---|
| | 3-7 | 8-12 | 13-18 | Adult Males | Adult Females |
| Feet: | | | | | |
|   Plantar flexion | 7.75 | 8.82 | 9.20 | 10.00 | 10.00 |
|   Dorsal flexion | 3.20 | 3.00 | 2.86 | 2.85 | 2.90 |
|   Inversion | 2.21 | 2.14 | 2.07 | 1.90 | 1.95 |
|   Eversion | 2.28 | 2.07 | 2.20 | 1.80 | 1.90 |
| Hips: | | | | | |
|   Aduction | 1.55 | 1.55 | 1.63 | 1.50 | 1.70 |
|   Abduction | 1.47 | 1.43 | 1.42 | 1.40 | 1.45 |
|   Extension | 2.91 | 2.92 | 2.77 | 3.70 | 3.40 |
|   Flexion | 3.41 | 3.24 | 3.07 | 3.20 | 2.70 |
| Knees: | | | | | |
|   Extension | 3.04 | 3.20 | 3.15 | 3.30 | 3.15 |
|   Flexion | 1.73 | 1.67 | 1.64 | 1.75 | 1.30 |

quoted by her, that the smaller the ratio between the strength of trunk flexors and trunk extensors, the better the alignment of the trunk and its contribution to good antereo-posterior posture.

The human organism begins life with a high degree of muscular imbalance. The fetal position, which the human has maintained for approximately nine months, has been one of neck and lumbar spine flexion, hip and knee flexion. Through crawling, an infant assists in developing strength in the antigravitational extensor muscles. It is not until he stands up for the first time that flexion begins to change to extension. In crawling, the curve of the spine is primarily a single dorso-lumbar kyphotic curve (upper-lower back); on standing, the lumbar spine moves into a lordotic (inward) curve and all the normal curves of the spine begin to appear. Stretching of the leg and hip flexors to full extension of the hip joints continues for the first five or six years of live.

At birth, the flexor muscles, favored by acting with and not against gravity as their opponent extensor muscles must do, have a position of advantage and during infancy and early childhood are stronger than the antigravity extensors. As soon as the child stands, the trunk extensor (lower back), knee extensor (front thigh), and plantar flexor (calf) muscles began to gain strength and soon surpass the opponent flexor muscles. In contrast, the hip flexor muscles tend to overbalance the antigravity hip extensor muscles (buttocks) up to the age of 11 or 12. The flexor muscles of the front neck and chest are much stronger at birth than the neck extensors (rear) and shoulder adductors (upper back), and tend to maintain their superiority up to adulthood and, in far too many cases, throughout life. This shoulder girdle muscular imbalance is manifested in the round-shouldered posture observed in so many persons, including athletes.

In addition, it has been well established by corrective physical education and physical fitness authorities that in the great majority of people, after early childhood, the trunk flexors (abdominals) begin to weaken and stretch, due to the weight of the internal organs, while the trunk extensors (lower back) contract and become stronger.

## CAUSES OF IMBALANCE

Causes such as pathological diseases of neurological origin resulting in atrophy, dystrophy, or spasticity of muscles; severe congenital (inborn) deformities; abnormalities of the skeleton; and traumatic injuries resulting from body contact, terrain, or other external factors are not discussed here, as they are beyond the control of the individual, his parents, or teachers during his developmental years of early childhood and pre-adolescence.

## BIRTH, GROWTH, AND DEVELOPMENTAL CAUSES

1. *Intrauterine life and birth delivery:* Michelle's book *Orthotherapy* is devoted exclusively to muscle imbalance, its causes, results, and correction, and is a first of its kind in the Western world.[21] He maintained that muscle imbalance may begin in the fourth month of pre-natal life. It is at this time that the leg and spinal rotation of the unborn infant begins. If the turning is inadequate and the legs fail to cross, a deformity of the feet known as talipes calcaneovarus may occur. If one or both legs overcross, a tibial torsion syndrome may begin. A severe form of tibial torsion developing in the unborn child results in a clubfoot deformity.

Fahey pointed out that human beings during birth and delivery must rotate through a hazardous 180-degree turn with a normal driving force of 30 to 40 pounds per square inch.[7] This force on the head, shoulders, and pelvis can be the cause of a "pressure syndrome." In cases where a woman's pelvis is rigid and the ligaments inelastic, obstetricians have noted a delivery force of 70 to 80 pounds per square inch. This tremendous torque generated at birth results in developmental defects in the hip that show up later in life as a "retarded leg syndrome." Fahey maintained that low back pain and injuries to ankle, knee, and hip may be due in part to this syndrome.

2. *Environmental:* Some cultures are characterized by a rigid posture, others by kyphosis (rounded upper back) or lordosis (inward curve of lower back), which are postural faults or defects that create muscular imbalance in the body. These cultural posture traits can often be traced to differences in nutrition, climate, or training.

3. *Sleeping and Sitting Habits:* Kite, more than any other authority, has emphasized the importance of faulty sleeping and sitting habits in the small child that create muscle imbalance in the lower legs and feet and lead to various deformities and faults in the feet.[12] With the exception of the relatively few due to congenital causes, these conditions are produced in the first few months of childhood. Kite also pointed out that many mothers place large bulky diapers on children that force the legs into a right angle to the body, with legs flexed at the knees, the legs rotation laterally (outwards) at the hips, which creates a "frog" or "spread eagle" position. Most babies are placed on their stomachs to sleep, for safety in case they should regurgitate. When placed on his stomach, with the legs in the "frog" position, the baby's big toe rests on the mattress and his foot is pushed around into a valgus (outward) position, with the inner side of the foot from the heel to the toe resting on the mattress. In this position, the outer calf muscles (peroneals) are contracted and the posterior and anterior calf muscles that support the medial arch of the foot are stretched and weakened, which leads to the onset of the acquired flat foot. The legs, being rotated laterally, develop a lateral femoral (upper thigh) and tibia (shin bone) torsion.

Other children when placed on their stomachs assume a prayerful posture on their knees with their feet turned inward toward each other. This position stretches and weakens the outward lateral rotator muscles of the hip and the outer calf muscles, and contracts and shortens the medial hip rotators and the posterior and anterior calf muscles, leading to a medial (inward) torsion of the upper and lower leg—and pigeon-toes. There is a tendency for this prayerful posture to continue in the child as he sits-up and plays games between two and eight years of age. He will sit back on his heels, knees bent, and his feet will be turned inward in the pigeon-toed position. This position is also favored by the child who has a short Achilles tendon.

The slouched round-shouldered position of older children of grammar school age either at home or at desks in school that are too low for them leads to muscular imbalance in the upper spine and shoulder girdle. Those who sit with one leg under them develop muscle imbalance in the hips and spine and in the lower leg and foot of the turned-under leg.

4. *Parental Influence:* Many overprotective mothers, due to their fear that a small child may hurt himself (or to keep the child from getting under their feet), confine the child to a playpen. Invariably, such a child will stand before the muscles of his lower extremities are strong enough to keep the leg and foot in good alignment. The child pulls himself to a standing position, since his chest and arm flexors are the strongest muscles of his body at this stage of life. If, in standing, he continually raises on his toes, he will tend to develop a short Achilles tendon and short calf muscles, leading to various foot deviations.

Encouraging a child to stand and walk before his muscle strength is developed is a strong contributing factor to poor leg alignment Knock-knees is a common aftermath of efforts to stand without adequate muscular strength. Also, because his sense of balance is poor, the child spreads his feet and the forefoot outward for stability. Because the extrinsic muscles of the calf and shin are weak, the forefeet in an outward position will cause the foot and ankle to go into pronation (ankle and foot bent inward) and the tendency toward development of muscular imbalance in the feet is under way.

5. *Nutrition:* Poor nutrition or malnutrition has been closely associated with general body slump, fatigue posture, and scoliosis (lateral curvature of spine) in growing children. Cobey commented that an excess of free sugar in the diet of children and young adolescents will interfere with epiphyseal growth of the spine, resulting in wedging of the dorsal (upper back) spine, a round back, and eventually kyphosis.[4] This posture, which stretches the upper back muscles and shortens the anterior shoulder and chest muscles, is highly conducive to a permanent imbalance in the muscles enclosing the shoulder joints.

Carey pointed out that with chronic inanition (exhaustion) and malnutrition there is a decrease in muscle weight and a persistence of skeletal growth in length.[2] The extent of muscle degeneration varies greatly, not only in the fibers of some muscles, but also in muscles in different regions of the body. This leads to a form of scoliosis (lateral curvature of spine) due to the imbalance of the bilateral musculature of the spine.

6. *Play Habits:* When scooters, speed wagons, and skates are used constantly with one leg only, such continual action can result in a shortening of one leg, a lateral tilt of the pelvis, and overdevelopment of one side of the body.

Katznetsov pointed out that in the child between the ages of one and two, the use of the left hand and right hand are at a reasonable balance in the arm movements of various activities.[11] However, due to parental urging, 95 percent are righthanded by the time they reach first grade. He cited this right hand usage as a cause of functional and later anatomical asymmetry (imbalance) in the muscles of the arm, shoulder, chest cavity, back, and hips, and stated that 60 percent of cuts, burns, bruises, and traumatic injuries occur in the left arm.

7. *Psychological Attitudes and Disease Conditions:* Habitual emotional traumas, such as fear, anxiety, frustration, and anger, keep muscles and fascia in a constant state of tension, which can result in a permanent shortening through thickening of the muscle fascia. Kraus maintained that the majority of low back pains are due to muscle imbalance and habitual tension.[17] Other writers in the corrective physical education field have commented on psychological feelings of shyness, bashfulness, modesty, self-consciousness, insecurity, depression, and inferiority that are expressed in body slump and fatigue posture with a round upper back, forward head, inward curve of lower back, and forward thrust of hips, all contributing to muscular imbalance in the shoulder girdle, lower back, and hips.

Cyriax maintained that in addition to the traditional list of causes of development of lateral muscle imbalance and lateral curvature of the spine in children and adults, diseases of the abdominal organs and chest cavity should be added as a precipitating cause.[6] He pointed out that these diseases, through localized contraction of muscles from reflex nerve irritation (pain), force their victims to adopt vicious attitudes in order to relieve the pain. This is particularly true with regard to the muscles and nerves of the spinal column. The reflex contraction takes effect through the visceral nerves and anterior divisions of the spinal nerves, i.e., the inter-costals. He provided examples of abdominal, liver, gallbladder, and heart disease bringing about conditions of scoliosis in the spine. The scoliosis was eliminated when the disease was cured.

8. *Standing Habits:* It is usual for children when they first stand up to space their feet apart, with the feet in an abducted (outward) position, which is a natural adjustment for the purpose of widening their base of support. Their sense of balance is undeveloped at this time. The longer they take to attain a sense of balance with the feet in the abducted position, the greater the probability that they will use that foot position when they begin to walk.

In the process of growing up, most people stand on one foot in the resting posture. Generally, the non-supporting foot is in a relaxed position with the foot abducted. A study made in Japan by Masaki of the standing rest posture of people waiting on a train platform reflected the following: Slightly less than four percent stood with both feet parallel and pointing straight ahead.[20] Nearly 75 percent stood on one foot, with the relaxed leg placed some distance ahead of the standing leg. Masaki commented that these two types of standing posture were the most comfortable for the average person, but that all those so standing showed signs of asymmetry (bilateral muscular imbalance) in the lower extremities.

Rasch and Burke pointed out that relaxed standing on one foot is usually accompanied by relaxation of the gluteus medius which, along with the tensor fascia latae, is considered the most important postural thigh muscle in the adjustment to sideways postural sway.[23] This relaxation of the gluteus medius results in a hip drop on the opposite side. If the position is habitually assumed, lateral ligaments of the hip and spine are stretched unilaterally, which predisposes the person to habitual lateral curvature of the spine. This observation was confirmed by Fitzgerald, who found that standing easy with the weight on one leg and the other forward resulted in a lateral tilt of the pelvis, which was lowered on the side of the forward leg.[9] The spine therefore takes a convex curve to the same side as the lowered hip tilt.

Klein, in a test for quadricept (front thigh) strength, tested 13 of 15 persons who stood in an unbalanced posture position (mainly on one leg) and 12 to 15 persons who stood in a balanced posture position (both legs).[13] Based on Wolf's law of body development—that muscle structure growth is influenced by the way body weight is borne—he found the following: Of those tested who favored the unbalanced posture standing position, most showed considerably more strength in the leg that bore the weight than in the opposite leg; of those tested who favored the balanced standing posture position, a large majority showed a balanced quadriceps development between both legs. He concluded that there appears to be a positive relationship between balanced standing position, bilateral quadriceps muscle strength, and the physiological laws of body development.

Fahey commented as follows on the retarded leg syndrome:[7]

Few people realize they go through life with one underdeveloped or retarded leg. During early creeping, crawling, and later walking, one foot—usually the left—everts, as a preference develops for the other foot. Because most persons favor one foot when walking and the other when standing, one leg underdevelops. With one everted foot, walking cannot be properly accomplished and chronic strain on the medial ligaments of the knee and undue stress on the sacroiliac (lower back) develop.

9. *Walking and Running Habits:* Patterns of muscular action in movement generally follow established habit patterns. A child who stands in a slouched and round-shouldered position, with a forward-tilted pelvis and a lordotic (inward) curve in the lumbar region, will continue that habitual postural position for the rest of his life unless he is trained in proper postural, walking, and running habits and his basic muscular imbalance is corrected.

Muscular imbalance caused by slumping posture affects the antereo-posterior or lateral tilt of the pelvis, which puts abnormal stress on the joints of the lower extremities. When in running the weight is shifted to the balls of the feet, the fascia tension on the bottom of the feet is so increased that it equals approximately twice the body weight. A young person with a forward tilt of the pelvis and lumbar lordosis will produce an unfavorable angle of foot strike, in which the magnitude of force exerted on the ball of the foot is considerable, which leads to further weakening of the intrinsic foot muscles.

By far the greatest stress to which the vulnerable knee joint and arches of the feet are subjected comes from the abducted toes-out-foot type of walking and running. From a mechanical standpoint, muscles pulling on a straight line are stronger than those that pull around the corner. In the toed-out position, the peroneals pull on a straight line, while the posterior tibialis and flexor hallucis longus of the calf pull around the corner. The latter are the main extrinsic (calf) muscles supporting the intrinsic (foot) plantar flexor muscles in maintaining integrity of the medial longitudinal arch. Not more that 15 to 20 percent of the tension stresses in the longitudinal arch are borne by the extrinsic muscles of the calf. The major support of the arch is provided by the intrinsic plantar (foot) ligaments, plantar aponeuroses, and short plantar muscles.

The intrinsic plantar flexors in themselves, without any support from the extrinsic muscles, cannot completely maintain the integrity of the medical longitudinal arch against the tremendous pull of the triceps surae (calf) whose action in contracting and raising the heels tends to flatten and depress the medial longitudinal arch.

The muscular imbalance between peroneals (evertors) and the invertor muscles, which are stretched by the splay foot position, and the weakening of extrinsic muscles supporting the plantar flexors of the arch lead eventually to a pronation (inward curve) of the foot and ankle. In the splay foot position of running, the line of drive is out and across the metatarsal arch. This unnatural stress repeated many times over in walking and running is one of the primary causes of stress fractures in this arch (forefoot).

10. *Occupation:* Corrective physical education authorities have consistently pointed out the effects of occupation in the development of muscular imbalance and the resultant postural deviations. Among the occupations frequently mentioned as causing over-development of one side of the trunk or body extremities are plastering, painting, hod carrying, brick laying, mail and news-paper delivery, and violin playing. Lateral curvature of the spine is a hazard in all of these.

Attention has also been called to the one-sided development of coal miners, stokers, heavy laborers, agricultural workers, accountants, stenographers, etc., who labor or sit at desks in round-backed stooped-over positions which shorten the muscles on the front side of the upper body and stretch those of the upper back, leading to a round-shouldered posture and eventually some degree of kyphosis.

Salespeople, policemen, and others continually on their feet tend to stand on one foot and over a period of time can develop a lateral tilt of the pelvis and lateral curvature of the spine.

11. *Miscellaneous Causes:* Postural correction authorities have mentioned several environmental factors that create poor posture and resulting muscular imbalances, particularly in children and young adolescents. Among these are improper shoes, narrow or short socks, clothing that does not fit the growing youngster properly, overwork and overfatigue, and such items of furniture as short beds, sagging beds, and poor mattresses. Of these, clothing and overwork no longer present serious problems in Western civilization. Fatigue, however, as a result of poor diet leading to minor malnutrition, is still a major factor, and one which is intensified by the emotional problems prevalent among a high percentage of today's children.

Cobey stated: "It is a conceded fact among orthopedic surgeons that the innerspring mattress is a victory of advertising over common sense and good judgment. A soft bed permits harmful curves of the spine to develop."[4] Children sleeping on their backs with high pillows can start the development of a stoop-shouldered forward head position.

The most common environmental cause of postural imbalance today is poorly-fitting and tight shoes. The modern shoe, due to its rigidity, has to a large extent eliminated the flexion action of the toes, which sacrifices the power of the flexor muscles of the foot and weakens the ligamentary structure that supports the medial longitudinal arch.

Equipment manufacturers have conducted intensive research and, in general, produced well-designed shoes for various types of athletes. However, despite the progress made, thousands of athletes will use shoes that are too short for their feet or do not fit properly. Wearing them results in a breakdown of the muscular structure of the foot and can cause numerous types of external injuries to the foot and toes. This observation is confirmed by the studies of Conway, a podiatrist.[5] A study of college basketball players in the Rochester area during 1969 reflected that 25 percent of the players were wearing the wrong size sneakers. In a further study of 17 college players in the same area, 12 of them, after a complete foot examination, were given sneakers at least one-half size larger than those they had been wearing, indicating that they had been improperly fitted in the past. Sneakers of the correct size helped to minimize the number of digital problems encountered during the study. Conway concluded by stating:

> Whenever possible, athletic footwear should be modified for an
> individual's foot to allow him to function more efficiently. With a great
> number of black athletes in college and professional basketball, serious
> thought should be given to the design and fabrication of a sneaker for
> the low-arched flattened type of foot."

*N.B.*: This type of arch is common among Negroes.

## SPORTS RELATED CAUSES

Up to this point, we have been discussing developmentally
acquired muscular imbalance. The prevention of a high degree of
muscular imbalance in the person's earliest years is largely the
responsibility of his family doctor, parents, and school teachers. Now
let us look at muscular imbalance in the light of physical education
and preparation for and participation in sports. These activities can
increase developmentally acquired muscular imbalance at a rapid
rate, due to the stresses on the body incurred during such activities.

1. *Improper Care or Treatment of Minor Injuries:* It has been well
established that muscular imbalance can be a natural outgrowth of
athletic injury, particularly if the injury is severe enough to require
surgery or immobilization. This is recognized by athletic trainers,
orthopedic doctors, and physical therapists, who recommend that
appropriate corrective and rehabilitative exercises be instituted as
soon as possible after the occurrence of an injury.

The basic problem with respect to the development of further
muscle imbalance, however, lies in those minor strains and sprains
that do not require surgery or immobilization. There is a natural
desire on the part of the athlete to return immediately to normal
activity. In doing so, the athlete will either protect the slightly
strained muscle or sprained joint by altering his style of walking,
running, or throwing or, in total body movement, by substituting
non-injured muscle action for action of the injured muscles. The injured muscles become weaker, and the substituting muscles become
stronger, creating a muscular imbalance that predisposes the
athlete to further injuries to the muscle or joint.

This alteration in style can also create problems in other joints of
the lower extremities. Travers related a case that clearly illustrates
the point.[24] A runner with constant knee problems over a period of a
year was brought to his attention. An examination of his running
style revealed a gross inequality in pace length and almost a
complete loss of mobility in the ankle of the leg that troubled him.
Investigation disclosed he had experienced a slightly sprained ankle
in that leg six weeks prior to the beginning of the knee problem.

The alteration of style caused by the ankle injury had created an overstress on the bones and musculature of the knee joint.

A strained foot, for example, will many times lead to a habit of limping onto the uninjured foot, adding overstress effects to that foot through a shift of balance and body weight distribution on the feet. When the habit persists, muscle weakness develops in the injured foot, ankle, and leg.

Ferguson and Bender pointed out what may occur when an athlete suffers a severe muscle bruise that does not hinder his capablities.[8] The athlete inadvertently substitutes other muscle groups for the injured group. This causes a pronounced muscle weakness to occur in the bruised muscle, which may be responsible for more severe injuries in the future.

Muscle weakness and imbalance are only two of the problems that can result from minor soft tissue injuries. Burry, in an article on the late effects of neglected injuries of this type, commented:

> Neglect of an injury may be the responsibility of the patient or the doctor. On the one hand, the player may regard his symptoms as trivial in the early stages, as he often does with lesions of the adductor origin, or may, in his anxiety to return to training before his hard-won fitness is lost, disregard his doctor's advice. On the other hand, the advice he receives may be poor—ill-informed, unenthusiastic or, not uncommonly, both.[1]

2. *Participation in Sports*: Sports predispose an athlete to unilateral and imbalanced muscular development. These are activities leading to a considerable overdevelopment of muscles on one side of a joint or of the body. The resulting imbalance is manifested in postural deviations as the body seeks to reestablish itself in relation to the center of gravity, and in deviations in the feet and ankles, both of which place abnormal stresses on the joints of the lower back and extremities. Muscular imbalance resulting from sports participation may begin at that level or may represent further development of a pre-existing muscular imbalance in the body structure.

Boxers, baseball players, golfers, tennis players, fencers, javelin throwers, shot putters, and other athletes who consistently use one side of the body in application of skills related to their sport will eventually develop some degree of lateral curvature of the spine and asymmetry of the shoulder, trunk, and hip muscles Various authorities have written that wrestling tends to develop the muscles of the chest and anterior shoulders at the expense of the shoulder adductors.

Two intensive research studies made in the Soviet Union prove conclusively that participation in competitive sports creates muscular imbalance in the body. It should be kept in mind that all athletes involved in the studies engaged in supplementary strength development programs during the training process.

Mirzamukhamedov and his associates studied the relative width of the psoas (hip flexor), quadratus lumborum, and sacrospinalis muscles (back extensors) in 329 persons from 17 to 30 years of age, of whom 279 were sportsmen (89 wrestlers, 107 soccer players, 53 men gymnasts and 30 women gymnasts) and 50 (control group) were non-sportsmen.[22] The mean number of years in participation for soccer players was 5.3; for wrestlers and gymnasts, 3.8; and for all the sportsmen studied, 4.4.

Measurement results reflected that the group of muscles studied was expressed more evenly in gymnasts than in soccer players, wrestlers, or the control group. Such muscular development corresponded to the character of the physical exercises which were specifically worked on in the various sports. In soccer players, the psoas muscles (hip flexors) and in wrestlers, the sacrospinalis muscles and quadratus lumborum (low back muscles) received a greater load and were thus much better developed than they were in the two other groups.

With regard to asymmetrical development, the results reflected symmetrical sacrospinalis muscle development in soccer players and gymnasts, and less symmetrical development in wrestlers and the control group. In the latter two cases, the right side was more developed than the left. The quadratus lumborum was better developed on the right side in wrestlers and on the left side in soccer players and gymnasts The psoas muscle in most cases was asymmetrical; in almost all groups studied, it was better developed on the right side. Researchers concluded that in sportsmen, as in non-sportsmen, the muscles of the right side are better developed than those of the left side and that this is especially noticeable in measurements of the psoas muscles.

The second study was of particular importance. First, it has generally been accepted in the sports world that wrestling is one of the best, if not the best, sport for all-round development of the body. Second, the athletes tested had all engaged in heavy weight training in their conditioning programs. Martirosov and Ribalko conducted laboratory tests on 212 amateur wrestlers, involving over 6,000 measurements of strength in various muscle groups.[19] The test groups comprised the national competitive teams and the strongest first class and Master of Sport wrestlers in Moscow. Results of the testing reflected the ratio of strength between various muscle groups in the two groups of wrestlers:

| *Master of Sports and First Class* Confidence limits | | *Competitive* Confidence |
|---|---|---|
| Forearm flexors | 3.8 | 5.0 |

| | | |
|---|---|---|
| Forearm extensors | 4.4 | 4.6 |
| Shoulder flexors | 9.6 | 5.8 |
| Shoulder extensors | 6.8 | 12.2 |
| Trunk flexors | 5.4 | 5.8 |
| Trunk extensors | 14.5 | 25.0 |
| Thigh flexors | 2.8 | 6.8 |
| Thigh extensors | 5.8 | 15.0 |
| Foot (sole) flexors | 10.8 | 12.8 |

The researchers concluded that the strongest groups of muscles are the extensors of the thigh and trunk and the sole flexors of the foot, and that the weakest are the posterior flexors of the foot, the flexors of the knee, and the flexors of the trunk. The tremendous emphasis placed on strength development of the antigravity muscles (extensors) through weight training, and the length of time the training was used, were reflected in the increase in strength in the shoulder, trunk, and knee extensors as compared to the lowered ratio of strength in the antagonists, the shoulder, trunk, and knee flexors, between the first class competitive team athletes and the first class wrestlers.

3. *Pre-conditioning Programs*: Coaches and trainers are in an ideal position to detect and start correction of the basic muscular imbalances the prospective athlete brings with him to the field of competitive sports participation. Few give attention to postural or foot deviations or to testing for muscular imbalance around the joints of those athletes who are under their supervision at the outset of their careers. Yet coaches will consistently devise conditioning programs that further existing muscular imbalances or create ones. This is particularly true with respect to strength development programs which have followed upon recognition by the athletic world that strength is a basic physical requirement of sports participation and important in injury prevention through increasing the stability of body joints. Based on the advice of weight-training and conditioning authorities, they design their training programs to emphasize development of strength in the prime mover muscles involved in the sport for which the athlete is preparing himself, but devote little if any attention to specifically strengthening the antagonist muscles.

Many of the exercises incorporated into conditioning programs by coaches, weight-training authorities, and experts on conditioning are contra-indicated for correction of muscular imbalance and further existing muscular imbalance, regardless of the flexibility exercises also included in the programs.

An example occurs in the case of athletes who have highly-developed anterior shoulder and chest muscles in a shortened condition, and develop a round-shouldered posture due to the weakened and stretched adductor and extensor muscles of the upper back. As part of a general or specific conditioning program, they are given floor push-ups or bench presses that create a greater muscle imbalance in the shoulder girdle. No attention is given to strengthening their upper back muscles, particularly the shoulder adductors and posterior deltoids.

Athletes with a minor inward curve of the spine (lordosis), overstretched hamstrings, and a forward-tilted pelvis are given straight leg sit-ups and leg raises that further shorten and strengthen the hip flexors. Such movements fail to strengthen the buttock muscles to offset the lordosis and forward tilt of the pelvis.

Athletes with foot weaknesses and slight pronation of the ankles are automatically given toe raises, with or without weights, that futher depress the longitudinal arches and do nothing to correct the already-existing imbalance.

Further, in this writer's opinion, most athletes—unless they are recovering from an acute injury and under the supervision of a physical therapist—misuse weight training both in conditioning and reconditioning work. This misuse is based on failure to determine the difference between strength conditioning and power conditioning and the correct use of weights in developing strength.

The writer has observed hundreds of athletes swinging heavy weights with some degree of velocity, instead of completing the movement at a slow controlled pace to develop strength throughout the entire range of the muscle group. The maximum resistance of a power movement is, at its outset, to overcome the forces of gravity. For the rest of the movement, velocity compensates in overcoming resistance. Most athletes, in performing their exercises, rarely complete a full flexion and extension of the body joint being exercised. This misuse of strength conditioning exercises is of little value to the athlete, if his objective is to strengthen the muscles, tendons, and ligaments around vulnerable body joints. The incomplete flexion and extension also lessen the extensibility limits of the muscle fibers and fascia.

In summarizing the results of studies on imbalance, and the opinions of authorities from various disciplines presented above, five conclusions can be drawn:

1. There can never be an absolute muscle balance in the body.
2. A definite muscular imbalance of the muscles surrounding body joints exists from childhood through old age.
3. The goal of training and conditioning from the standpoint of injury prevention should be to reduce the ratio of imbalance to as small a differential as possible.
4. The reduction in the ratio of imbalance should be directed toward the shoulder girdle, trunk and pelvis, knees and ankles.
5. The lateral side (abductor muscles) of the ankle and foot should

be strengthened considerably, but should never exceed the strength of the adductor muscles on the medial side of the ankle and foot.

## REFERENCES

1. Burry, Hugh C., "Late Effects of Neglected Soft Tissue Injury," *Proceedings of the Royal Society of Medicine*, Vol. LXII, September 1962.
2. Carey, Eben J., "Scoliosis," *Journal of the American Medical Association*, January 9, 1932.
3. Clarke, H. Harrison, *Muscular Strength and Endurance in Man* (Englewood Cliffs, N.J.: Prentice-Hall, Inc., 1966).
4. Cobey, M. C., *Postural Back Pain* (Springfield, Illinois: Charles C. Thomas, 1956).
5. Conway, David H., "Podiatry's Role in Basketball," *Journal of Podiatry*, Vol. 60, No. 10, October 1970.
6. Cyriax, Edgar F., "Some Hitherto Unrecognized Causes of Spinal Curvatures," *Journal of Scientific Physical Training*, Vol. 4, No. 12, Summer 1912.
7. Fahey, J. F., "Some Hitherto Unrecognized Causes of Spinal Curvatures," *Journal of Scientific Physical Training*, Vol. 4, No. 12, Summer 1912.
7. Fahey, J. F., "The Retarded Leg Syndrome," *Abstracts of Joint Meeting of A.C.S.M. and C.A.S.S., Toronto, 1971.*
8. Ferguson, A. B. and Bender, Jay, *The ABC's of Athletic Injuries and Conditioning* (Baltimore: The William and Wilkins Co., 1964).
9. Fitzgerald, Gerald, "Standing Easy with the Weight on One Leg," *Journal of Scientific Physical Training*, Vol. XIII, 1918.
10. Hutchins, Gloria L., "The Relationship of Selected Strength and Flexibility Variables to the Antereo-Posterior Posture of College Women," *Research Quarterly,* Vol. 36, No. 3, October 1965.
11. Katznetsov, Z. I., "Short Items of Importance," *Theory and Practice of Physical Culture,* 10:8, 1965.
12. Kite, J. H. "Torsion of the Lower Extremities in Small Children," *Journal of Bone and Joint Surgery,* Vol. 36-A, No. 3, June 1954.
13. Klein, K. K., "A Comparison of Bilateral Quadricepts Muscle Strength of Individuals in Good or Poor Standing Posture," *The Physical Educator.*
14. Klein, K. K., "Flexibility—Strength and Balance in Athletics," *Journal of N.A.T.A.,* Summer 1971.

15. Knapp, Miland E., "Exercises for Poliomyelitis," *Therapeutic Exercise* (Baltimore: Waverly Press, Inc., 1969.)

16. Korobcov, A., "The Biological Principles of Physical Training," *Proceedings of International Congress of Sport Sciences, Tokyo, 1966* (Tokyo: University of Tokyo Press, 1966).

17. Kraus, Hans, *Backache, Stress and Tension* (New York: Simon and Schuster, Inc., 1965).

18. Martin, E. G., "Tests of Muscular Efficiency," *Physiological Review,* July 1921.

19. Martirosov, E. G. and Ribalko, B. M., "The Dependence of Achievement in Wrestling on Strength Preparation," *Theory and Practice of Physical Culture,* 9:13-15 (Moscow), 1966.

20. Masaki, Takeo, "Electromyographic Study of Rest Standing Posture in Man," *Proceedings of International Conference on Sports Sciences, Tokyo, 1964* (Tokyo: Japanese Union of Sports Sciences, 1964).

21. Michelle, Arthur A., *Orthotherapy* (New York: M. Evans and Co., Inc., 1971).

22. Mirzamukhamedov, A. G., "Development of Several Muscles in the Lumbar Region in Sportsmen," *Theory and Practice of Physical Culture,* 5:27-28 (Moscow), 1969.

23. Rasch, Philip J. and Burke, Roger K., *Kinesiology and Applied Anatomy* (4th ed.) (Philadelphia: Lea and Febiger, 1971).

24. Travers, P. R., "Injuries Due to Faulty Style," *Track Technique,* No. 11.

# 7

# Effects of Muscular Imbalance

In discussing the effects of muscular imbalance on the musculo-skeletal structure of the body, a question arises as to whether muscular imbalance causes postural and foot deviations or is itself caused by them. The answer is that although either one can cause the other, muscular imbalance is the precipitating cause in most cases.

In 1741, Nicolas Andry, Professor of Medicine at the University of Paris, who is recognized as the creator of the word "orthopedics" and the founder of that branch of medicine, expressed the opinion that skeletal deformities resulted from muscular imbalance in childhood.[1] He was the first member of the medical profession to note the active participation of the muscles in producing deformities of the skeletal system, and he became an ardent advocate of exercises as a prophylactic measure to prevent the development of such deformities in children.

## POSTURAL DEVIATIONS

In 1941, Cureton wrote that most authorities in corrective physical education work believed that poor posture was caused by unbalanced pull of muscles.[5] He reported that in 1927 Stafford had analyzed the posture of 1,940 college freshmen at the University of Illinois. His findings indicated the percentage of postural deviations of a moderate or severe degree to be as follows: Kyposis, 88.3-31.5 percent; Scoliosis, 71.7-14.1 percent; Lordosis, 81.2-14.1 percent.

Specializing in the treatment of postural disorders, the Kendalls have long maintained that muscle imbalance is a major cause of postural faults, and that the effects of such faults include: low back pain, sciatic nerve symptoms, sacroiliac strains, and slipping of the fifth lumbar vertebra.[7]

Michelle commented that round back, round shoulders, and the so-called "growing pains" of young adolescents are all symptoms of muscle imbalance.[14]

Riddle and Roaf, in electromyographic studies of the spinal muscles in cases of scoliosis (lateral curvature) not caused by congenital deformities, pointed out that the onset of scoliosis is due to muscular imbalance in the deep rotator and transverse muscles of the spine.[16] This is in contrast to the traditional concept of its being caused by muscular imbalance in the superficial longitudinal muscles (spinal erectae) of the back. They defined scoliosis as a rotational deformity.

## FOOT FAULTS

Lewin credits Duchenne, who in 1855 conducted his classic studies on the physiology of motion, with being the first to observe a specific relationship between muscular imbalance in the leg and eversion and pronation of the foot.[12] Osgood, in 1908, verified Duchenne's findings in his studies of weak and flat feet.[15] Osgood and his colleagues found the most common intrinsic predisposing cause of weak, strained, and flat feet to be muscle imbalance.

Dickson and Dively have reported that loss of muscle balance in the foot and lower leg muscle groups will disturb the normal balance of the leg and the foot, thereby causing a breakdown of postural and structural stability of the foot.[6]

In 1951, Todd and his associates, orthopedic surgeons, expressed the opinion that the basic cause of pes cavus (high arch) was a lack of balance between the flexors and extensors of the foot, with relative weakness of the extensors leading to depression of the forefoot.[19] The intrinsic foot muscles were not at fault, and shortening of the Achilles tendon was not a responsible factor. Clawing of the toes was secondary to the pes cavus.

## SKILL, COORDINATION, FLEXIBILITY, AND ENDURANCE

Coaches, trainers, and physical therapists place great emphasis on optimum flexibility in body joints. It is extremely difficult to acquire any degree of flexibility in a joint when there is a great disparity in the ratio of strength between the muscles on both sides of the joint. The antagonist muscles and ligaments are already in a stretched and weakened condition, and the overdeveloped prime mover agonist muscles in a shortened condition. In addition, the ligaments on the agonist side of the joint have shortened. The antagonist muscles and underlying ligaments must first be strengthened and the ratio of imbalance between the opposing muscles reduced before an appreciable degree of stretching of the agonist muscles can be achieved.

Many authorities have pointed out that in our daily activities, whether in play, work, or sport, we tend to use some muscles more than others. Unless this is recognized, there is a great tendency to develop imbalance between the antagonist and the agonist muscles. This results in the shortening of those muscles that are used the most, effecting limitations of motion that are detrimental to sports efficiency.

Constantly overstretched muscles on one side of a joint due to imbalance created by the stronger muscles on the opposite side result in weakness and loss of power in the stretched muscles. A weak atrophic muscle is easily fatigued and is exposed to loss of elasticity sooner than a strong non-fatigued muscle. A tired muscle loses some of its ability to relax. This interferes with the process of reciprocal innervation which requires the antagonistic muscles to relax completely, while the prime mover muscles move the joint in one direction, if optimum speed and coordination are to be attained. As muscular imbalance increases, excess work is required of the central nervous system, because uncoordination results more quickly and is a definite indication of the onset of fatigue. When adjustment and improvement in the strength of opposite groups of muscles around a joint have become a habit of reflex action, fatigue will generate more slowly.

Klein commented on this, stating: " ...but in all of this, there is a tendency to forget that the antagonists control the prime muscle movement and should also be conditioned to maintain balance so as to prevent the "fatigue syndrome."[9] He went on to say: "Not to be repetitive, but for emphasis, the antagonists control prime mover muscle action and unless these muscles are considered in the training program for balance and flexibility, muscular coordination will suffer due to the earlier fatigue of the antagonist."

It has been well established that fatigue and a lack of skill, coordination, or flexibility which are the symptoms or results of hidden causes are primary apparent causes of athletic injuries.

## PREDISPOSING CAUSE OF INJURIES

In the writer's opinion, there is more than sufficient evidence obtainable by research to support the hypothesis that muscular imbalance is a major predisposing and causative factor that results in muscle and fascia strains, ligament sprains, and various overuse syndromes in the lower back, legs, and feet.

Over 30 years ago, the famous Dr. Charles Lowman wrote about the effects of muscular imbalance on postural deviations. He described the effect of postural deviations on athletic prformance and the injuries and overuse syndromes resulting from muscular imbalance and postural deviations.

During the fifties, in his monumental studies on the causes of knee injuries, Klein proved that muscular imbalance was a major predisposing factor in such injuries.[10]

In the early sixties, two orthopedic physicians at the University of Oregon, Slocum and Bowerman, emphasized the importance of postural deviations and muscular imbalance as predisposing factors in soft tissue injuries and overuse syndromes in running.[18]

During the past five years, Burkett[2] and Christensen and Wiseman[3] have proven that muscular or bilateral imbalance is a predisposing factor in hamstring injuries; Merrifield and Cowan[13] have proven the same with regard to thigh adductor strains.

Corrigan and others have suggested that muscular imbalance is one of the causes of the troublesome problem of "shin splints" that plagues athletes.[4]

Unfortunately, the valuable contributions of these authorities did not make a large impact on coaches, trainers, and athletes because the majority of their writings appeared in professional journals associated with the orthopedic, physical therapy, and physical education professions.

With respect to the foot and its contribution to lower leg overuse syndromes, Dr. George Sheehan, a cardiologist and also a runner, has been instrumental in showing the effects of muscular imbalance in the feet in this regard.[17] Sheehan listed some of the leg problems associated with foot weaknesses and deviations: Achilles tendonitis, stress fractures, pain on inside of leg, chondromalacia of the knee, and pain in the back of the knee. He stated: "It goes without saying, that muscle weakness and imbalance contribute to the foot and leg syndrome, and exercises to strengthen foot and shin (antigravity) muscles should be performed. In thigh, groin, and back injuries, weakness is often noted in the hamstrings or abdominal muscles."

Michelle stated that muscular imbalance is a leading cause of sports-connected injuries.[14] LaCava coined a term, "enthesitis," which describes a group of conditions characterized initially by inflammatory reactions and subsequently by fibrosis and calcification around the tendons, ligaments, and muscle insertions.[11] Klafs and Arnheim, discussing overuse syndromes, pointed out that as a result of muscular imbalance, severe strain may be exerted on the insertions with enthesitis resulting.[8]

The problem of athletic-related injuries caused by muscle imbalance has been recognized and discussed by school and professional coaches, as well as by physicians. At a recent meeting of the American Medical Association, the New York Jets' physician, Dr. Jim Nicholas, urged exercise programs to compensate for muscle imbalance and help prevent the 15 to 20 million sprains and dislocations that Americans suffer every year in sports and school activities.

Recently, Joseph Zohar, a physiotherapist, in an article on preventive conditioning, commented on the many investigations that have been made into the causes of sports injuries.[20] He maintained that these investigations have focused on the external causes of injuries (playing surfaces, protective equipment, poor training set-ups, etc.), and that very few have examined the subject himself—the athlete. He asked: "Why can't his body withstand the external stresses imposed upon it?" Zohar contended that the approach to the athlete's body is being ignored in the conventional conditioning program, and that coaches fail to condition athletes' muscles equitably to see that not a single muscle weakness remains uncorrected. Zohar went on to comment that several studies have indicated that any imbalance in muscle strength greatly increases the odds on an injury to the weaker muscles, and concluded: "The large number of muscle pulls sustained by the most 'superbly' conditioned sprinters, football players, and even basketball players is living proof of that fact."

## REFERENCES

1. Andry, Nicolas *Orthopaedia,* facsimile reproduction (Philadelphia: J. B. Lippincott Co. 1961).
2. Burkett, L. M., "Causative Factors in Hamstring Injuries," *Medicine and Science in Sports,* Vol. 2, Spring 1970.
3. Christensen, C. S. and Wiseman, D. C., "Strength, the Common Variable in Hamstring Strain," *Athletic Training,* Vol. 7, No. 2, 1972.
4. Corrigan, A. B., "The Aetiology of Recent Muscle Injuries," *Australian Journal of Sports Medicine,* Vol. 1, No. 9, 1966.
5. Cureton, Thomas K., "Bodily Posture as an Indicator of Fitness," *Supplement to the Research Quarterly,* Vol. 12, No. 2, May 1941.
6. Dickson, Frank D. and Diveley, Rex L., *Functional Disorders of the Foot* (Philadelphia: J. B. Lippincott Co., 1953).
7. Kendall, Henry O. and Kendall, Florence P., "Study and Treatment of Muscle Imbalance in Cases of Low Back and Sciatic Pain," *The Physiotherapy Review,* Vol. 16, No. 5, 1936.
8. Klafs, C. E. and Arnheim, D. D., *Modern Principles of Athletic Training* (St. Louis: C. V. Mosby, 1963).
9. Klein, Karl K., "Flexibility—Strength and Balance in Athletics," *Journal of N.A.T.A.,* Summer 1971.
10. Klein, Karl K. and Hall, William L., *The Knee in Athletics* (Washington, D.C.: American Association for Health, Physical Education, and Recreation, 1963).

11. LaCava, Giussepe, "Enthesitis—Traumatic Disease of Insertions," *Journal of the American Medical Association,* January 17, 1959.

12. Lewin, Philip, "The Foot and Ankle" *Minnesota Medicine,* November 1938.

13. Merrifield, H. H, and Cowan, R. F. "Bilateral Force, Torque and Power Imbalances as Contributory Factors in Hip Joint Adductor Strains in Selected Ice Hockey Players," *Abstracts of Joint Meeting A.C.S.M. and C.A.S.M., Toronto, Ontario, 1971.*

14. Michelle, Arthur A., *Orthotherapy* (New York: N. Evans and Co., Inc., 1971).

15. Osgood, Robert B., "The Comparative Strength of the Adductor and Abductor Groups in the Foot," *American Journal of Orthopaedic Surgery,* January 1908.

17. Sheehan, George, "Medical Advice," *Runner's World,* September 1972.

18. Slocum, D. B. and Bowerman, W., "The Biomechanics of Running," *Clinical Orthopaedics,* Vol. 23, 1962.

19. Todd, A.; Jones, A. Rocyn; and Martin, D. J.; "Orthopaedic Miscellany," *British Medical Journal,* May 5, 1951.

20. Zohar, Joseph, "Preventative Conditioning for Maximum Safety and Performance," *Scholastic Coach,* May, 1973.

# 8

# Body Mechanics and Posture

Traditionally, the word "posture" has expressed status and position of the body in an upright standing position. Throughout history, this concept has been molded at various times by the opinions of artists, anatomists, the military, physical education teachers, the kinesiologist, and the clinician.

The idea expressed by the term "body mechanics" involves movement of the body. Body mechanics is an outgrowth of kinesiology (science of body movement) based upon mechanical principles. It refers to both the static and the functional relationships between body parts and the body as a whole. The interrelationships of the more than 200 bones and 600 muscles of the body are subject to the same mechanical laws and forces which control any other machine.

The modern viewpoint manifests less interest in an upright erect body position *per se*. It places greater stress on integration of body segments during movement. Within this concept, posture is the natural way a person stands. Good body mechanics is a functional balance and poise of the body in all positions: standing, lying, sitting, and during movement.

## CORRECT POSTURE AND GOOD BODY MECHANICS

Correct posture in the upright stance according to modern conceptions is an alignment of maximum physiological and biomechanical efficiency. This stems from a balanced action of muscles to maintain all segments of the body in a position which does not involve excessive stress on joints, muscles, and ligaments, and from which coordinated action of any body part is possible.

With respect to the prevention of injuries and manifestations of overuse syndromes, the most adequate definition of correct posture is that provided by the Posture Committee of the American Academy of Orthopedic Surgeons (Chicago, Illinois), reprinted here with their permission:

> Posture is usually defined as the relative arrangement of the parts of the body. Good posture is that state of muscular and skeletal balance which protects the supporting structures of the body against injury or progressive deformity, irrespective of the attitude (erect, lying, squatting, stooping) in which these structures are working or resting. Under such conditions the muscles will function most efficiently and the optimum positions are afforded for the thoracic and abdominal organs. Poor posture is a faulty relationship of the various parts of the body, which produces increased strain on the supporting structures and in which there is less efficient balance of the body over its base of support.

## BODY TYPES AND POSTURE

W. H. Sheldon, physical anthropologist, classified three extreme body types based upon the type of cell layer that dominated the specific body type and the temperament of each type.[3]

1. *Mesomorphic:* Muscular cell tissue predominates. Displays efficient and relatively effortless body movement, efficient sugar metabolism, and easy recovery from fatigue. Is better adapted structurally, organically, and neurologically to meet the stress of life situations than the other two types. Has a dominant, aggressive, competitive temperament. This type thrives on physical activity.

2. *Endomorphic:* Fat cell tissue predominates. Body is soft and well-rounded and muscles lack strength. Physiological processes emphasize the internal or visceral functions. This type has an extremely effective absorption of maximum nutritional value from food eaten. Shuns physical activity and fatigues easily. Has a placid, social, tolerant, and phlegmatic type of temperament.

3. *Ectomorphic*: Low muscle and relatively few fat cells. Long and lean muscles and internal organs. Bones are prominent. Predominate in surface or ectomorphic cell tissue. Usually lacks strength and endurance for contact and many other strenuous sports. Body type tends toward quickness and agility of movement. Has a high-strung, tense, and sensitive temperament.

4. *Somatotype*: The extremes of body type are in the minority. Most people are a blend of the three types, with one of the three extreme types predominating. Sheldon's studies showed that those persons with a dominance of mesomorphic body tissue were predominant in athletics. His system of classification (Somatotyping) rated the body type blends. The ectomorphic-mesomorphic body type tends to dominate sporting activities such as

running and hurdling, that require speed and/or endurance. The endomorphic-mesmorphic tends to dominate sporting activities requiring strength and power. The mesomorphic body type is found in all fields of physical activity.

## BODY BUILD AND POSTURE

Human beings are also classified for posture evaluation purposes by types of body build based on the length, diameter, and weight of the bony structure and the weight distribution on the skeletal structure.

1. The lean slender body build has long, light, and small-diameter skeletal bones. Generally has a shallow chest and pelvis from front to back and slender (gracile) feet.

2. The stocky broad body build has short to long, heavy, and long-diameter bones. Generally has a deep chest and pelvis structure from front to back.

3. The intermediate body build has short to long, medium-heavy, and medium-diameter bones.

4. Many people display an irregular body build. They will have a slender bony structure in one part of the body and a stocky heavy bone structure in another part.

## BODY BUILD AND STRUCTURAL VARIATIONS

The vertebrae normally are thicker in front in the cervical (shoulder) and lumbar (lower back) regions and thicker in back in the dorsal or thoracic (chest) region (Figure 1). These differences comprise the three typical curves of the human spine. Variations in the thickness of the vertebrae at different regions of the spine will influence the depth of the spinal curves, as will variations in the anteroposterior depth of the chest or pelvis.

The angular measurement of the femoral (thigh bone) head in its relation to the shaft of the bone and to the acetabulum (socket that holds head of thigh bone) display wide differences between persons of the same age groups. These relations affect the degree of lordosis (inward curve) in the lower back and the degree to which the feet toe in or toe out.

Short clavicles or particularly large shoulder blades, combined with a relatively narrow chest, will give the impression of round-shulderedness even though the body is not out of alignment.

Orthopedic texts and journals generally class these structural variations as congenital anomalies. They may or may not have a serious effect on the antereo-posterior posture curves of the spine.

## BODY BUILD AND PROPENSITIES TO POSTURAL FAULTS

Slender athletes, due to suppleness of muscle and ligaments, muscular imbalance, and weakness in the upper body, are prone to easily develop faults in the antereo-posterior curves of the spine and shoulder girdle. During adolescence, they tend to develop the common fatigue posture. This posture is manifested by a forward head, a sway back with increased lordosis of the lower spine, a slumped chest, and round upper back. The fatigue posture fault leads to a forward tilt of the pelvis, which will affect leg and foot alignment and place abnormal stresses on the joints of the knee, ankle, and foot. This body build is also subject to development of a flat back lumbar posture profile.

With the exception of sprinters up to 440 yards, an overwhelming number of competitive runners are of slender build and fall within the ectomorphic-mesomorphic classification.

The intermediate body build with a higher proportion of mesomorphic tissue is less apt to develop serious antereo-posterior postural faults. However, when postural faults in the spine do develop, this body build has much greater difficulty in overcoming them. The intermediate build can develop the upper round back posture due to muscular imbalance in the shoulder girdle body area and, as is the case with most athletes, the tendency to relax into a slumped position between movement activities in order to conserve energy.

The stocky mesomorphic-endomorphic body build generally is subject to a restricted mobility of the spine, and is less likely to show serious antereo-posterior faults in the spine. If such a person tends to slump, however, due to poor postural habits, he may develop a round hollow back—but with much less forward tilt of the pelvis than is found in the slender type. He may also develop a backward extension of the spine and trunk at the hip or the dorso-lumbar junction of the spine. He is also prone to more serious faults in the lower extremities and feet.

All body builds are subject to lateral curvature of the spine. Lateral curves are generally due to unilateral muscle development resulting from participation in play and sports activities. This is particularly true of athletes participating in throwing sports. The other major cause of lateral spine curvature is the short leg syndrome or a flat foot, which will be discussed later in this volume.

## CORRECT POSTURE FOR ATHLETIC PERFORMANCE

At this point, the reader may well ask the following question: What is good posture? Morrison and Chenweth, in *Normal and Elementary Physical Diagnosis*, maintained that three conditions must be met before posture can be classified as good.[2] They are: (1) Does the posture make for mechanical freedom? (2) Is the posture true to anatomical fact? (3) Does the posture provide for a more efficient functioning of one or more internal organs (heart, lungs, intestines)?

There are two basic elements in correct posture, whether it be in the non-athlete or the athlete—skeletal alignment and muscle balance. These elements are dependent on normal muscle tonus, muscle balance, adequately developed postural reflexes, and normal development of the antigravity (postural) muscles.

Charles Sherrington, a great neurosurgeon early in this century, demonstrated conclusively that the correct upright posture of the body is being maintained when continuous tonic reflex muscular activity over long periods of time does not produce fatigue. Tonic reflexes, a nervous system activity, are acquired and developed through habit and repetition. This activity requires voluntary conscious effort during the early childhood developmental growth stage, but it eventually becomes an involuntary automatic reflex habit. Tonic reflexes are the antigravity (extensor) postural reflexes and muscle tonus discussed in Chapter 2.

Whether tonic postural reflexes develop in a manner that results in correct body alignment during adolescence and adult life or fail to develop, resulting in poor body alignment, is the crux of the problem. Proper body alignment contributes to effective body mechanics and the prevention of non-contact injuries and overuse syndromes, while poor body alignment is a major predisposing cause of injuries and overuse syndromes and interferes with maximum efficient performance in running and jogging.

In 1951, Anderson, a Scottish physiotherapist whose interest in body mechanics over the preceding 25 years was first stimulated by his experience in the field of athletic and occupational worlds, wrote a book called *Human Kinetics*, in which he commented that the character of a correct body movement, in respect to athletic performance or occupational activity, is determined by fundamental *lock, check,* and usually *evasive actions.*[1] The most important, in relation to posture and movement in the upright position, is the *lock* action.

Anderson defined *lock* action as "putting a part into a position which will automatically stabilize other parts of the body and lead to more efficient action with the minimum of effort." The *lock* action position of certain body joints reduces to a minimum the amount of muscle work in maintaining upright erect posture. In it, the body is substituting mechanical forces and fibrous muscle tissue tonic tension for stabilization of body joints, instead of relying on ligaments to maintain the joints in proper weight alignment.

The two most important *lock* actions are the foot and neck *lock* actions. A correct foot *lock* action is based on a straight ahead foot position that activates the all-important plantar reflex, which in turn activates all the postural reflexes of the antigravity (extensor) muscles above the foot. A correct neck *lock* action involves the "tucking in" of the chin to elevate the head and straighten the upper spine. These two key *lock* actions are interdependent and together they open the door to erect posture and correct application of body movements in the upright position.

Some 20 years later, Bowerman, Slocum, and James of the University of Oregon, in writing about the biomechanics of running, emphasized the principle of the upright posture and the straight ahead foot position for effective running performance and the avoidance of overuse syndromes in the lower extremities and feet.

It is interesting to note Anderson's observations concerning the problem of relaxation. Athletic writers stress the importance of relaxation in the training of athletes, including, to conserve energy, the relaxation of antagonist muscles while prime mover muscles perform their functions of moving the joints without restriction and relaxation between body movements. His important findings on *lock* actions and relaxation continue below:

> The idea that a body which is allowed to "sag" is relaxed is, unfortunately, common among athletes. Allowing the body to sag certainly relieves the muscles which maintain the erect position from the tension caused by actual contraction, but the tension caused by stretching of the muscles when the body sags will retard free circulation. Sagging or slouching when in the upright position has the further disadvantage of relatively increasing the load on the spinal joints and the deeper-seated back muscles and also restricting movement of the respiratory organs.

> Many athletes have the idea that by allowing certain parts of the body to sag during movement they are conserving energy. This is a false conception for two main reasons: (1) It relatively increases the load on the deeper-seated postural muscles in all parts of the body. (2) The joint instability which it produces seriously undermines muscular efficiency. The efficiency of a muscle depends to a great extent upon the stability of one of its attachments. For example, instability of the shoulder girdle will undermine the efficiency of biceps in moving the forearm. On the other hand, when its upper attachment is properly stabilized by fixation of the shoulder girdle, biceps can control the forearm more accurately and efficiently. Further, when the body is well-balanced in the erect position and *lock* action positions are utilized, less energy is expended in postural muscle work—which is the most energy-taxing type of muscle work.

Working parallel to Anderson in time, Tucker, an eminent British orthopedic physician, was developing his concept of *active alerted posture* in the upright position, in contrast to what he termed *inactive slumping posture*.[4] In a lecture presented in England, he pointed out that many athletic injuries occur and re-occur because the athlete has not been taught the essentials of good body mechanics.

Tucker maintained that the *active alerted posture* was dependent on the balanced action of muscle groups on both sides of body joints at six fixing levels: (1) ankle joints; (2) knee joints; (3) hip joints; (4) lumbo-sacral joints (lower back); (5) occipto-atlantoid joints (head and neck); and (6) shoulder girdle joints. The weight of the mobile parts is carried by these muscles and there is no chronic strain upon the ligaments or other components of the body joints.

*Inactive slumping posture*, however, involves support of weight-bearing mobile parts by ligaments only. This type of posture places progressive strain on the joints and the soft tissue structures surrounding them. This shows itself first as a fibrosis (muscular rheumatism) of the involved muscles with subsequent muscle spasm, and finally leads to joint degeneration and the onset of osteo-arthritis in the joints. In addition, when movement occurs in athletic activities, injuries to muscle and joint structures are more likely to occur, because the movement takes place on slack muscles with the corresponding joints unprotected.

The qualifications of an *active alerted posture*, described by Tucker, are as follows:

1. At the ankle and joint level, weight should be carried on the outer side of the foot and toes to form an inverted Gothic arch in a straight ahead foot position.

2. At the knee joint level, the knee is held very slightly flexed so there is balanced action between hamstrings at back and the quadriceps in front.

3. At the hip and lumbo-sacral joint levels, abdominal muscles are held up, the buttock muscles are tucked in, and the lumbo-sacral articulations are firmly fixed.

4. At the head and neck joint level, an erect position of the head on the neck is maintained by the balanced contraction of the muscles on both sides of the neck with the chin well tucked in.

5. At the shoulder girdle level, there must be a fixation of the shoulder girdles by continuous tonic muscular activity of the upper back muscles to oppose the downward sagging force of gravity.

Tucker has long held that, contrary to the general opinion, *active alerted posture* is a relaxed posture. The different fixing levels are fixed by just enough tonic muscle activity to hold the muscle groups around each joint in perfect balance, with the body in correct alignment. He contended this is highly important to the runner, as it permits the prime mover muscles to work continuously with the minimum formation of waste products of metabolism (lactic acid) which bring on fatigue prematurely.

Concluding his lecture, Tucker stated:

Each week I see two or three injured athletes, who have had first-rate treatment for their injury up to the time of examination, but are still not symptom free. Their injury does not get better or keeps on recurring. They have not been taught *active alerted posture* and simple body mechanics. As soon as they master these, their symptoms disappear and the chances of recurrence are lessened.

## REFERENCES

1. Anderson, T. McClung, *Human Kinetics and Analyzing Body Movements* (London: William Heinemann Medical Books, Ltd., 1951). Excerpts reprinted by permission of publisher.
2. Morrison, W. R. and Chenoweth, L. B., *Normal and Elementary Physical Diagnosis*, 5th edition (Philadelphia: Lea & Febiger, 1955).
3. Sheldon, W. H.; Dupertuis, C. W.; and Dermott, E. H.; *Atlas of Men, A Guide for Somatotyping the Adult Male at All Ages* (New York: Harper and Bros., 1954).
4. Tucker, W. E., "Postural Training in Athletes," Lecture presented at Royal Northern Hospital, England, 1974.

# 9

## Structure and Anatomy
## of Spinal-Pelvic Girdle Complex

The athlete and jogger should possess a basic knowledge of the skeletal and musculo-ligamentous structure of the spinal-pelvic girdle complex. The interrelationships of the two body segments are important for two reasons: (1) Their combined structural integrity and correct vertical alignment determine the posture of the upper body and play an important role in determining correct leg alignment and the positioning of the feet. (2) Their effects, from a positive or negative standpoint, on the efficiency of running, hurdling, and jogging are considerable.

### DEFINITIONS

There are several medical terms used in the structural description of the spine and pelvis:

*Acetabulum*—a large cup-shaped cavity on the lateral surface of the ilium bones of the pelvis, in which the head of the femur (thigh bone) articulates as a ball and socket joint.

*Kyphosis*—a convexity (outward curve) in the dorsal segment of the spine as viewed from the side, becoming an abnormality when the convexity is increased beyond the normal.

*Lordosis*—a concavity (inward curve) in the lumbar or cervical segment of the spine when viewed from the side, becoming an abnormality when the concavity is increased beyond the normal.

*Scoliosis*—an appreciable lateral deviation or curve of the normal straight vertical line of the spine.

### THE SPINE

The spine is a single weight-bearing column that is still adapting itself to the upright position of the human being (Figure 3A). It is

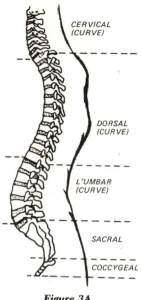

**Figure 3A**
THE SPINE

comprised of 33 vertebrae, 24 of which are known as the flexible spinal column, separated by elastic disks of cartilage called inter-vertebral disks. The five vetebrae immediately below and attached to the flexible column are fused together in a pyramidal or wedge shape to form the sacrum (Figure 3B). Immediately below are the four fused-together vertebrae, called the coccyx.

The 24 vertebrae of the flexible column number 7 in the neck, called cervical vertebrae; 12 in the region of the chest, called dorsal vertebrae; and 5 in the lower back, called lumbar vertebrae. The skeleton of the chest (thorax) includes the sternum (breast bone) and 12 pairs of ribs, a pair for each of the dorsal vertebrae to which they are attached. The flexible column vertebrae are joined together by ligaments, the anterior and posterior ligaments running from the base of the skull to the sacrum and short lateral ligaments joining the bodies of the adjacent vertebrae.

The three curves of the spine are formed by the shape of the inter-vertebral disks during structural growth. They form a normal lordosis in the lumbar and cervical segments of the spine and a normal kyphosis in the dorsal segment of the spine. The three curves transect a straight vertical line in the upright position in order to maintain balance. The curves gradually merge into one another. The only sharp angle is where the fifth lumbar vertebra joins the sacrum and the top (sacral table) of the sacrum slants forward on an incline of about 45 degrees from the horizontal.

89

## SPINAL MOVEMENTS

Movements of the spine take place by the compression of the inter-vertebral disks and by the gliding of the articular (vertebrae) surfaces upon each other. The movements of the spine are illustrated in Chapter 2. It should be noted that lateral flexion of the spinal column always involves some degree of spinal rotation. Spinal rotation always involves some degree of spinal flexion.

## ANATOMY OF SPINE

The spine is entirely supported by muscles and ligaments. Anatomical illustrations of the major muscle groups, supporting and involved in the movements of the flexible spine and shoulder girdle, are illustrated in Figure 4 (upper back, chest), Figure 5 (abdomen-lower back), and Figure 6 (antereo-posterior hip).

## PRIME MOVER MUSCLES AFFECTING SPINAL MOVEMENT

*Upper Back and Shoulder Joint*—The shoulder joint is a highly complicated joint with numerous muscles participating in its various movements. However, the major muscles keeping the shoulder in an erect posture are those of the upper back (rhomboids, trapezius, posterior deltoid) and chest (pectoralis major, anterior deltoid). In most humans, particularly of slim body build, the muscles of the anterior shoulder and chest are more strongly developed than those of the posterior shoulder and upper back.

*Dorsal and Lumbar Spines*—Forward flexion: abdominals, external and internal obliques. Extension: erector spinae group and deep posterior spinal group. Lateral flexion: external and internal obliques, erector spinae group. Rotation to the same side: internal obliques, erector spinae group. Rotation to opposite side: external obliques, rotators, and multifidus muscles of deep posterior spinal group.

The primary action of the abdominals (flexors) and spinal erectae (extensors) is to keep the body above the pelvis upright and, whatever the pelvic inclination below may be, to vary the curves of the spine. The erectae spinae muscles are in the lumbar area, which is the strongest area. The weakest part of the erectae spinal group is in the upper lumbar and lower dorsal areas of the spine. Weakness in this area of the spine, which is very common, allows the entire weight of the upper part of the body to come onto the spine. This produces one of the most prevalent of postural faults, dorso-lumbar kyphosis, more commonly known as round back posture.

## THE PELVIC GIRDLE

The pelvic girdle (Figure 4) is comprised of two hip bones firmly attached to the sacrum at the sacroiliac articulations. Each hipbone is made up of three bones—the ilium, ischium, and pubis. These bones became fused together into a single bone at about the time of puberty.

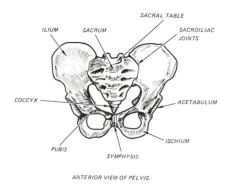

SACRAL TABLE
ILIUM
SACRUM
SACROILIAC JOINTS
COCCYX
ACETABULUM
PUBIS
ISCHIUM
SYMPHYSIS

ANTERIOR VIEW OF PELVIS.

**Figure 3B**
SACRUM
THE PELVIC STRUCTURE

The sacrum (Figure 3B) is firmly bound to the two iliac bones by means of the three sacroiliac ligaments, reinforced by spinal ligaments and the lower end of the spinal muscles. Due to its firm attachments, the sacrum might well be considered a part of the pelvis structure in terms of function. The lumbar portion (fifth vertebra) of the flexible spine rests upon the sacrum and is known as the lumbo-sacral joint. The top of the sacrum is called the sacral table. From an antereo-posterior view, the fifth lumbar vertebra rests on the sacrum (Figure 3B), which is on an inclined (forward and downward) plane. The friction of the two normally prevents a sliding action. When there is a sliding action down the inclined plane due to malalignment, it will create a shearing stress. As the downward angle of incline increases, the greater the shearing stress. At an angle of 30 degress, the shearing stress will be 50 percent of superimposed body weight; at 40 degrees, 65 percent.

From below, the pelvic girdle is supported by the bones of the lower extremities and the feet. The upper end of the femur (thigh bone) is attached to the pelvis at the acetabulum.

## PELVIC MOVEMENTS

The joints at which the movements of the pelvic girdle take place are the two hip joints and the joints of the lumbar spine—the lumbo-sacral junction in particular. The manner in which the

# ANTERIOR UPPER BODY

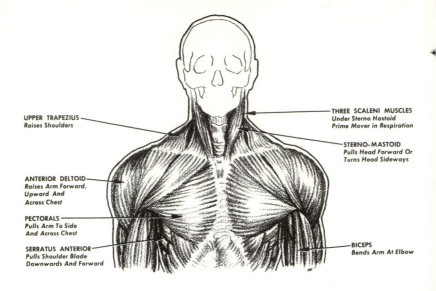

**UPPER TRAPEZIUS**
*Raises Shoulders*

**THREE SCALENI MUSCLES**
*Under Sterno Hastoid*
*Prime Mover in Respiration*

**STERNO-MASTOID**
*Pulls Head Forward Or*
*Turns Head Sideways*

**ANTERIOR DELTOID**
*Raises Arm Forward,*
*Upward And*
*Across Chest*

**PECTORALS**
*Pulls Arm To Side*
*And Across Chest*

**SERRATUS ANTERIOR**
*Pulls Shoulder Blade*
*Downwards And Forward*

**BICEPS**
*Bends Arm At Elbow*

# POSTERIOR UPPER BODY

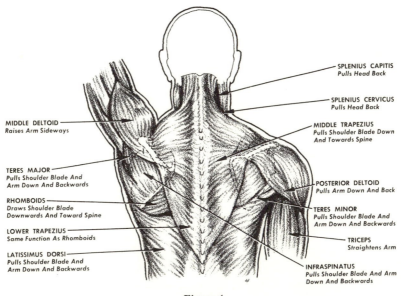

**SPLENIUS CAPITIS**
*Pulls Head Back*

**SPLENIUS CERVICUS**
*Pulls Head Back*

**MIDDLE DELTOID**
*Raises Arm Sideways*

**MIDDLE TRAPEZIUS**
*Pulls Shoulder Blade Down*
*And Towards Spine*

**TERES MAJOR**
*Pulls Shoulder Blade And*
*Arm Down And Backwards*

**POSTERIOR DELTOID**
*Pulls Arm Down And Back*

**RHOMBOIDS**
*Draws Shoulder Blade*
*Downwards And Toward Spine*

**TERES MINOR**
*Pulls Shoulder Blade And*
*Arm Down And Backwards*

**LOWER TRAPEZIUS**
*Same Function As Rhomboids*

**TRICEPS**
*Straightens Arm*

**LATISSIMUS DORSI**
*Pulls Shoulder Blade And*
*Arm Down And Backwards*

**INFRASPINATUS**
*Pulls Shoulder Blade And Arm*
*Down And Backwards*

*Figure 4*

# ABDOMINAL AND SIDES

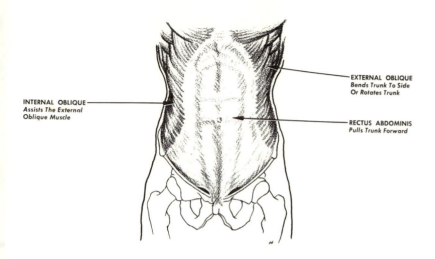

INTERNAL OBLIQUE
*Assists The External
Oblique Muscle*

EXTERNAL OBLIQUE
*Bends Trunk To Side
Or Rotates Trunk*

RECTUS ABDOMINIS
*Pulls Trunk Forward*

# LOWER BACK AND SIDES

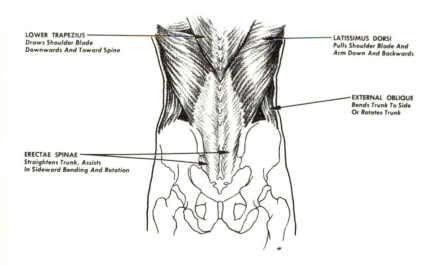

LOWER TRAPEZIUS
*Draws Shoulder Blade
Downwards And Toward Spine*

LATISSIMUS DORSI
*Pulls Shoulder Blade And
Arm Down And Backwards*

EXTERNAL OBLIQUE
*Bends Trunk To Side
Or Rotates Trunk*

ERECTAE SPINAE
*Straightens Trunk, Assists
In Sideward Bending And Rotation*

*Figure 5*

93

# ANTERIOR HIP

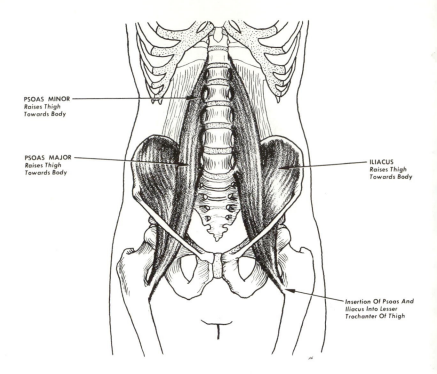

PSOAS MINOR
*Raises Thigh
Towards Body*

PSOAS MAJOR
*Raises Thigh
Towards Body*

ILIACUS
*Raises Thigh
Towards Body*

Insertion Of Psoas And
Iliacus Into Lesser
Trochanter Of Thigh

*Figure 6A*

sacrum articulates with the fifth lumbar vertebra and the ilium bones determines the efficiency of the pelvis as a base or platform for the support of the superincumbent weight of the trunk, head, and upper extremities. The movements of the pelvis depend upon the movements of the hip joints and lower spine. These movements are limited by the tension of the very powerful ilio-femoral ligament (thigh bone and ilium bone of the pelvis) and are influenced by alternations in gravity (leaning forward or backward).

## ANATOMY OF PELVIS

The heaviest muscle masses of the body surround the pelvic girdle. The bones of the pelvis are also held together by some of the most powerful ligaments in the body. Anatomical illustrations of the major muscle groups supporting and involved in the movement of the pelvic girdle are illustrated in Figure 6.

94

# POSTERIOR HIP

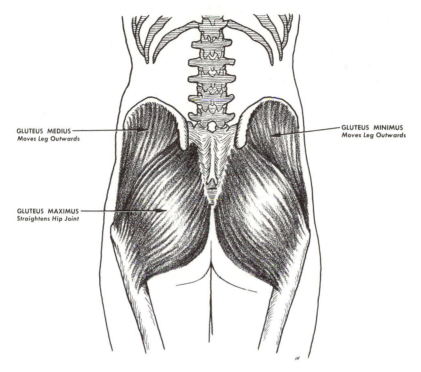

GLUTEUS MEDIUS
Moves Leg Outwards

GLUTEUS MINIMUS
Moves Leg Outwards

GLUTEUS MAXIMUS
Straightens Hip Joint

*Figure 6B*

## PRIME MOVER MUSCLES AFFECTING HIP MOVEMENT

*Flexors*—Iliopsoas, rectus femoris, pectineus.

*Extensors*—Gluteus maximus, hamstrings.

*Abductors*—Gluteus medium—assisted by tensor fasciae latae, gluteus maximus and minimus, satorius, and rectus femoris.

*Adductors*—Pectineus; gracilis; adductor longus, brevis, and magnus.

*Inward Rotators*—Tensor fasciae latae, gluteus minimus assisted by hamstrings.

*Outward Rotators*—Gluteus maximus and the six outward rotators, and assisted by posterior fibres of the gluteus medius and minimus.

The pelvis is balanced on the femoral (thigh) bones. The pelvic angle of inclination is dependent on the balanced posture of the hip joints and the muscles controlling the pelvis and maintaining the

95

balance. In the upright erect position, the thighs are the fixed points from which the muscles act.

Contraction of the hip flexors (iliopsoas, rectus femoris) increases the pelvic inclination, and contraction of the hip extensors (three gluteal muscles, hamstrings) will decrease the inclination.

Tests on several hundred persons in various age groups by Martin and Rich,[1] and on a group of adult females by Mosher,[2] reflect the strength level of the muscles controlling the forward and backward inclination of the pelvis.

| Muscle Group | Age | Age | Age | Adult Male | Adult Female |
|---|---|---|---|---|---|
|  | 3-7 | 8-12 | 13-18 |  |  |
| Extension | 2.91 | 2.92 | 2.77 | 3.70 | 3.40 |
| Flexion | 3.41 | 3.24 | 3.07 | 3.20 | 2.70 |

*N.B.:* Note the dominance of the flexors in the early years of life and the period of time taken by the antigravity extensor muscles to overcome the inborn advantage of the flexor muscles.

The important function of the hip abductors in maintaining lateral pelvic balance will be discussed in Chapter 12. The role of the hip rotators will be covered in Chapter 14.

## REFERENCES

1. Martin, E. G. and Rich, W. H., "Muscular Strength and Muscular Symmetry in Human Beings," *American Journal of Physiology,* Nos. 46 and 47, 1918.
2. Mosher, Clelia and Martin, E. G., "The Muscular Strength of College Women," *Journal of the American Medical Association,* January 19, 1918.

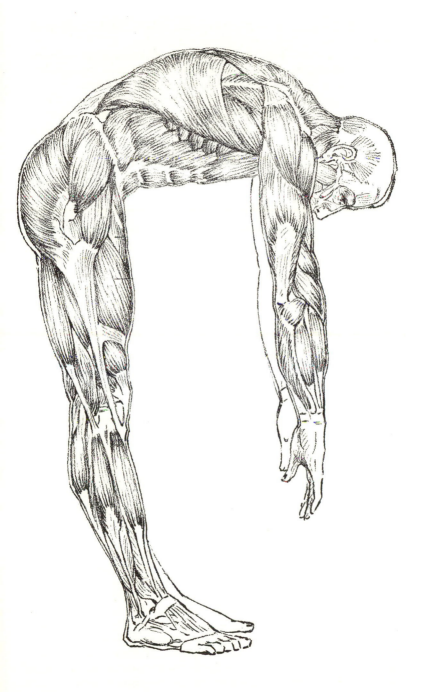

# 10

## Antereo-Posterior
## Upper Body Postural Faults

Numerous studies of elementary, high school, and college students over the past 70 years have disclosed that correct body alignment in relation to standing posture is found in less than 20 percent of the total population. Those who emphasize the concept of dynamic posture tend to overlook the importance of the static standing posture. The athlete spends more time each day standing, sitting, or walking than he does in training.

It is the continued strain on muscles, ligaments, and body joints that is the basic predisposing factor in degenerative breakdown of the musculo-skeletal structure. Training and competition magnify the stresses. In addition, habitual faulty posture in everyday activities is carried over into training and competition.

### DEFINITIONS

*Postural Fault*—a malalignment of a body segment which is immediately correctible by the athlete's own volitional movement or positioning and has not yet affected the skeletal structure of the body. These faults are known as functional divergencies. As Hines pointed out, they can be corrected or lessened by proper exercise.[2]

*Postural Defect*—a malalignment of a body segment which has affected the skeletal structure of the body and cannot be corrected by the athlete's own volitional movement or positioning. These are known as resistant or structural divergencies. All such cases must be referred to an orthopedic specialist or, when the segment involved is the foot, to a podiatrist. A great many of these cases can be corrected only by surgery, bracing, or the use of orthotic appliances. Once the correction has been made, however, exercise becomes a valuable therapeutic tool in strengthening the muscles, tendons, and ligaments.

## PELVIC INCLINATION AND ANTEREO-POSTERIOR POSTURE

Orthopedic and physical education postural authorities all agree that in the static upright position the pelvic inclination plays a highly important part in determing the normal antereo-posterior alignment of the upper body. In fact, many maintain that the pelvis and its degree of inclination is the key to the entire antereo-posterior body posture, because it is the foundation upon which the spinal column rests.

This viewpoint was highlighted by the intensive studies made by Wiles, the English orthopedic specialist, in 1937.[3] Wiles came to the conclusion that up until 1937 no direct method existed either by instrumentation or visual observation for accurately measuring the degrees of variation in the normal spinal curves. It was his opinion that this could be accomplished by an indirect method, through measurements of the forward and backward inclination of the pelvis.

His studies reflected that in individuals of normal posture the average forward inclination of the pelvis from the horizontal was 31 degrees in males and 28 degrees in females. A variation of four degrees on either side of the average was classed as being within the normal average range.

In a group being treated for lordosis, the average angle of pelvic inclination was 39 degrees—with a range of 34 to 41 degrees. In a group being treated for a sway back condition, the average angle of pelvic inclination was 37 degrees—with a range of 35 to 41 degrees.

## CAUSES OF ANTEREO-POSTERIOR POSTURAL FAULTS

Postural faults have been attributed to many causes. Most of them are identical to those previously discussed as factors in the development of muscular imbalance. To them should be added the following: (1) rapid growth in the presence of faulty nutrition, heavy labor, or general lack of muscular development; (2) growth divergencies in the skeletal structure; (3) pathological diseases affecting the organic, skeletal, and neurological structures of the body; (4) poor posture habits; (5) poor development of correct postural reflexes; (6) muscular imbalance in the pelvis creating an increase or decrease in the tilt of the pelvis; (7) inward rotation of the thighs due to pronating and relaxed feet; and (8) congenital defects in the skeletal structure of the spine.

Due to the interrelationship between the spine and pelvis, deviations from normal antereo-posterior pelvic tilt can arise from conditions in the upper body, from the pelvis itself, or from the lower extremities and feet. The sway back posture in the upper body automatically projects the pelvis forward and tips it downward. Muscular imbalance in the muscles controlling the pelvis will increase or decrease its tilt. Pronated and flat feet will create an upper leg inward rotation and pull on the rotator muscles of the thigh, which pull the pelvis forward and downward.

## EVALUATION OF ANTEREO-POSTERIOR FAULTS

The conductor of an evaluation of deviations from the normal static upright posture should keep two factors much in mind:

1. Extreme variations in the normal static erect posture are readily recognizable. Minor variations—particularly the sagging round-shouldered posture of the slim ectomorphic individual—are not too difficult to recognize. Minor variations in mesomorphic (muscular) and endomorphic (fat) individuals, however, are difficult to recognize. With these body builds, roentgenography (X-ray) is the only accurate method of determination. Minor faults in the lower or middle spine can be concealed by heavy well-developed spinal muscles or subcutaneous fat. The apparent round shoulders of the athlete may indicate nothing more than short clavicles or a high degree of muscular imbalance.

2. Postural faults in the antereo-posterior spinal curves rarely occur by themselves alone without affecting other segments of the spine, the pelvis, the lower extremities, or the feet. Any fault in one segment of the spine throws the body out of antereo-posterior alignment and almost invariably creates a fault in the opposite direction to bring the upper body back into vertical alignment.

## EXAMPLES OF ANTEREO-POSTERIOR SPINAL FAULTS

Figure 7 illustrates the normal upright posture and the more common variations, classed as faults or defects, along with the pelvic inclination associated with each variation.

*Normal*—line of gravity passes vertically through the mastoid process, down through the shoulder joint, in front of the sacroiliac joint, the knee joint, and the ankle joint. Pelvic inclination: 30 percent. (Figure 7A)

*Lordotic back*—increased pelvic inclination (40 percent) and inward curve of lumbar back. The inward curve is compensated for by a backward shift of the upper body and a slight kyphosis of the dorsal spine and, in many cases, drooped shoulders and a forward position of the head. With these three faults present, the condition is commonly termed kypholordosis. (Figure 7B) The lumbar back and hip flexor muscles are shortened and contracted, causing the pelvis to tip forward and leading to obliquity of the hip joints, internally rotated legs, and pronation of the feet. If the abdomen is prominent, the abdominals are also stretched and weakened. In the

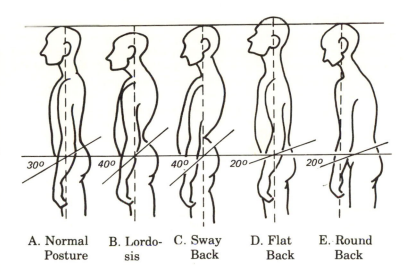

| A. Normal Posture | B. Lordo-sis | C. Sway Back | D. Flat Back | E. Round Back |

**Figure 7**

NORMAL POSTURE AND FOUR POSTURAL FAULTS

(after Wiles and Tucker)

muscular mesomorphic body build, the main fault is in the lower back and there may be evidence of faults in the spinal curvatures above.

*Sway Back*—increased pelvic inclination (40 percent) and a sharp inward curvature in lower lumbar region to restore the center of gravity. (Figure 7C) Accompanied by a dorso-lumbar kyphosis (long curve), flattened chest, drooped and rounded shoulders, and forward head position. Lower abdomen and pelvis generally project forward beyond the line of gravity, leading to internally rotated legs and pronated feet. The muscular imbalance in the pelvis and hips is similar to that found in the lordotic back.

Burt maintained that there are two types of sway back: (1) the short round back, where sway and curve of the lumbar dorsal spine begins in the upper lumbar segment; and (2) the long round back described in the previous paragraph.'

Sway back is the common "fatigue posture" observed in too many of today's adolescents. It occurs much too often in the slim ectomorphic athlete.

*Flat Back*—the pelvic inclination is decreased (20 percent) and the lumbar spine is flattened in compensation. (Figure 7D) This is sometimes known as the "weak back" posture. The lumbar spine loses its mobility. Athletes with this postural fault are subject to backache and sacroiliac strains, and extremely prone to acute low back strains.

101

*Round Back*—decreased pelvic inclination (20 percent) associated with a dorso-lumbar kyphosis, drooped shoulders, and forward head. (Figure 7E) In one type (Figure 3A), the upper body is bent forward in the lower lumbar region and most of the entire body is behind the vertical line of gravity—though in a bent forward position. This postural position is commonly observed in persons suffering from a ruptured inter-vertebral disk and attempting to ease the pain.

The second type of round back (not illustrated) is similar in posture to the short round back posture (dorso-lumbar kyphosis) described by Burt.

## POSTURAL FAULTS OR DEFECTS

The following faults or defects (not illustrated) in the upper back or shoulder area, while existing alone at their onset, may eventually cause variations in the spinal curves below.

*Dorsal Kyphosis*—an alteration of the skeletal structure which is hereditary characteristic in many families or is sometimes due to disease of the inter-vertebral disks or Scheurmann's disease (epiphysis of the vertebrae bodies). It can arise from poor postural habits, psychological states of depression, and an excess of sugar in the diet (associated with muscular weakness) during developmental growth. Dorsal kyphosis is generally accompanied by forward shoulders and a forward head position.

*Round or Forward Shoulders*—a forward projection of the points of the shoulders, although the dorsal spine retains its normal curve. This may be due to congenital anomalies (short clavicles or widely-spaced scapulae); but more often it is caused by muscular imbalance. It is commonly found in gymnasts, wrestlers, football linemen, i.e., mesomorphic body builds.

## REFERENCES

1.  Burt, H. A., "Effects of Faulty Posture," *Proceedings of the Royal Society of Medicine,* Vol. XLIII, 187.
2.  Hines, Thomas F., "Posture," *Therapeutic Exercise,* Sidney Light, ed. (New Haven: Elizabeth Light, 1965).
3.  Wiles, Philip, "Postural Deformities of the Antereo-posterior Curves of the Spine," *The Lancet,* April 17, 1937.

# 11

## Effect of Antereo-Posterior Postural Faults

Minor postural faults in the body's antereo-posterior plane can affect the athlete and jogger in many ways. Their effects on the musculo-skeletal structures are manifested in soft tissue injuries and stress or overuse syndromes. Their effects on the internal (visceral) organs of the body, particularly in the thoracic (chest) cavity, can seriously hamper optimum performance. Their effects on the neurological system of the body result in pain and interference with neuromuscular response and coordination. They can appreciably affect performance in athlete or jogger by causing inability to relax muscles, diminished agility, and limitation of movement in the spine and pelvis. Indirectly, their effects will place abnormal stresses on the lower extremities and feet.

In an address before the Royal College of Surgeons in 1949, Burt commented that little attention had been given by orthopedic physicians in recent years to the relation between disturbances of posture and disorders of the locomotor system.[2] He attributed this to the recent discovery that a ruptured inter-vertebral disk was the most common cause of sciatica pain. According to him, the resultant assumption that the remaining 80% of low back pains were also the result of ruptured inter-vertebral disks was a wrong one.

Fortunately, most of today's orthopedic physicians indirectly realize that poor posture is a contributing factor to low back pain and a predisposing cause of the ruptured disk. Except in the most serious cases of sciatica pain, conservative treatment will be recommended and tried before surgery is considered.

## GENERAL MUSCULO-SKELETAL EFFECTS

Minor faults in the normal alignment of the body lead to more serious problems in three ways:

1. Minor malalignments, especially in weight-bearing joints, lead to overstretching and weakening of the supporting ligaments that bind the joints together. This, in turn, makes the joints more susceptible to sprains.

2. The muscles surrounding the joints slowly become fatigued and weakened. They no longer have a balancing muscular action in holding the body in correct alignment. They must then frequently act vigorously to keep the body in alignment against the constant force of gravity. Eventually, muscles on one side of a joint become stretched and lose strength, while muscles on the opposite side contract and lose extensibility (flexibility). Permanent weakness and relaxation of stretched muscles and permanent contraction of their antagonists may result.

3. They produce a slight incongruence in the articular (joint) surfaces. The opposing hyaline cartilages are no longer completely parallel; the pressure of body weight, the repetitive jars from continued activity, the stresses of balanced and unbalanced muscular pulls are all distributed unevenly upon the articular surfaces and other internal structures of the joints.

The long continued effects of minor postural faults, particularly under the repetitive stresses of modern training and competition, produce a number of changes in the joints, muscles, and ligaments. Degeneration and decreased elasticity are observed in the articular cartilages. Spur formation about the margin of the joints is an attempt by the body to make the joint more stable, but leads to osteo-arthritis. Weakening from overstretching and contractures from persistent relaxation result in the various overuse syndromes associated with the muscles, tendons, ligaments, and connective tissues of the body. The ability to tolerate ordinary stresses of activity in the upright position, let alone in running or jogging, decreases as the degree or duration of the faulty alignment increases.

Armstrong and Tucker have long maintained that chronic postural strain, the result of an *inactive slumping posture,* is one of the three basic causes of traumatic athletic and occupational injuries.[1] Tucker outlines the main effects of *inactive slumping posture:*[13]

1. When movement occurs, acute strains and sprains more easily occur to muscle and joint structures, because the movement takes place on slack muscles with the corresponding joints unprotected.

2. Progressive strain shows itself first as a rheumatic fibrotic tenderness of the involved muscles, proceeding as age advances or as the joints are subjected to repetitive stresses and joint strain with

subsequent muscle spasm. He commented that muscle tenderness giving rise to so-called "fibrositis" or muscular rheumatism from chronic postural strain, can be explained by the stagnation of waste products or metabolites in the interstitial and inter-cellular fluid circulation. Metabolites which should be eliminated, as they are by the active pumping action of the muscles in *active alerted posture,* remain in the muscle tissues. These metabolites are thought to consist of large protein molecules which cause pain and tissue tenderness if they are not eliminated through the circulation.

3. There are changes in the auricular cartilages, synovial membranes, and the joint capsule.

4. Strain finally leads to osteo-arthritis of body joints, particularly those that are subjected to constant repetitive stresses. The detrimental effects of chronic postural strain on the total skeletal structure are illustrated in Figure 8.

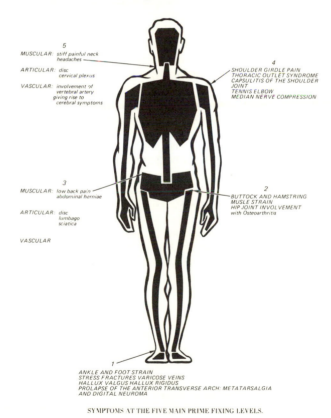

5
MUSCULAR: stiff painful neck
headaches
ARTICULAR: disc
cervical plexus
VASCULAR: involvement of
vertebral artery
giving rise to
cerebral symptoms

4
SHOULDER GIRDLE PAIN
THORACIC OUTLET SYNDROME
CAPSULITIS OF THE SHOULDER
JOINT
TENNIS ELBOW
MEDIAN NERVE COMPRESSION

3
MUSCULAR: low back pain
abdominal herniae
ARTICULAR: disc
lumbago
sciatica
VASCULAR

2
BUTTOCK AND HAMSTRING
MUSLE STRAIN
HIP JOINT INVOLVEMENT
with Osteoarthritis

1
ANKLE AND FOOT STRAIN
STRESS FRACTURES VARICOSE VEINS
HALLUX VALGUS HALLUX RIGIDUS
PROLAPSE OF THE ANTERIOR TRANSVERSE ARCH: METATARSALGIA
AND DIGITAL NEUROMA

SYMPTOMS AT THE FIVE MAIN PRIME FIXING LEVELS.

**Figure 8**

## UPPER BODY MUSCULO-SKELETAL EFFECTS

The points on the spine which are most exposed to chronic postural strain are the lumbo-sacral, sacroiliac, and dorso-lumbar joints, because they represent junction points between fixed and flexible portions of the spine. Next in order are the effects on the cervico-vertebral (head and neck) joints and the shoulder joints.

## LOWER AND MIDDLE (LUMBAR AND DORSAL) BACK

Athletes in general are prone to minimize or disregard low back pains of a minor nature. In many cases, the low back pains appear only after a day's activity and disappear after a night's rest in bed. Other types of low back pain are felt on arising in the morning, but diminish with activity and increased blood circulation.

Ochsenhirt *et al,* in a wide survey of athletic injuries, found that injuries to the lower back were common and that 82 percent of the cases were of soft tissue origin.[10] They commented: "We have observed that lordosis 'sway back' with tight erector spinae is by far the most consistent finding in the amateur and professional athlete. Tired, sore backs, pain across the small of the back are the most common complaints." At the 57th annual meeting of the Clinical Orthopaedic Society in 1969, a symposium on the tight back syndrome noted that this syndrome was frequently seen in athletes.

In the incorrect position of lordosis, the sacrum (Chapter 9, Figure 4) is more horizontally placed than it normally is, so that the sacroiliac joints derive less support from the shape of the joints. The sacrum is left hanging by its posterior ligaments, with the result that they become relaxed and strained. The position of extreme hyperextension of the lumbo-sacral joint causes the articular processes of the fifth lumbar vertebra to slide down, until they rest against the sacrum, and painful bursae may develop beneath them. If the fifth lumbar vertebra slips down too far, we have the "true slipped disk" problem, which in medical parlance is termed spondylolisthesis. The upper body weight is transmitted to the sacrum by way of the spinal arch, instead of by way of the vertebral body. The inter-vertebral foramina are narrowed and nerve root compression can occur that may result in sciatic pain radiating down the leg. The ilio-lumbar, lumbo-sacral, and all other ligaments supporting the joint are strained and eventually stretched. Conditions are similar at the dorso-lumbar junction (Chapter 9, Figure 3A), with resultant ligamentous strain and, in addition, the last rib (lowest) may be approximated to the transverse processes of the first lumbar vertebra, thus making possible compression of the intercostal nerve.

Tucker commented on the effects of bad posture on the upper body as follows:

Athletes are very prone to back strains and with a slumping slack posture, the abdominal, back, and buttock muscles tend to contribute to these strains. In alerted posture, abdominal muscles are held up, the buttock muscles are tucked in, and the lumbo-sacral articulations are firmly fixed. Movement of the trunk on the pelvis takes place on a firm base. In a slumping posture, leaning forward is carried out as a passive slump, the weight of the trunk is the activating force. The slack abdominal muscles are not producing even abdominal pressures, and strains and sprains, with or without disc involvement, keep on occurring and recurring with involvement of all the structures that go to make up a spinal segment, that is to say, the muscles, ligaments, discs, and the facet or apophyseal joints. Flexion of the spine must take place by either bending the hips and knees, or if there is a forward bend, there must be active contraction of the abdominal muscles, so that the intra-abdominal pressure is kept constant, with the result that the discs do not compress in the anterior parts, thus tending to press the nucleus pulpsus backwards in the action of forward flexion of the spine. The Apophyseal or facet joints are so shaped that in the action of flexion there is also a certain amount of rotation and if an athlete bends forward slightly off balance, there is often a locking of the facet or apophyseal joints with a production of severe muscle spasm. The ligaments of the apophyseal joints are also attached to the tranverse fibres of the inter-vertebral disc. Traction of these causes disturbances of the disc mechanism. Also, in the slumping posture, the abdominal muscles are slack and in bending, stress is put on the various apertures of the abdominal muscles and can lead to inguinal or umbilical herniae.

Many athletes have come to me over the past 40 years with a suggestion that they were developing early herniae in relation to the abdominal muscles, and it has been possible to check the progress of these herniae by the athlete learning to hold his abdominal muscles up and slightly contracted.[13]

Upper Back, Shoulder, Neck (Thoracic and Cervical) Tucker also stated:

Chronic postural strain of the forward drooping head on the neck produces the so-called "fibrositis" of the cervical muscles and will gradually lead to strains of the cervical-vertebral joints, with symptoms of pain and limitation due to eventual disc degeneration and involvement of the facet or apophyseal joints. At the upper cervical level, that is to say, the head on neck, occipital neuritis and pain in the distribution of the cervical plexis may occur. At the lower shoulder girdle level the incorrect position of the shoulder girdle and the upper extremity (arm) will produce a strain on the lower cervical joints with radiculitis and brachial neuritis that result in pains down the arm. There is often also pain in relation to the shoulder joint itself.

Johnson, in commenting on cervio-brachial pain syndromes that affect the upper back and shoulder areas of the body, noted that the myriad syndromes reported in the orthopedic literature were due to the fact that each was treated as a specific clinical entity.[7] He pointed out that the common factor in a variety of cervio-brachial syndromes is poor posture, and the correction of postural stress will contribute to the relief of symptoms. In a review of the orthopedic literature, he quoted numerous authorities who found that in the scalenius anticus muscle, costo-clavicular, scapulo-costal, and first rib syndromes poor posture was the primary cause of disability. These syndromes all apply to pains due to pressure on nerve roots that affect the neck, upper back, and shoulder joints and to radicular pains down the arm. Johnson closed by stating: "In an effort to develop a more practicable clinical approach to the problem of cervio-brachial pain and acroparathesia, it seems justifiable to define a diagnostic category based on the factor common to so many cervio-brachial syndromes, i.e., the postural factor. Postural myoneuralgia is a descriptive term for this category."

## CHEST AND ABDOMINAL CAVITIES

Depression of the ribs due to the slumping posture restricts the free movement of the lungs, heart, and diaphragm. Abdominal stagnation also results from depression and limited movement of the diaphragm. The effects on the internal organs will be covered more thoroughly in the discussion of the visceral functions.

## LOWER BODY MUSCULAR EFFECTS

Spinal postural faults also affect the joints of the hip and can eventually affect the structure of the feet.

### HIP JOINTS AND FORWARD PELVIC TILT

The flexion contractures of the hip muscles result in a slight flexion of the knees and an inward rotation and adduction of the thighs. This reduces the weight-bearing stability of the hip joints and imposes an unnecessary amount of postural work on the hip joint rotator and extensor muscles. The constant excess tension on the deep rotator muscles interferes with the nutrition (blood supply) of both the muscle structure and hip joints. The contraction, as it was referred to by Frieberg,[4] or stretching, as it was termed by the Kendalls,[8] of the piriformis muscle, a deep-seated outward hip and femur rotator muscle, can impinge on the sciatic nerve and create the painful condition of sciatica.

The total effect on the skeletal and cartilage structure of the hip joint is manifested eventually in degeneration and osteo-arthritis. The latter condition is frequently observed among middle-aged joggers.

## THE LOWER EXTREMITIES AND FEET

Wiles discussed a form of foot valgus (pronated or flat) usually beginning in childhood and resulting from poor upper body antereo-posterior posture which he termed postural pes valgus.[14] He pointed out that faulty trunk posture—with forward head position, compensatory rounded back (dorsal kyphosis), and lumbar lordosis, along with anterior pelvic tilt—shifts the body weight forward to the forefoot. Flexion contractures of hip muscles occur from the habitual forward pelvic tilt, causing the lower extremities to assume the position of a flat-footed person—femurs rotated inwards, hip and knees flexed, and feet pronated. Along with the abnormal stresses imposed by the forward body weight, the pronation of the foot predisposes to longitudinal arch strains and stress fracture of the metatarsal bones.

## CONGENITAL ANOMALIES

If the athlete does not display a faulty antereo-posterior posture with lordosis and forward tilt of the pelvis, a short leg, lateral tilt of the pelvis, scoliosis, chronic tension, muscular imbalance, or pathological disease, then the cause of low back pain can be a congenital anomaly. These can be identified only by X-ray. They may or may not eliminate a competitive runner from competition. Rose pointed out that two of the most common congenital anomalies are bilateral pedicle defects and spina befida occulta.[11] He has banned many athletes from competition in body contact sports because of these. Another anomaly which sometimes causes low back pain is spondylolysis (bony defect in the pars inter-articularis of affected vertebra). Frequently, this leads to spondylolisthesis (slipped disk), which occurs when the separated anterior portion of the vertebra slips forward onto the body of the vertebra below.

Medical explanation of these anomalies is unnecessary in this discussion. However, the coach, athlete, and trainer should be aware that they do exist in a small number of cases of faulty posture.

## EFFECT ON VISCERAL FUNCTIONS

Downing, an osteopathic physician, commented in the *Journal of the American Osteopathic Association* on the effects of faulty posture, stating: "Malnutrition, chronic fatigue of nervous and muscular systems, congenitive disturbances and circulatory vagaries, mechanical retardation in somatic (body) functions, diminished respiratory activities and interference with heart action, and derangement of visceral functions of pelvic organs may be attributable to postural disorder."[3]

Goldthwait, an orthopedic physician, and his associates, between 1900 and 1930, did a great amount of research on the effects of faulty antereo-posterior posture on the functioning of the internal organs in the thoracic and abdominal cavities of the body and its contribution as a cause of organic disease.[5] Dividing body types into two basic categories, they found that faulty posture and its effects on the musculo-skeletal structure and the functioning of the internal organs affected the slender individual far more than his counterpart, the stocky individual. The majority of middle and long distance runners are of slender build.

From the standpoint of the competitive runner and jogger, the major effects of faulty antereo-posterior posture on the efficiency of the visceral functions involve the respiratory and cardiovascular body systems.[6] Secondary effects on the efficiency of the digestive and excretory body system may be manifested in competitive runners, but appear more often in middle-aged joggers.

## RESPIRATORY SYSTEM

The lungs in themselves are incapable of expansion and contraction. It is the elasticity of their tissue that allows the inspiration (intake) and expiration of air and interchange of gases. The effectiveness of the lungs depends upon the muscles that control the elevation and depression of the rib cage and increase or decrease the thoracic (chest) capacity.

The most important muscle of inspiration is the diaphragm muscle, a musculo-tendinous tissue that separates the thoracic and abdominal cavities. Its efficiency in respiratory inspiration is dependent on the inter-costal muscles of the ribs, and the sterno-mastoid (front) and scaleni (side) muscles of the neck. These muscles increase the capacity of the chest and permit maximum mechanical efficiency of the diaphragm by raising the thoracic cavity upwards and increasing its diameter and capacity during inspiration.

The working effectiveness of the neck muscles, as accessory muscles of respiration, depends on the strength of the rear neck muscles and shoulder adductors in holding the shoulders and head in an erect position. When the thoracic wall is depressed and the efficiency of the diaphragm is limited by poor posture, total respiratory capacity for intake of oxygen is greatly decreased. The residual air volume, (amount in lungs after expiration) is increased due to the limited chest movement. The athlete with faulty posture soon builds up an oxygen debt, with resultant anoxia (reduction of oxygen in body tissues).

In addition, such decreased capacity of the chest places the inter-costal muscle arteries, veins, and nerves in poor functional relationship, and nutrition of the important marrow of the ribs and sternum is jeopardized. The ribs and sternum harbor a large portion of the red blood marrow; hence, normal circulation to these bones is necessary to maintain the normal production of red blood cells that transport oxygen to the working muscles.

## CARDIOVASCULAR SYSTEM

The heart is the prime source of the energy which drives the blood through the vascular systems. The right side of the heart is occupied with driving the blood through the relatively short pulmonary (lung) system, while the left side of the heart must propel an equal volume of blood through the extensive general circulation of the body. The velocity of the blood stream remains fairly constant until the capillary structure of organs and muscles is reached, at which point it decreases considerably. Postural defects which cause increased pressure upon internal organs or muscular tissue embarrass by further slowing down or even stopping capillary circulation. Since the right side of the heart can pump into the pulmonary circulation only that amount of blood which reaches it from the general circulation, and since the output of the left side of the heart is controlled by the amount of blood reaching it through the pulmonary circulation, it follows that circulatory stasis (slowing down or stopping) anywhere in either the pulmonary or the vascular system will influence the total circulation in both systems.

## DIGESTIVE AND EXCRETORY SYSTEMS

In faulty posture, the stomach is forced down from its normal position—which leads to distension, impairment of peristaltic activity, and altered emptying time. The depression and crowding of the lower abdominal organs (vicertoposis) interferes with normal peristaltic activity of the intestines and leads to constipation, as well as to impaired portal circulation and return of venous blood to the heart.

## EFFECTS OF FAULTY POSTURE ON NERVOUS SYSTEM

As postural strain increases to the stage of inflammatory reaction, the sensory nerves about the joints begin to register the discomfort and pain, which provokes a protective spasm or increased tension in the muscles that surround the joint.

When ligaments and muscles on one side of a joint are stretched, then antagonists are shortened and neuromuscular response to emergency situations and quick movements suffers.

In faulty antereo-posterior posture, inter-vertebral muscles and ligaments are shortened and restricted movement in the joints retards absorption from the spinal canal. Accumulation of waste products in the spinal canal lowers the vitality of spinal nerve centers and increases the fatigue state, which leads to postural depression.

## EFFECTS OF FAULTY POSTURE ON PERFORMANCE

The eminent Dr. Charles Lowman, America's pioneer in calling the attention of the athletic and physical education world to the deleterious effects of malposture both on performance and on the musculo-skeletal structure of the body, wrote:

> It should be self-evident that a machine with properly aligned working members acts efficiently and, with care, lasts much longer than one that is out of line. In the malaligned machine, wear and tear on the bearings increases, and stress and strain on working members produce general structural depreciation. Our bodies are just like other machines and, when maximum good performance is desired, attention to the alignment of their bearings (joints) is essential. The maintenance of alignment is affected by the balance of all muscles activating, or acting on, any bearing (joint).[9]

Slocum and James commented that when the mechanics of running are disturbed by postural abnormalities, errors in alignment, or restriction of joint motion, the normal pattern of the stride is altered, performance is decreased, and joints may become painful.[12] As Slocum and Bowerman pointed out (see Chapter 5), the position of the pelvis is the key to postural control in running and jogging.

Intimately related to the correct posture of the pelvis are trunk deviations, such as round back, round hollow back, flat back, and lordosis (Figure 7). Lumbar lordosis is the most common condition affecting the use of the lumbar spine-pelvic unit. With a long round back, there is generally a sharper shorter lordotic curve, with a more acute flexion at the hip joints and shortness of the hip flexor and lumbar spinal extensors. With a round hollow back, the same effect is manifested in the pelvic unit—although the stresses are lessened because of more equal compensation. With a flat back (a less common trunk deviation), there is interference with forward flexion of the spine. Simple lordosis, not associated with any of the above trunk malalignments, generally results in the competitive runner from muscular imbalance and in the middle-aged jogger from obesity.

The forward tilt of the pelvis that accompanies lordosis creates an adaptive shortening of the hip flexors, the adductor muscles of the thighs, and the low back extensor muscles. The hip extensors (buttocks), the hamstrings, and the abdominal muscles stretch and weaken.

The lordosis places the more mobile segments of the spine in an extended position, which decreases the amount of spinal extension available for backward thrust of the trailing leg at take-off. If lordosis becomes habitual, the contracted lumbar fascia prevents full flexion of the lumbar spine. The forward tilt of the pelvis with the adaptive shortening of the hip flexors serves to limit the forward extension of the leading leg.

During running or jogging, hip rotation permits the forward and backward oscillation of the pelvis. When the muscles on the front of the hip become shortened due to forward pelvic tilt, the rotation range of the hip joints is reduced. If internal rotation is restricted, the full backward movement of the trailing leg cannot be carried out, and if external rotation of the hip joint is limited, forward placement of the leading leg will be affected.

The rotation of the runner's or jogger's trunk is highly important in coordinating arm and shoulder movements with lower leg movements. The lifting action of the lateral loin muscles holds the leg of the same side up during the forward swing phase, while the rotator action of the internal and external oblique muscles brings that side forward. The alternating action of the opposite oblique muscles must relax sufficiently to permit the shoulder girdle to be rotated backwards. With shortened low back extensors and stretched abdominal muscles, the rotation of the trunk is limited to some degree. Interference with trunk or hip rotation and restriction of the extension and flexion of the spinal-pelvic complex due to postural faults and muscular imbalance will drastically alter attempts at hurdling and increasing the stride length of the runner or jogger.

Kyphosis (rounded upper back) and/or forward head position create a forward displacement of the upper body similar to the forward lean of the runner due to fatigue. The center of gravity is shifted forward, which causes more weight to be placed on the ball of the foot, limits the height of hip flexion, decreases the functional range of spinal extension, and interferes with the working efficiency of the important breathing muscle, the diaphragm.

## REFERENCES

1. Armstrong, J. H. and Tucker, W. E., *Injury in Sport* (London: Staples Press, 1964).
2. Burt, H. A., "Effects of Faulty Posture," *Proceedings of the Royal Society of Medicine,* Vol. XLIII, 187.
3. Downing, Carter H., "Mechanical Control of Posture," *Journal of the American Osteopathic Association,* Vol. 38, No. 4, December 1938.
4. Freiberg, Albert H. and Vinke, T. H., "Sciatica and the Sacroiliac Joint," *Journal of Bone and Joint Surgery,* Vol. XVI, 126.
5. Goldthwait, Joel E., "An Anatomic and Mechanistic Conception of Disease," *Boston Medical and Surgical Journal,* June 17, 1915.

6. Hansson, R. G., "Body Mechanics and Posture," *Journal of the American Medical Association,* Vol. 128, No. 13, July 28, 1945.

7. Johnson, Donald A., "Posture and Cervio-brachial Pain," *Journal of the American Medical Association,* Vol. 159, No. 16, December 17, 1955.

8. Kendall, Henry O.; Kendall, Florence P.; and Boynton, Dorothy A.; *Posture and Pain* (Baltimore: Williams and Wilkins Co., 1952).

9. Lowman, Charles L., "Faulty Posture in Relation to Performance," *Journal of Health, Physical Education, and Recreation,* April 1958.

10. Ochsenhirt, Norman C.; Chambers, Clifford D.; and Ferderber, Murray B.; "Prevention and Management of Athletic Disabilities," *Archives of Physiology, Medicine, and Rehabilitation,* March 1953.

11. Rose, Kenneth D., "Congenital Anomalies of the Low Back," *Medical Times,* Vol. 89, No. 10, October 1961.

12. Slocum, Donald B. and James, Stanley L., "Biomechanics of Running," *Journal of the American Medical Association,* Vol. 205, No. 11, September 9, 1968.

13. Tucker, W. E., "Postural Training in Athletes," Lecture presented at Royal Northern Hospital, England, 1974.

14. Wiles, Philips, "Flat-feet," *The Lancet,* November 17, 1934.

# 12

## Lateral Asymmetry

Lateral asymmetry (imbalance) includes any dissimilarity, whether skeletal, anatomical, or morphological, between the two equal halves of the body when viewed from an anterior or posterior vantage point. It includes lateral curvature of the spine (scoliosis), lateral pelvic tilt, the short leg syndrome, muscular imbalance of spinal or pelvic (hip) muscles, and bilateral strength imbalance of the lower extremities.

### LATERAL CURVATURE OF SPINE

Lateral curvatures of the spine are classified under three designations:

1. *Functional (postural or first degree):* The curvature has affected the alignment of the body and the balanced pull of the muscles supporting the spine, but has not affected the spinal skeletal structure.

2. *Transitional (second degree):* The muscles and ligaments are becoming permanently shortened or stretched and the skeletal structure is beginning to become rigid and lose its lateral mobility.

3. *Structural (third degree):* The skeletal structure has become rigid (has completely lost mobility), and the structure of the spinal processes is changed.

Lateral curvatures of the spine always involve some degree of rotation of spinal vertebrae. Rotational effect is greater in the thoracic (dorsal) spine than in the lumbar spine, where it is somewhat limited by the bony processes. The rotational effect in the more severe cases of dorsal scoliosis will drastically affect the thoracic rib cage. The ribs on the convex side of the curve bulge backwards, while the ribs on the concave side of the curve move forward. This makes it appear that the entire thoracic rib cage is twisted.

In lateral curvatures, the muscles on the concave (inner) side shorten and contract, while on the convex (outer) side they lengthen and stretch. In the majority of cases, the muscles on the convex side are stronger than those on the concave side. An opposite effect would occur if the curvature were due to the unopposed action of the surface spinal muscles. This situation results from the fact that imbalance of the deeper spinal muscles (rotators of the spine) is the major reason for the appearance of this curvature early in life.

When the large superficial muscles of the back are dominantly imbalanced, the result is a definite lateral deviation of the spine with relatively slight rotation of the vertebrae. When the deep intrinsic muscles of the spine are dominantly imbalanced, there is a definite rotation of the spine with relatively slight lateral displacement.

Very few spines are absolutely straight in the lateral plane. Numerous studies have shown that evidence of one of the three stages of curvature (scoliosis) exists in from 35 to 40 percent of the population. Many authorities believe the stages are progressive in nature and lead eventually to severe deformity of the spine. However, a great many first stage postural curvature cases appear to make a spontaneous recovery during growth. Compensating curves bring the upper body back into vertical alignment, which offsets the pull of gravity on the original curvature. The structural processes become set and the curvature progresses no further.

## CAUSES OF LATERAL CURVATURE

The causes of lateral curvature of the spine, which are many, can be divided into two broad classifications:

1. *General:* Includes hereditary or acquired defects in spinal structure, pathological diseases affecting spinal processes or muscles, general muscular weakness, malnutrition, chronic fatigue, psychological factors, bad postural habits, sleeping postures, etc.

2. *Unilateral:* Includes one-sided play, recreational, athletic, or occupational habits; faulty hearing or vision on one side; right- or left-handed dominance; lateral pelvic tilt; short leg syndrome; unilateral flat or pronated foot; muscular imbalance in the spinal or hip muscles; and habitual one-legged standing posture.

The overwhelming majority of postural or structural spinal curves in the lower back are due to lateral pelvic tilt, short leg syndrome, one-legged standing posture, or unilateral foot faults.

## CHARACTERISTICS AND SIGNS OF LATERAL CURVATURES

The direction of a lateral spinal curvature is designated by its convexity (outer side):

1. *Single Curve ("C" Curve):* The long "C" curve may extend through two areas of the spine, generally the lumbar and thoracic (dorsal). The short "C" curve is found in only one spinal area. The "C" curve is the most common type of curve observed in lateral curvatures. Most people are right-handed. The muscles on the right side are stronger than those on the left. The spine is pulled to the right. Therefore, the left "C" curve is encountered most frequently.

2. *Compound or Compensatory Curve ("S" Curve):* This is a combination of two curves—the original, and the curve that develops above or below the original in a compensatory action to restore the spine to a balanced vertical alignment.

There are distinctive signs that should prompt the coach or trainer to at least suspect the existence of a minor postural curve that may progress into a more serious structural curve. Recognizing such a condition is particularly important in the case of young adolescent athletes, because at their age postural faults can be corrected.

These signs are: (1) one shoulder higher than the other (generally convex side); (2) uneven scapula: (3) one hip more prominent than the other; (4) lateral pelvic tilt; (5) head tilted to one side; and (6) unequal distance between the arms and sides. Figure 9 illustrates various degrees of lateral spinal curvature and pelvic tilt. If any of these signs is present, or if visual observation discloses a possible curve, the athlete should be referred to an orthopedic specialist for X-ray examination of the spine. It is the only method for accurately determing whether a suspect curve is a minor postural curve, a transitional, or an actual structural curve.

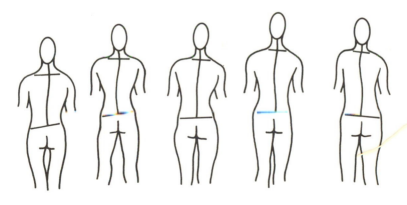

**Figure 9**
VARIOUS DEGREES OF SCOLIOSIS AND LATERAL PELVIC TILT

## LATERAL PELVIC TILT

Authorities estimate that approximately 50 percent of the population display a lateral tilt of the pelvis of one-quarter inch or greater. Rothburt commented that a tilt of more than one-quarter inch is structurally abnormal.[12]

Excluding congenital defects of the pelvic structure, structural variations in the size of pelvic bones, pathological diseases affecting the skeletal or muscular structure of the pelvis, and injuries, the major causes of lateral pelvic tilts are muscle imbalance, habitual one-legged standing posture, the short leg syndrome, and unilateral divergencies and faults in the lower extremities and the feet.

## ANATOMY AND FUNCTION OF HIP ABDUCTOR MUSCLES

Martin and his associates conducted extensive strength tests on hip adduction and abduction muscles among various age groups.[7]

| MUSCLE GROUP | 3-7 yrs. | 8-12 yrs. | 13-18 yrs. | Adult Males | Adult Females |
|---|---|---|---|---|---|
| Adductors | 1.55 | 1.55 | 1.63 | 1.50 | 1.70 |
| Abductors | 1.47 | 1.43 | 1.42 | 1.40 | 1.40 |

In the normal population, the hip adductors are consistently stronger than the hip abductors. The adductor muscles (pectineus, gracilis, three adductors) are illustrated in Figure 17. Movements of hip adduction and abduction are illustrated on Page 138.

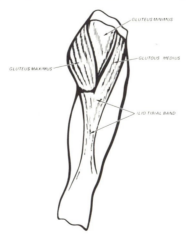

*Figure 10*
Hɪᴘ Aʙᴅᴜᴄᴛᴏʀs

118

Three of the four principal hip abductor muscles are illustrated, the other being the tensor fascia latae. The gluteus medius is the prime mover in abduction, providing 55 percent of the total muscle power, the other three muscles being classed as assistant movers. The posterior fibers of the gluteus medius are covered by the gluteus maximus and the anterior fibers by the tensor fascia latae. The latter two muscles blend into the ilio-tibial band which runs down the lateral side of the knee, and inserts into the tibia bone of the lower leg.

The function of the abductor muscles is to abduct the leg upon the pelvis or the pelvis upon the fixed leg. In the standing position, wth the fixation of the leg and foot on the ground, the adduction or abduction of the leg on the pelvis is a misappearance. In reality, there is in this position an actual adduction or abduction of the pelvis on the legs, created by the pelvis tilting laterally on the legs.

The gluteus medius muscle, assisted by the other abductors, is the major muscle involved in maintaining the lateral balance of the pelvis and counteracting postural sway in standing and walking. The function of the gluteus medius in standing, walking, or running is to pull the pelvis down laterally towards the hip and maintain the lateral balance of the hip.

## PELVIC MUSCLE IMBALANCE

Muscle imbalance in the pelvis can occur between abductor-adductor and/or internal or external rotator muscles of the hip on one side of the pelvis, and bilaterally between the two psoas (hip flexor) muscles on both sides of the pelvis.

1. *Imbalance of Adductors-Abductors:* If the downward lateral pull on the pelvis by the gluteus medius on one side of the pelvis is affected by a *slight* weakness and it results in an apparent adduction and internal rotation of the leg on that side of the body. The medius on the opposite side will remain normal in length or slightly contract, and the leg will go into abduction and external rotation. With a high and prominent hip on the side of the weak gluteus medius, there is usually compensation through a lowering of the shoulder on the same side. Additionally, the lumbar spine is thrust into a functional "C" curve towards the side opposite the slightly weak gluteus.

If the downward lateral pull on the pelvis by the gluteus medius on one side of the pelvis is affected by a *severe* weakness in the muscle, the pelvis will be tilted laterally downward on the side of the weakness. The leg on the weak side is thrust into a position of apparent abduction (outward rotation) and is slightly extended in a locked position at the knee. There is an apparent adduction (inward rotation) of the leg on the opposite side. This eventually results in a secondary weakness developing in the gluteus medius muscle on that side. The lumbar spine is carried towards the weak side in a postural "C" curve that soon develops into a compensatory structural curve.

Atkins pointed out the effect on the lower extremities and feet when the pelvis tilts to one side:

> The relative abduction of the thigh on the lower side of the pelvis and the relative adduction of the thigh on the high side create disturbances in the knee mechanism by changes in muscle lengths. The abducted thigh forces the knee into extension and the adducted thigh is forced into flexion. The abducted leg in external rotation turns the foot outward more than the opposite leg, and the ankle loses some of its mobility. The foot shows a tender plantar fascia and restricted movements.[1]

2. *Internal-External Rotator Muscle Imbalance:* This is closely associated with abductor-adductor imbalance. It may be secondary to the abductor-adductor imbalance or primary, due to a unilateral pronated or flat foot or knock-knee. Internal rotation due to a pronated foot stretches the external hip rotators, resulting in a lateral pelvic tilt on that side of the hip.

3. *Imbalance of Psoas Flexor Muscles:* The psoas muscle—the most powerful hip flexor—on one side will occasionally overdevelop from either a postural stress or occupational or athletic overuse. A contracted overdeveloped psoas muscle can lead to lateral pelvic tilt and lumbar spine rotation. Michelle has long maintained that this is the most important muscle imbalance syndrome found in the body.[9] He pointed out that a short ilio-psoas muscle pulls on the femus (thigh bone), forcing it into outward rotation. The ilio-psoas passes over the anterior rim of the pelvis, and if it becomes overdeveloped and shortened, it tilts the pelvis downward and to the side of the shortened muscle. In their extensive study of 329 persons reported on in Chapter 6, Russian researchers included statistics on the relative width of the psoas muscles in the 279 sportsmen and 50 non-sportsmen involved.[10] In all the groups studied, they found the psoas muscle well-developed on the right side, less developed on the left side. They concluded that in sportsmen as in non-sportsmen, the muscles of the right side of the body are better developed than those on the left side, and that that fact is especially noticeable in measurements of the psoas muscle.

## ONE-LEGGED STANDING POSTURE

When children first stand up, it is natural for them to space their feet apart, with the feet in an abducted (outward) position. Their sense of balance is undeveloped at this time, and this is a natural adjustment for the purpose of widening their base of support. The longer they take to attain a sense of balance with the feet in the abducted position, the greater the probability that they will use the abducted foot position when they begin to walk.

In the process of growing up, most people in resting posture stand on one foot. Masaki's earlier mentioned study of resting posture in people waiting on a train platform in Japan revealed that slightly less than 20 percent stood with both feet parallel and pointing straight ahead.[8] Approximately 30 percent stood on one foot, with the relaxed leg placed some distance ahead of the standing leg. Masaki commented that these two types of standing posture were the most comfortable for the average person, but all of the 80 percent showed signs of asymmetry (bilateral muscular imbalance) in the lower extremities.

In 1920, Fitzgerald, commenting on the stand-easy position with weight on one leg, maintained that habitual posture of this type induced lateral pelvic tilt and curvature of the spine.[4]

In 1938, Wesson, discussing types of malposture, described a type which he named "shop girl's hip." (Figure 11).[14] He pointed out that in this form of malposture the leg upon which the weight rests is locked into adduction, the opposite leg is in an abducted position, the pelvis is rotated, and there is a secondary functional scoliosis, as well.

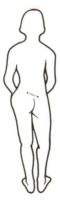

*Figure 11*

Relaxed standing on one foot is usually accompanied by relaxation of the gluteus medius muscle of the hip on the standing leg side. This results in a hip drop on the opposite side, with an abduction of the leg and foot.

Habitual standing on one leg over a period of time can lead to unilateral stretching of the ligaments of the spine and hip, which predisposes the person to a habitual lateral pelvic tilt and curvature of the spine.

Commenting on the retarded leg syndrome as a cause of athletic injuries, Fahey stated:

> Because most persons favor one foot when walking and the other when standing, one leg underdevelops. With one everted foot, walking cannot be properly accomplished and chronic strain on the medial (inner) ligaments of the knee, and undue stress on the lower back develop.[3]

The reader is also referred to Klein's study of the same subject covered in Chapter 6.[5]

## SHORT LEG SYNDROME

In 1950, Beal presented a review of 81 studies made between 1862 and 1950 (and in all involving several thousand persons) pertaining to the short leg syndrome and its relationship to low back pain.[2] In his summary, he commented:

> X-ray studies show the short leg has an incidence of 70 percent in the population. The importance of this factor in the etiology of backache is demonstrated by the fact that 65 to 95 percent of the patients presented for postural X-ray studies showed a difference in leg length. A short right leg is observed more frequently than the left; about half of the short leg cases have the accommodation mechanism of short leg, sacral tilt, and convexity of the lumbar curve on the same side.

Klein, noted for his monumental studies on the cause and prevention of knee injuries in American football, has devoted a substantial portion of his time to the study of lateral asymmetry among growing school children. In a three-year study of 187 elementary school children, 211 junior high school students, and 187 students from a senior high school, he found a 92 percent incidence of lateral asymmetry in the senior high school group.[6] Klein concluded that lateral asymmetries are progressive in nature during the period of skeletal growth. The greatest change appeared to take place between the elementary and high school age levels.

Pearson, in a study of 830 school children from 8 to 13 years of age, determined that 93 percent displayed some degree of lateral asymmetry.[11]

*Etiology of the Short Leg:* The causes of the short leg syndrome can be divided into two groups: intrinsic and extrinsic.

*Intrinsic*—Involves the skeletal structure of the leg itself, the pelvis, or the foot. A large percentage of cases result from trauma sustained during periods of growth in the skeletal centers responsible for the longitudinal growth of the long bone of the leg. These centers are the junction of the diaphysis (compact shaft between extremities) and the epiphyses (ends of long bone composed entirely of cartilage or separated from shaft by cartilage disk). The epiphyses ossify (convert into bone) with the shaft during puberty. Trauma (overstress, nutritional deficiencies, or injury) can affect the ossification process and retard or stimulate lengthening growth of the legs.

Structural anomalies in the foot represent a contributing factor in the development of a short leg. Swift found that in 97 percent of the cases she studied involving the short leg, there were structural anomalies in the foot.[13] The anomaly most frequently found was a short first metatarsal (big toe).

Growth divergencies or congenital anomalies in the pelvis at the juncture of the femur (thigh bone) with the acetabulum of the hip can also create a short leg.

*Extrinsic*—Includes fractures or dislocations of the legs or hipbones, knee angulations (knock-knees or bowlegs), poliomyelitis, paralysis, muscle imbalance in the pelvis, pelvic side shift or rotation, one-legged standing posture, unilateral low or flattened longitudinal foot arch, or pronated foot.

## REFERENCES

1. Atkins, Charls E., "Pelvic Imbalance as Causative Factor in Foot Disturbance," *Clinical Osteopathy,* July 1938.
2. Beal, Myron C., "A Review of the Short-Leg Problem," *The Journal of the American Osteophathic Association,* Vol. 50, No. 2, October 1950.
3. Fahey, J. F., "The Retarded Leg Syndrome," *Abstracts of Joint Meeting of A.C.S.M. and C.A.S.S., Toronto, 1971.*
4. Fitzgerald, Gerald, "Standing Easy with the Weight on One Leg," *Journal of Scientific Physical Training,* Vol. XIII, 1918.
5. Klein, Karl K., "A Comparison of Bilateral Quadriceps Muscle Strength of Individuals in Good and Poor Postural Balance," *The Physical Educator,* Vol. XI, No. 2, May 1954.
6. Klein, Karl K., "Progression of Pelvic Tilt in Adolescent Boys from Elementary Through High School," *Archives of Physical Medicine and Rehabilitation,* Vol. 54, 1973.
7. Martin, E. G., "Tests of Muscular Efficiency," *Physiological Review,* Vol. I, 1923.
8. Masaki, Takeo, "Electromyographic Study of Rest Standing Postures in Man," *Proceedings of International Conference on Sports Sciences* (Tokyo: The Japanese Union of Sports Sciences, 1964).
9. Michelle, Arthur A., *Orthotherapy* (New York: M. Evans and Co., Inc., 1971).

10. Mirzamukhamedov, A. G., "Development of Several Muscles in the Lumbar Region in Sportsmen," *Theory and Practice of Physical Culture,* (Moscow), Vol. 5, 1969.

11. Pearson, W. M., "Early and High Incidence of Mechanical Faults," *Journal of Osteophath,* Vol. 41:18, 1954.

12. Rothburt, Brian A., "Phasic Activity of Muscles Within the Lower Extremities," *Journal of American Podiatry Association,* Vol. 63, No. 4, April 1973.

13. Swift, L. F., "Brief Survey of 90 Roentgenposturgraphs," *Clinical Osteopathy,* Vol. 37, March 1941.

14. Wesson, A. S. and Douthwaite, A. H., "Discussion on Manipulation in Rheumatic Disorders," *Proceedings of the Royal Society of Medicine,* Vol. 23, 273, 1938.

# 13

## Effects of Lateral Asymmetry

There is a strong interrelationship between dorsal-lumbar or lumbar lateral curvatures, the lateral pelvic tilt, and a short leg. This relationship does not apply to the localized curvature that affects only the upper portion of the spine. This localized curvature of the upper spine is observed among many athletes who specialize in the one-sided sports (throwing, tennis, golf, etc.). The over-development of the superficial muscles on one side of the upper body creates a muscular imbalance and lateral displacement of the head and shoulders.

### EFFECTS OF LATERAL CURVATURE OF THE SPINE

In all cases of lateral curvature, the vertebrae are tilted. This causes an approximation of the joint facets on the concave (inner) side of the curvature with a concentration of weight on the concave side of the spinal joint. There is a separation of joint facets on the convex (outer) side of the curvature.

*Effects on Vertebrae*—On the concave side of the curve, the concentration of weight on one side of the joint results in a wearing away of the articulating surface of the vertebrae on that side. In addition, there is a compression of the inter-vertebral disk on the concave side. The wear and tear on the spinal joints takes place unequally. Eventually, an inter-vertebral disk on the concave side of the curve becomes permanently compressed. The malalignment of the joint surfaces and inter-vertebral disk eventually impinges on the nerves emanating from the spinal column. The result is constant pain.

The rotational effect imposed on the spine, which is added to the compression resulting from the tilting of the vertebrae, creates further tension on the joint surfaces. Klafs and Arnheim pointed out that in addition to suffering chronic pain, the scoliotic athlete may be subject to severe epiphysitis or bursitis of the spine.[2]

## EFFECTS ON MUSCLES, LIGAMENTS, AND FASCIA

The muscles, ligaments and fascia on the concave side of the curvature shorten and contract, while those on the convex side stretch, weaken, and lose tone. Some muscles can become so contracted as to be tendinous in nature. The imbalance of the deep spinal muscles in lumbar scoliosis can be sufficient enough to change the balanced line of the pelvis from horizontal to oblique (lateral pelvic tilt) and cause pelvic and low back instability.

Due to the muscular imbalance that is the cause or result of lateral curvature, the lateral mobility of the spine is restricted and the muscles, ligaments, and fascia are highly susceptible to acute strains from sudden movement.

## EFFECTS OF LATERAL PELVIC TILT

Yonders clearly demonstrated that lateral pelvic tilt is a direct cause of lateral curvature of the spine.[8] Commenting that with the pelvic tilt there is an associated lateral tilt of the sacrum (Chapter 12, Figure 9) and the fifth lumbar vertebra, he stated:

> The tendency to lumbo-sacral and sacroiliac joint strain is inevitable, this being caused by the abnormal oblique direction of weight pressure on these articulations. Hypermobility of the lumbo-sacral joint may develop. Also, there is frequent development of separation of the sacroiliac joint on the higher side of the pelvic tilt, with resultant hypermobility. On the lower side of the tilt, this joint is subject to jamming and strain because the center of gravity of the pelvis is often shifted toward that side and it therefore takes more than its normal half share of the weight imposed from above.

There is always a slight degree of rotation of the pelvis on the thigh bones associated with a lateral pelvic tilt. The pelvis tends to rotate forward on the side of the high hip. The body will tolerate relatively little change in the lateral or rotatory (tortipelvis) position of the pelvis before symptoms of strain in the lower back and pelvis are noted. The low back pain associated with a lateral pelvic tilt generally appears as a one-sided lumbo-sacral strain. This is due to the abnormal compression at the articulating surfaces of the spinal joints on the high side of the lateral pelvic tilt. The main effects of this abnormal compression are reflected by pain in the area of the fifth lumbar vertebra.

In addition, on the high hip side of the lateral pelvic tilt, there is a compensatory change in the shoulder area through a lowering of the shoulder on the side of the high hip. This can cause a stretch strain and fatigue of the lateral neck muscles on the lowered shoulder side.

With a lateral hip tilt, the leg on the high side will go into adduction and inward rotation, while the leg on the low side will rotate outward. Muscle imbalance develops, with posterior lateral trunk muscles and lumbo-dorsal fascia tight on the high side and the tensor fascia latae muscle (Chapter 14, Figure 17) tight on the low side. The gluteus medius muscle shows weakness on the high side, while the adductor muscles of the leg on the high side shorten and contract. The tightness of the tensor fascia latae can result in severe pain on the outside of the thigh.

Constant tension on a point of tendinous or ligamentous attachment may excite periosteal (bone covering) irritation and thickening of the bone at that point. With a lateral pelvic tilt, the psoas (hip flexor) and pyriformis (outward hip rotator) muscles that connect the thigh with the spinal column are placed under constant tension at both their origin and insertion, enough to eventually produce irritation at their points of attachment. The constant irritation can eventually form extoses (bone spurs) either at the crest of the iliac (pelvis bone) or the inner femoral (thigh) condyle.

The sacrosciatic ligaments binding the sacroiliac joint begin to lose tone and stretch, which allows the ilium on the one side of the pelvis to drop down on the muscles passing between the spinal column and the greater trochanter of the thigh bone. As was pointed out in Chapter 11, the tension on the pyriformis muscle can impinge on the sciatic nerve with resultant pain down the leg.

Osteo-arthritis of the hip joint is many times found in runners and joggers of middle age due to their long years of walking and running with a slight lateral tilt of the pelvis.

Lowman, in 1912, proved conclusively that internal rotation of the thigh in anterior pelvic tilt or lateral pelvic tilt places abnormal stresses on the joints of the knee, ankle, and foot.[5] The inward rotation of the thighs throws the knees out of line and produces or accentuates valgus ankles and pronation of the feet. He found that by rotating the thighs outward a person rotated his heel outward and threw his body weight on the outer border of the foot. Outward thigh rotation also took the tension off the muscles of the hip below, in the region of the hip joint, and above, along the lumbar vertebrae and the crest of the ilia.

## EFFECTS OF THE SHORT LEG SYNDROME

In 1950, Beal wrote an extensive review of the literature relating to the short leg problem, citing 81 references from 1862 through 1950.[1] He noted that one of the obvious results of short leg is poor body mechanics, which results in various types of postural disturbances—the outstanding one being scoliosis. The most common symptom associated with short leg is backache. Other orthopedic problems which have been shown to be influenced by short leg are compressed and ruptured inter-vertebral disks, foot disturbances, psoas muscle fibrositis, and shoulder pain. Beal cited the comment of Goldthwait and his associates that postural disturbances are directly related to arthritis. Increased stress of postural imbalance may in time lead to the development of osteo-arthritis in the hip joints and spinal column.

The accommodations to a short leg result in a lateral tilt, a sideways shift, and rotation of the pelvis. Lateral curvature of the lumbar spine results from compensating efforts to offset the lateral pelvic imbalance.

Beal concluded his paper by stating that X-ray studies have shown that short leg has an incidence of 70 percent in the population. Redler, in a study of 99 adult cases with average difference in leg length from about one-half to five-eighths of an inch, found the common complaints in short leg were: (1) low back pain; (2) sciatic pain; (3) pain about the knee; (4) pain in the ankle or foot, usually the heel.[6] In a group of 21 children, Redler found the following complaints: (1) peculiar or awkward type of gait or posture; (2) pain in the hip on the shorter side; (3) pain in the legs; (4) pain in the heel; (5) pain in the foot and ankle. In both the adult and juvenile cases, the one common factor was the short leg syndrome.

Yonders maintained that the major cause of lateral pelvic tilt is the short leg syndrome.[8] It is found in over 50 percent of the cases of lateral pelvic tilt.

Larson commented that probably the most common cause of chronic and recurrent sacroiliac lesions is the presence of difference in leg length.[4] With a difference in stress applied through the two femurs to the pelvis, there will be a constant attempt to compensate. The result is chronic irritation in pelvic and lumbar joints. He pointed out that the type and direction of compensatory changes in the spine are dependent upon the type of compensation in the pelvis. The changes in the pelvis in relation to the midline of the body (lateral displacement) occur in rotation of the pelvis as a whole, the extent of lateral flexion, and rotation of the sacrum.

In a study of lateral asymmetry of the pelvis and legs (lateral tilt and short leg) as a causative factor in knee injuries, Klein found the short leg abducted and toed outwards, and ankle pronation as the foot was placed on the ground, as well as a valgus position of the knee as the leg was carried forward.[3] This placed abnormal stresses on the medial ligament of the knee and the medial ankle. In a four-year study of 150 cases of knee injury, Klein found a consistent pattern of injury occurrence to the short leg side (80 to 82 percent). This was the result of the basic mechanisms of injury being put into motion: inward rotation of the femur, outward rotation of the tibia, and the knee inside of the foot in weight bearing.

## EFFECTS OF LATERAL ASYMMETRY ON PERFORMANCE

Lateral balance for good running form depends on correct foot position, straight leg alignment, a horizontal pelvis in the frontal plane, straight leg alignment, a horizontal pelvis in the frontal plane, straight alignment of the upper body and head, synchronized action of arms and shoulders with rotation of the hip joints, and arms held close to the sides of the body. Lateral curvature of the spine, lateral pelvic tilt, and the short leg all result in lateral displacement of the body in the frontal plane, and interfere with running efficiency.

*Lateral Curvature of the Spine*—Lateral curvature of the spine in the lumbar or dorsolumbar area of the spine reduce spinal motion, shorten the length of the stride, and decrease balancing movements of the trunk. Restriction of spinal motion and decreased performance parallel each other and necessitate the use of energy-consuming compensating movements of the extremities to maintain lateral body balance.

*Lateral Pelvic Tilt*—Slocum and James maintained that the lateral oscillations of the pelvis in running should be kept at a minimum to lessen the burden borne by the postural muscles in maintaining lateral balance of the body.[7] Lateral tilting of the pelvis causes asymmetrical muscle lengths in the pelvic structure and a tilt in the hip joints' axis that produces an eccentric motion between the two hip joints instead of opposite and equal motion, i.e., the transmission of weight and thrust on the legs and feet will be different on one leg than on the other. Therefore, wear and tear on the ligaments and joints will be different, particularly if there is any deviation in leg alignment (knock-knee, tibia torsion, valgus ankle). With a lateral pelvic tilt, there is asymmetrical action of the lower trunk muscles due to pelvic torque and the compensating curvature and torque of the lumbar spine.

When there is a combined lordosis of the lumbar spine and lateral pelvic tilt, one hip socket will be further forward than the other, due to the rotational torque of the twisted lumbar spine. This will result in eccentricity in two planes which will influence the stride. The hip joint will be flexed due to the forward tilt. The hip joint flexors are shortened and the muscles of the lumbar spine are contracted into a position of lordosis. The forward trajectory of the leading leg on one side will not be similar to the one on the opposite side. The discrepancy must be offset by adapting the swing phase differently to obtain a rhythmic and equal action. The difference in muscle length in all three planes must be adjusted to the asymmetry. This condition creates a greater lateral oscillation of the hip joints than is required for good running form and which, in turn, disturbs the lateral balance of the body.

*Short Leg Syndrome*—Klein, in discussing the short leg syndrome, wrote:

> Now, what is the possible effect of this lateral asymmetry on the distance runner who uses the heel-toe technique? Every time he steps on the short leg side, the length of the step is shorter than that of the long leg side. So in a mile run, of alternating a short and long step, it should take more time to travel the course. Although there is little evidence of any postural balancing work being done in this area, it seems logical that lateral postural balancing to equalize the gait pattern would result in a new world record or two, and reduce the veering tendencies of gait action.[3]

## REFERENCES

1. Beal, Myron C., "A Review of the Short Leg Problem," *Journal of the American Osteopathic Association,* October 1950.
2. Klafs, Carl E. and Arnheim, Daniel D., *Modern Principls of Athletic Training* (St. Louis: The C. V. Mosby Company, 1963).
3. Klein, Karl K., "Flexibility—Strength and Balance in Athletics," *Journal of N.A.T.A.,* Summer 1971.
4. Larson, Norman J., "Sacroiliac and Postural Changes from Anatomic Short Lower Extremity," *Journal of the American Osteopathic Association,* October 1940.
5. Lowman, Charles L., "The Relation of Thigh and Leg Muscles to Malposture of the Feet," *Boston Medical and Surgical Journal,* January 18, 1912.
6. Redler, Irving, "Clinical Significance of Minor Inequalities in Leg Length," *New Orleans Medical Journal,* Vol. 104, 1952.
7. Slocum, Donald B. and James, Stanley L., "Biomechanics of Running," *Journal of the American Medical Association,* Vol. 250, No. 11, September 9, 1968.
8. Yonders, H. H., "Tilted Pelvis," *Journal of the American Osteopathic Association,* July 1947.

# 14

## Leg Alignment

The close interrelationship between separate postural faults in the total body structure is nowhere better illustrated than in the relationship between the pelvis, legs, knees, and feet. Any fault of alignment in the pelvis is expressed downward through the legs to the feet. Any fault in foot alignment is transmitted upward through the legs to the pelvis. Deviations in knee joint alignment may be transmitted upwards or downwards to the pelvis or feet.

### IMPORTANCE OF LEG ALIGNMENT

If we exclude deviations in the skeletal structure, but have a proper muscle balance in the hips, legs, and ankles, the weight line of the body in the frontal plane (from the front view) lies midway between the first and second metatarsal bones, and passes upwards bisecting the ankle joint, patella of the knee, and antereo-superior spine of the ilium (Figure 3B). This straight and correct vertical alignment of the leg results in a mechanically straightforward position of the feet during walking and running. The straight-ahead foot position allows the most efficient and powerful action of the lower leg and foot muscles in forward propulsion of the body.

From a postural, mechanical, and injury prevention standpoint, the importance of a straight leg and foot position cannot be over-estimated. Any deviation from the straight vertical line in the frontal plane imposes abnormal stresses on the joints, tendons, ligaments, and muscles of the lower extremities and feet.

### DEFINITIONS

*Genu Valgum or Valgus*—knock-knees.

*Genu Varum or Varus*—bowlegs (may be in the thigh or lower legs, or both).

*Genu Recurvatum*—back or hyperextended knee.

*Rotation*—movement of a body about its axis.

*Torsion*—the condition of being twisted.

*Tibial Torsion*—twisting of the tibia on its long axis (shaft) so that the proximal end appears to be inwardly or outwardly rotated.

The terms "rotation" and "torsion" are many times interchanged in the literature and this leads to confusion. Rotation pertains to the turning, either internal or external, of the long shaft of a bone within a body joint at either end of the shaft, such as the knees and hips, and involves muscle action. Torsion pertains to the twisting of the long shaft of a bone within itself.

The emphasis in this discussion will be placed on rotation rather than torsion. Torsion is a highly complicated orthopedic problem.

## STRUCTURE AND ANATOMY OF THE LEGS

The skeletal structure of the legs is illustrated in Figure 12. The major muscles supporting the skeletal structure are illustrated in Figure 17 and in Chapter 17, Figure 30.

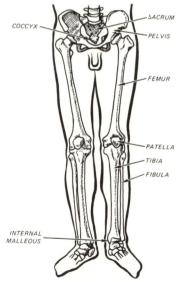

**Figure 12**
STRUCTURE OF UPPER AND LOWER LEG

## MUSCLES AFFECTING HIP ROTATION

*Inward prime movers:* tensor fasciae latae and anterior fibers of gluteus minimus.

132

*Outward prime movers:* gluteus maximus and six outward rotators (not illustrated).

The adductor and abductor muscles of the hip assist the rotators in internal or external rotation of the hip. Internal and external movements of the hip are illustrated in Chapter 2.

## MUSCLES AFFECTING KNEE ROTATION

*Inward prime movers:* biceps femoris.

*Outward prime movers:* semi-tendinosus, semi-membranous, and popliteus (not illustrated).

The power ratio between the prime mover muscles in hip rotation is strongly in favor of external rotation. Inward rotation of the hip is practically always a secondary function to adduction of the hip. However, the combined action of the powerful adductors and internal rotators, favored by the action of gravity and the superincumbent body weight, favors internal femoral (thigh) rotation.

The knee joint cannot be rotated if the leg is extended. Tests for lower leg rotation at the knee joint are conducted in the seated position. Several recent studies have shown that the power ratio between internal and external rotation strongly favors internal rotation.[2,5]

## GROWTH CYCLE IN LEG ALIGNMENT

The normal child passes through a growth cycle in respect to the development of leg alignment. Children are born with moderate bowlegs and some degree of medial torsion. When they first stand up, they will spread their feet to obtain a wide base of balance. The wide stance is compensated for by development of a knock-knee defect, although the bowlegs (tibia) may still be present. If the foot itself is normal, a child will then toe inwards in an effort to correct the knock-knees. Children tend to rotate the thighs internally at the hips, and the outer side of the knee faces more to the front. In walking, one leg at a time is firmly fixed on the ground. As they take a forward step, the forward thrust of weight through the knee tends to straighten out the knock-knees. The toeing-in foot position also raises the inner border of the foot and the longitudinal arch is formed. After the knock-knees are corrected and the arch has formed, the child will naturally begin to toe more directly ahead with the feet slightly abducted.

This growth cycle follows the normal pattern unless it is interfered with by obesity, malnourishment, muscle imbalance, congenital flat feet or other foot defects, tibial torsion, or internal or external contracture of the hip rotator muscles.

The normal correct alignment of the legs in the frontal plane is illustrated in Figure 13.

With respect to the competitive runner and hurdler, the most commonly found faults in frontal plane leg alignment result from: (1) internal or excessive external rotation of the legs at the hip joint; (2) an abducted toes-outward foot position; and (3) pronated feet, whether in an abducted foot position or pointed straight ahead. It should be noted that normal leg alignment displays a slight outward rotation of the leg at the hip joint.

With the exception of joggers, rarely does one find an athlete in running or hurdling events displaying excessive deviations in leg alignment resulting from knock-knees, bowlegs, or tibial torsion. Minor faults of this type do not affect running or hurdling performance.

Knock-knees (genu valgus), bowlegs (genu varus), or tibial torsion (internal or external twisting of the tibia) are complicated orthopedic problems. After eight to ten years of age, these defects can be corrected only by surgery.

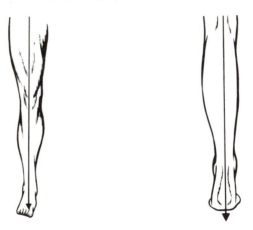

*Figure 13*
NORMAL LEG ALIGNMENT FRONTAL AND POSTERIOR PLANES

## LEG ROTATION

The relationship between the two ends of the entire leg lever from the hip to the foot, in respect to internal (medial) or external (lateral) rotation of the leg at the hip joints was first pointed out by Lowman in 1912.[4] He described his efforts in correcting pronation of the feet (Figure 9). Despite the use of orthotic appliances (arch supports) and corrective foot exercises, the pronation of the foot persisted. In a series of 300 cases suffering from flat pronated feet, he found in each case femoral (thigh) internal rotation at the hip joints. He designed an exercise to develop the external rotator muscles of the leg and hip which automatically raised the medial longitudinal arch of the foot and brought the foot into a normal weight-bearing position.

## ROTATION AT THE HIP

With the leg extended and the knee joint locked in a weight-bearing position, rotation of the entire leg can occur either at the hip joint or by a change in foot position (abduction, adduction, pronation).

If the leg is extended and the foot is prevented from moving due to the pressure on the ground, internal rotation may cause the foot to go into pronation, whether the foot is pointed straight ahead (Figure 15) or abducted outwards (Figure 14). In both foot positions of internal rotation or foot pronation, the weight line will fall to the medial (inner) side of the foot. When the foot pronates, the medial longitudinal arch will drop towards the ground, and the outer edge of the foot will evert (raise upwards) with the heel deflected outwards (Chapter 18, Figure 46).

If the feet are turned toward each other (pigeon toes) due to internal rotation of the leg, the feet do not pronate.

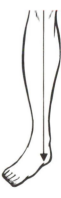

**Figure 14**
OUTWARD THIGH ROTATION
ABDUCTED AND PRONATED FOOT

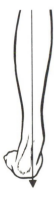

**Figure 15**
INWARD THIGH ROTATION
PATELLA FACES INWARD-
PRONATION OF FOOT

Excessive outward rotation of the leg at the hip joint may cause a toed-out foot position (abduction).

In a weight-bearing position, turning of the foot in an outwardly flaring position (abduction) will cause the leg to rotate externally at the hips. Turning the foot into an adducted position (pigeon toes) or pronation of the foot in a straight ahead toe position will cause the leg to rotate internally at the hip joint.

## ROTATION AT THE KNEE JOINT

Internal rotation of the knees is often seen as the result of knee hyperextension (Figure 16B) or in combination with it. The knee position of internal rotation of the femur, with the patella facing inwards and external rotation of the lower leg accompanying knee hyperextension, is due to stretching of the popliteus muscle at the rear of the knee. This small muscle has the function of rotating the lower leg inward on the upper leg. Hyperextension or flexion of the knee permits the lower leg to rotate outwards on the femur if the popliteus muscle is weakened or stretched. This cannot happen when the leg is extended, as anatomically the knee joint cannot rotate in the extended position.

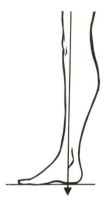

*Figure 16A*
NORMAL LEG ALIGNMENT
SAGITTAL PLANE

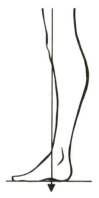

*Figure 16B*
HYPEREXTENSION
SAGITTAL PLANE

## LEG DEVIATIONS—SAGITTAL PLANE

The normal weight line in the sagittal plane is illustrated in Figure 16A. Hyperextension of the knee, which is a postural fault in sagittal leg alignment, is illustrated in Figure 16B.

Hyperextension, in the absence of structural defects, results from poor habit patterns of walking, muscular imbalance, and compensation for apparent bowlegs.

1. Overweight people tend to walk with the legs in hyperextension to maintain antereo-posterior upper body alignment. Walking in this position does not involve much quadriceps action. The

136

quadriceps weaken and the knee finally goes into forced hyper-extension.

2. When the foot strikes the floor in a fixed position, both the quadriceps and hamstrings extend the knee. If the knee joint opposing muscle groups are not balanced in strength, the knee goes into forcible hyperextension. The imbalance can result from weak quadriceps and strong hamstrings, or vice versa.

3. Internal rotation of the legs at the hip when accompanied by some hyperextension of the knees is the cause of apparent bowlegs in children and adults.

### TIBIAL TORSION

As stated previously, the emphasis in this chapter is on rotation of the leg rather than the torsion of the lower leg (tibia). Tibial torsion is a highly complicated orthopedic problem as it involves torsion (twisting) of the bone structure itself.

Many excellent athletes display evidence of internal tibial torsion that does not appear to affect their performance in any manner or become a cause of minor injuries. However, tibial torsion can play a big part in foot imbalance. For this reason, the coach and athlete should have a basic knowledge of the subject.

Internal tibial torsion is found in approximately 90 percent of the newborn. In the normal child, the tibia displays a slightly outward tibial torsion (2 percent) at birth. This increases during the first year to an average of 10 percent and then remains stationary for two to three years. At approximately four years of age, the outward tibial torsion increases to an average of 20 percent—which approaches the adult average of 23 percent.

Internal tibial torsion in the adult can be due to a congenital clubfoot, internal or external rotation of the entire leg at the hips, flat feet, or bowlegs. Internal tibial torsion is many times associated with a pigeon-toed position of the feet. In an attempt to cope with this problem and bring the feet into a straight ahead position, many young children will hyperextend the knees (Figure 16B).

Excess external tibial torsion, which is rare, is generally associated with knock-knees or highly arched feet (pes cavus). Hines maintained that external torsion is due to the bad habit of walking with the feet externally rotated (abducted) during childhood.[1]

In Chapter 5, we mentioned Kite's finding that childhood sleeping and sitting positions were a cause of muscular imbalance in the feet that eventually leads to foot deviations.[3] Sleeping and sitting positions are also a direct cause of internal or excess external torsion developing in the tibia bone.

# ANTERIOR — POSTERIOR UPPER LEG

## Anterior Upper Leg

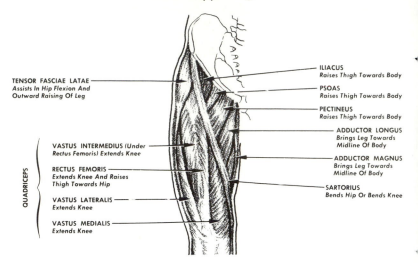

TENSOR FASCIAE LATAE
*Assists In Hip Flexion And
Outward Raising Of Leg*

ILIACUS
*Raises Thigh Towards Body*

PSOAS
*Raises Thigh Towards Body*

PECTINEUS
*Raises Thigh Towards Body*

ADDUCTOR LONGUS
*Brings Leg Towards
Midline Of Body*

ADDUCTOR MAGNUS
*Brings Leg Towards
Midline Of Body*

SARTORIUS
*Bends Hip Or Bends Knee*

VASTUS INTERMEDIUS (Under
Rectus Femoris) Extends Knee

RECTUS FEMORIS
*Extends Knee And Raises
Thigh Towards Hip*

VASTUS LATERALIS
*Extends Knee*

VASTUS MEDIALIS
*Extends Knee*

QUADRICEPS

## Posterior Upper Leg

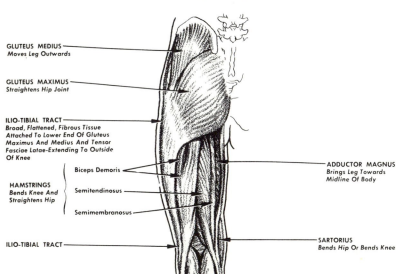

GLUTEUS MEDIUS
*Moves Leg Outwards*

GLUTEUS MAXIMUS
*Straightens Hip Joint*

ILIO-TIBIAL TRACT
*Broad, Flattened, Fibrous Tissue
Attached To Lower End Of Gluteus
Maximus And Medius And Tensor
Fasciae Latae-Extending To Outside
Of Knee*

Biceps Demoris

HAMSTRINGS
*Bends Knee And
Straightens Hip*

Semitendinosus

Semimembranosus

ILIO-TIBIAL TRACT

ADDUCTOR MAGNUS
*Brings Leg Towards
Midline Of Body*

SARTORIUS
*Bends Hip Or Bends Knee*

*Figure 17*

# REFERENCES

1. Hines, Thomas F., "Posture," *Therapeutic Exercise,* Sidney Light, ed. (New Haven: Elizabeth Light, 1965).
2. Jarvis, Dorothy K., "Relative Strength of the Hip Rotator Muscle Groups," *The Physical Therapy Review,* Vol. 32, No. 10, 500.
3. Kite, J. H., "Torsion of the Lower Extremities in Small Children," *The Journal of Bone and Joint Surgery,* Vol. 36-A, No. 3, June 1954.
4. Lowman, C. L., "Relation of Thigh and Leg Muscles to Malpostures of the Feet," *Boston Medical and Surgical Journal,* January 18, 1912.
5. May, Warren W., "Maximum Isometric Force of the Hip Rotator Muscles," *Journal of the American Physical Therapy Association,* Vol. 46, No. 3, March 1966.

# 15

## Effects of Faulty Leg Alignment

An anatomically and structurally straight leg is exceedingly rare among human beings. Deviations in leg alignment can result from faults at three points in the entire leg lever extending from the hip joints to the feet. If one end of the leg deviates, it will affect the other end. If the fault exists within the leg itself at the knee joint, it can affect the posture of the pelvis and position of the hip joints above, or the stability or position of the feet below.

### INTERNAL THIGH POSITION

This deviation keeps the external thigh rotator muscles, particularly the pyriformis muscle, under a constant state of tension which eventually stretches them. The psoas (hip flexor) muscles are also placed under constant tension. They begin to shorten and pull the anterior rim of the pelvis forward and downward. Eventually, the combined stretching and shortening lead to pain in the ilio-femoral ligament and weaken the sacroiliac ligaments, which causes pain in the lower back. The constant tension on the pyriformis muscle over a long period of time can lead to what the Kendalls called the "pyriformis syndrome," with sciatic nerve pain down the back of the leg.[4]

The internal thigh position ultimately produces symptoms of joint strain in the hips, knees, and feet manifested by changes in the joint linings. In the hip joints and pelvis, the changes result in hypertrophy of the joint fringes and spur formations, which cause pain in the sacroiliac notch, the hip joints, and the lower back. It leads to thickening of the iliac crest (Chapter 4, Figure 2) and spur formations due to the tension on the psoas muscles.

140

If the feet are pointed straight ahead with inward thigh rotation, the patellae (kneecaps) face inward towards each other. This appearance at the knee joint has been called "functional knock-knees." The weight line of the body is thrown to the medial side of the foot, placing great strain on the medial longitudinal arch with eventual pronation of the feet.

In 1912, Lowman described the effects of the combination of internal thigh rotation and pronated feet:

> In those cases complaining of "rheumatism" in feet and knees, "growing pains" at knee, cramps in thighs and legs, a sore place over the lower part of the back, and others just of a "continued tiredness," especially much worse on standing still than walking, with or without aching in feet, knees, or hips, I found nearly all showed a condition of inward rotation of the leg in relation to the weight line, and the knee cap pointing toward the opposite side, making the projected line from the antereo-superior spine through the knee fall on the floor to the inside of the knee.[7]

If the feet are pointed outward, the knee is thrown into a valgus (knock-knee) position with outward rotation of the tibia (tibial valgus), placing abnormal stresses on medial structures of the knee and compressing the lateral knee joint surfaces. The medial collateral ligaments (Figure 18) are stretched, and there is a slippage of the internal semi-lunar cartilage. In addition, the outward rotation of the tibia leads to pronation of the feet. Abnormal stresses are placed on the medial longitudinal arch and medial collateral ligaments of the knee. The effects of these lower leg deviations are similar to those described by Lowman when the foot is pointed straight ahead, but greater effects are seen in the knee joint with the feet pointed outward.

Internal thigh rotation combined with abducted (toed-out) foot position leads to malalignment of the quadriceps muscle and its tendon insertion, causing the patella (kneecap) to displace outward from its normal position in the groove between the two femoral condyles (Chapter 14, Figure 12). This results in a chronic subluxation of the patella (slippage) progressing to chondromalacia (degeneration of patella), and eventually to osteo-arthritis of the knee joint.

## KNEE HYPEREXTENSION (GENU RECURVATUM)

Hyperextension places undue compression on the anterior side of the knee joint and undue tension on the posterior ligaments (Figure 18 and Chapter 14, Figure 16B). It stretches not only the posterior ligaments, but also the popliteus muscle. This permits the lower leg to rotate outward on the femur in flexion or extension, throwing the knee into a valgus position at the time of foot strike. This places

# KNEE JOINT

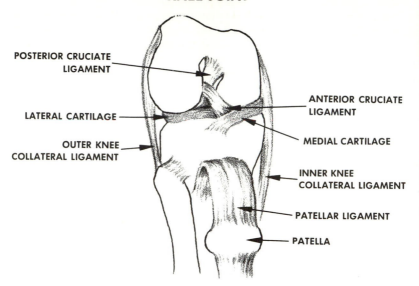

POSTERIOR CRUCIATE LIGAMENT

ANTERIOR CRUCIATE LIGAMENT

LATERAL CARTILAGE

MEDIAL CARTILAGE

OUTER KNEE COLLATERAL LIGAMENT

INNER KNEE COLLATERAL LIGAMENT

PATELLAR LIGAMENT

PATELLA

Ligaments Front View
(Knee Cap Has Been Peeled Back For Illustration)

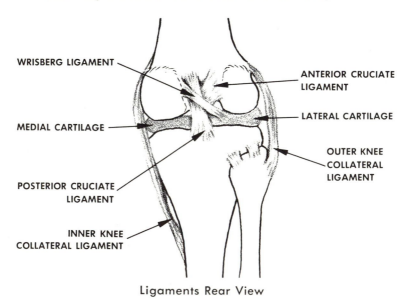

WRISBERG LIGAMENT

ANTERIOR CRUCIATE LIGAMENT

MEDIAL CARTILAGE

LATERAL CARTILAGE

OUTER KNEE COLLATERAL LIGAMENT

POSTERIOR CRUCIATE LIGAMENT

INNER KNEE COLLATERAL LIGAMENT

Ligaments Rear View

*Figure 18*

142

abnormal stresses on the medial collateral ligaments (Figure 18). With hyperextended knees, the thighs incline backward from the hip joints, creating tension on the ilio-femoral ligaments which, in turn, draws the anterior rim of the pelvis downward, increasing both forward pelvic inclination and lumbar lordosis. In addition, the hamstring muscles may stretch and weaken.

Pain in the popliteal space behind the knee joint is common among those who stand with hyperextended knees. In runners, the lower end of the quadriceps muscle tends to lose strength due to this condition—which further weakens the stability of the vulnerable knee joint.

The combination of weakened quadriceps and stretched popliteus muscle weakens knee stability, and merely stepping on a stone or into a slight depression in the ground can lead to a strained or sprained knee.

## BOWLEGS (GENU VALGUM)

This leg fault may be due to congenital factors, nutritional factors, or walking too early in life. Abnormal stresses are placed on the fibular collateral ligament (Figure 18) and the tendon insertion of the tensor fascia latae muscle (Chapter 14, Figure 17). It causes a compression of the medial joint surfaces and cartilage, forces the foot to pronate at foot strike, and eventually causes pain in both the knee and foot joints.

## KNOCK-KNEES (GENU VALGUS)

The valgus position of the knee, even though minor in nature, is one of the most troublesome faults of leg alignment in respect to distance runners and physical fitness joggers and, in particular, to women in all running sports. Women are more prone to genu valgum, due to their wider hips and greater angle of inward thigh inclination.

If the feet are rotated outward with a knock-knee position, the inner patella and internal coronary ligaments begin to stretch. Compression of the infra-patellar pads of fat and the inner parts of the synovial membrane results in a loss of resistance and cartilage deterioration. This predisposes the semi-lunar meniscus (cartilage) to tearing or rupture.

The valgus knee position stretches medial collateral ligaments (Figure 18) and shifts the line of pull of the quadriceps muscles and tendon insertion, which results in lateral displacement of the patella over the lateral femoral condyle. The subluxation of the patella leads to chondromalacia and eventual osteo-arthritis of the knee joint.

A valgus knee position of long standing may lead to a tight and shortened tensor fascia latae muscle on the lateral side of the thigh (Chapter 14, Figure 17), which can result in pain radiating down the lateral side of the knee at the muscle's point of insertion. In addition, due to compression of lateral joint surfaces, tendo-periostitis of the lateral femoral condyle may develop.

The increase in joint tension from the valgus knee posture may result in deterioration of the lower parts of the rectus femoris and vastus internus muscles (Chapter 14, Figure 17), whose strength is highly important to knee stability. The hamstrings may become shortened, particularly the leg biceps muscle (Chapter 14, Figure 17), predisposing the athlete to hamstring strains and rupture.

The valgus knee position throws the lower leg into a position of tibial varum with pronation of the feet that eventually leads to breakdown of the medial longitudinal arch and stretching of the medial ankle ligaments and tendons of the extrinsic muscles that assist the ligaments in supporting the foot arches.

## OTHER FAULTS IN LEG ALIGNMENT

Excessive external rotation of the thighs is associated with muscle imbalance at the hip joint. It is rarely found among track athletes, but is common among joggers. The outward rotation externally rotates the entire leg lever, forcing the feet into a duck-footed abducted position. Abnormal stresses are placed on the medial structures of the knee and the medial longitudinal arch.

Excessive internal tibial torsion moves the feet into pigeon-toed position, mainly affects the obliquity of the ankle joint, and causes instability in the heel at foot strike. If an attempt is made to correct the pigeon toes by rotating the feet to a straight ahead or slightly abducted position, the knee tends to go into hyperextension, which imposes abnormal stresses on the posterior aspects of the knee joint and eventually causes pain in the popliteal space and stretching of the cruciate ligament.

## THE KNEE JOINT

The effects of faulty leg alignment, whether it be due to forward tilt of the pelvis, internal rotation of the thighs, excessive external rotation of the thighs, knock-knees, bowlegs, or pronated or abducted foot positions, are centered on the largest and most complex synovial cavity in the body—the knee joint. No other joint in the body is so likely to suffer derangement of its function and its stability as this one.

The knee joint, because of its complex nature and due to its weight-bearing function, is highly susceptible to degenerative changes in its internal structure even after the most minor injury.

Smith, in discussing the aftereffects of minor injuries to the knee, stated: "There is no such injury as a minor injury to the knee, as all injuries to the knee are serious."[11] He pointed out that the term "strain," even if the strain is minor in nature, implies tissue damage—which, in turn, implies inflammation. Inflammation leads to exudation (inflammatory fluid) or, in the case of a joint, effusion (escape of liquid from the internal structure of the joint). Smith went on to state:

> There are three effects of effusion: (1) inhibition of the neuromuscular mechanism of the knee; (2) increase of intra-articular pressure when the joint is vigorously flexed; and (3) the escape of synovial fluid that lubricates the cartilage, leading to flaking and fissuring of the cartilage with consequent further mechanical derangement.

Klein, an outstanding authority on the prevention of knee injuries in contact sports, listed among other causes that predispose a knee to being injured pelvic imbalance and the short leg syndrome.[5] He pointed out that the psoas (hip flexor) muscles are usually overdeveloped in athletes, causing a forward pelvic tilt. Both shortened psoas muscles and short leg cause the thigh to rotate outward, forcing the feet—or one foot—into a "slue-footed" stance (abducted outward), and this foot position predisposes the knee to an increased torque action.

Lewin commented on the close relationship between internal and external derangements of the knee joints and mechanical (postural) faults in the pelvic area of the body which produce malalignment in the legs themselves (knock-knees, bowlegs, hyperextended knees).[6]

Orthopedic specialists since 1900, as well as modern podiatrists specializing in the foot problems of athletes, have called attention to the close relationship between defects and deformities of the feet and the internal derangement of the complex knee joint.

A flat or pronated foot that throws the knee into a valgus position tends to make the tibial collateral ligaments and medial meniscus (cartilage) more vulnerable to stress and strain. Osteo-arthritis of the knee can be affected by mechanical defects in the foot and ankle.

## INTERNAL DERANGEMENTS OF THE KNEE

Smillie stated that the term "internal derangement of the knee" is nothing more than a statement that there is something wrong with the joint.[10] He further pointed out that perfect muscles seldom control imperfect joints. Some wasting of the quadriceps muscle (Chapter 14, Figure 17) is the accompaniment of every internal derangement of the knee. Among the numerous disorders listed under this non-specific terminology in the orthopedic literature, those most closely associated with runners and joggers are medial collateral ligament (Figure 18) lesions, recurrent subluxation (slippage) of the patella (kneecap), and chondromalacia patella.

## MEDIAL COLLATERAL LIGAMENT LESIONS

Any time a joint, such as the knee, is out of alignment for whatever reason, the ligaments on one side of the joint are placed under a constant state of tension and stretch. Eventually, they permanently stretch and weaken. A minor tear (sprain) of a weakened ligament can result from a sudden or unexpected movement.

Minor acute sprains of the medial collateral ligaments result when the knee is in a valgus (knock-knee) position due to genu valgus (knock-knees), internal thigh rotation, pronated or flat feet, or poor foot position at foot strike (abduction), and are produced by a twist or sudden turn that results in a rotational strain. Situations of this type include stumbling, in stepping on or off curbs or stairs, and catching one's heel and stumbling, stepping into a small hole or on a rock such as those encountered by cross-country runners and joggers, and jumping from a height and landing with the knee in a valgus position as steeplechasers are apt to do in overcoming obstacles.

Smillie pointed out that partial sprain of the long parallel fibers of the medial collateral ligament at their attachment to the femur is one of the most common injuries to the knee joint.[10] Further, it possibly ranks third in frequency among minor injuries producing traumatic synovitis. He commented that not only does it occur frequently, it is frequently misdiagnosed. If not recognized, it gives rise to a "medial ligament syndrome," and the symptoms that follow are responsible for severe and prolonged disability.

Smillie went on to state that a history of major injury is no longer necessary for the diagnosis of meniscus (cartilage). In an aging population, an increasing number of lesions are of degenerative origin. A high proportion of patients have either a history of no injury or no more than a minor twist of rotational nature.

## RECURRENT SUBLUXATION OF THE PATELLA

Southwick *et al.* commented that chronic dislocation of the patella is relatively common, especially in women and girls.[12] They cited Smillie as stressing that every internal derangement of the knee joint of a young woman should be suspected of being a recurrent subluxation of the patella until it is proven otherwise. Smillie pointed out that in many mild cases the patella may slip momentarily over the edge of the lateral condyle of the patella, leading to feelings of insecurity or giving way of the knee, followed by recurrent synovial (fluid from inside the knee joint) effusion.

Hughston maintained that patella subluxation is the second most common cause of internal derangement of the knee in the athlete, torn meniscus (cartilage) being the first.[3] He went on to comment that chondromalacia of the patella and sometimes of the femoral condyles (Chapter 14, Figure 12) has been a frequent accompaniment of malalignment and malfunction of the extensor (quadriceps muscles) mechanism.

The patella is a sesamoid bone formed within the tendon of the quadriceps femoris (Chapter 14, Figure 17). This tendon continues over and on either side of the patella, and inserts in the tuberosity (upper end) of the lower leg tibia bone. At this point, it is known as the patellar ligament. The patella rides between the condyles of the femur. Watson-Jones pointed out that the direction of pull of the quadriceps above the patella is not the same as the direction of pull of the patellar tendon below the patella.[13] It passes downward and in a medial (inner) direction, while the ligament lies vertically. This means there is an inherent tendency toward lateral (outward) subluxation of the patella, particularly among women or among men with even the slightest degree of valgus (knock-knees). The patella has a thick cartilage, and its central part is poorly nourished.

There have been many causes listed in the orthopedic literature for recurring subluxation of the patella. Goldthwait commented in 1904 that recurrent dislocation of the patella is often associated with flat feet.[2] Valgus (knock-knee), either congenital or acquired, is a major cause. Others mentioned are hyperextended knees, weakness of the vastus medialis muscle (Chapter 14, Figure 17), internal rotation of the thighs with compensatory tibial torsion or lateral rotation of the tibia at the knee joint. It can be seen that faulty leg alignment, with the exception of a congenitally high or very small patella, is a major predisposing factor in recurrent subluxation of the patella.

Lewin poined out that chondromalacia of the patella is an almost constant accompaniment of subluxating patella.[6] Other pathomechanics in the knee joint due to subluxation are lesions of the articular cartilage of the patella and femur—leading to traumatic osteo-arthritis, pinching of the fat pads in the internal structure of the knee, and injuries to the cartilages of the knee. In chronic recurrent subluxations, severe osteo-arthritis may develop.

### Degeneration of the Patella (Chondromalacia)

Sheehan stated:

Runner's knee (chondromalacia) is the most frequent overuse injury in all of sports, and the most frequent complaint of runners. A *Runner's World* poll showed that 22 percent of runners had been sidelined for long periods of time with this problem. Sports podiatrist Dr. Richard Schuster reports that nearly 75 percent of runners seeking help have knee pain, although not always as the primary complaint.[8]

Sheehan listed the causes of runner's knee (chondromalacia) as pronated or flat feet, Morton's toe, postural instability, short leg syndrome, and environmental stresses such as inadequate shoes and running on slanted surfaces (roads)—which places further stress on the weak foot.

There are many other causes of chondromalacia listed in the orthopedic literature by authorities specializing in disorders of the knee. Among them are traumatic blows, habitual legs-crossed sitting posture that forces the knee joint—a hinge joint—to function as a universal joint, nutritional impairment of the patella cartilage as a result of knee sprains, repeated traumatization from abnormal mechanics at the patello-femoral junction (valgus knees, bowlegs, hyperextended knees), internal rotation of the thighs, and muscle imbalance in the quadriceps mechanism.

Classing chondromalacia patella as a disease of the active, Fulford commented that the patella is one of the earliest sites of wearing out of joint surfaces, and that several surveys have shown that simlilar changes are common in persons in their twenties and almost universal in those in their forties.[1] He listed several causes of the condition: (1) trauma; (2) congenital causes, such as a small or high patella or excessively valgus knees (knock-knees); (3) lateral subluxation or dislocation influenced by valgus knees or by imbalance of the extensor mechanism with weakness of the vastus medialis; and (4) meniscus (cartilage) lesions.

Fulford pointed out that the level of pressure on the patella during muscular activity is enormous. The compressive strain on the patella ligament can approach half a ton. The smallest abnormality of normal congruence and sliding function of the patella in its groove leads to local breakdown and damage to the joint surface. The resulting lesion is characterized by degeneration of the articular surface of the patella, manifested by fibrillation, with eventual fissuring and erosion of the cartilage. There is a definite effusion (escape of synovial fluid) and atrophy of the lower insertions of the quadriceps muscle. Synovitis may be present, and intense pain occurs within the joint.

## EFFECTS OF FAULTY LEG ALIGNMENT ON PERFORMANCE

In general, unless the faults in leg alignment are excessive, they do not interfere with performance of the track athlete as much as do faults in the pelvis or foot position. Slocum and James provided the best description of leg alignment faults and their effect on running performance.[9] They stated:

> While minor degrees of knock-knee, bowleg, and tibial torsion are consistent with good running performance, athletes with greater involvement do not run well.... The knock-kneed runner must either

run with a wide-based gait to avoid bumping his knees or must increase trunk shift to balance over the support foot. The bowlegged runner has a yawning gait due to increased side-to-side sway. When there is severe internal or external torsion of the tibia and the runner attempts to keep his foot straightforward along the line of progression in attempting to attain good running form, this places rotational strain on the knee which in turn may lead to increased joint wear.

## REFERENCES

1. Fulford, P., "Chondromalacia of the Patella," *Boston Medical and Surgical Journal,* Vol. 4, No. 3, August 1969.
2. Goldthwait, J. E., "Slipping or Recurrent Dislocation of the Patella," *Boston Medical and Surgical Journal,* February 1904.
3. Hughston, Jack C., "Reconstruction of the Extensor Mechanism for Subluxating Patella," *Journal of Sports Medicine,* September/ October 1972.
4. Kendall, Henry O.; Kendall, Florence P; and Boynton, Dorothy A., *Posture and Pain* (Baltimore: The Williams & Wilkins Co., 1952).
5. Klein, Karl K., "Muscular Strength and the Knee," *The Physician and Sports Medicine,* December 1974.
6. Lewin, Philip, *The Knee and Related Structures* (Philadelphia: Lea and Febiger, 1952).
7. Lowman, C. L., "Relation of Thigh and Leg Muscles to Malpostures of the Feet." *Boston Medical and Surgical Journal,* January 18, 1912.
8. Sheehan, George, "Taking Care of the Knees," *Runner's World,* January 1975.
9. Slocum, Donald B. and James, Stanley L., "Biomechanics of Running," *Journal of the American Medical Association,* Vol. 205, No. 11, September 9, 1968.
10. Smillie, I. W., "Diagnosis of Internal Derangement of the Knee," *American Journal of Orthopedics,* February 1961.
11. Smith, D. S., "The Late Effects of Injury to the Knee," *Boston Medical and Surgical Journal,* Vol. 4, No. 3, August 1969.
12. Southwick, Wayne O., Becker, George E., and Albright, James A., "Dovetail Patellar Tendon Transfer for Recurrent Dislocating Patella," *Journal of the American Medical Association,* Vol. 204, No. 8, May 20, 1968.
13. Watson-Jones, R., *Fractures and Joint Injuries* (fourth edition) (Edinburgh: E. and S. Livingstone, Ltd., 1955), Vol. 2.

# 16

## Importance of
## the Foot in Athletics

As was pointed out earlier in this volume, the importance of the foot in running, hurdling, and jogging has—with one exception—been recognized only in the past three years. The exception involves Dr. J. V. Cerney, Doctor of Podiatry, Doctor of Physical Medicine, and member of the National Athletic Trainers Association. In his outstanding textbook on athletic injuries, written in 1968, he devoted 64 pages to the treatment of foot injuries in athletes.[1]

Nowhere in athletic literature has the importance of the foot been so well-expressed as in his opening statement. Commenting that 80 percent of American athletes have weak feet, he wrote:

> An athlete is no better than the condition of his feet and as his feet and legs go, so goes his career. Since the momentum of any athletic action begins with the foot, every possible effort should be made to give the extremities specific, and not cursory, inspection and care.
>
> Power and speed begin in the feet, and the athlete who exerts the most power through utilizing locomotive force gains strength and accuracy through his degree of security on the ground.
>
> Stride emphasizes momentum. Throwing and plunging begins with a push of the toe. This power comes up through the limbs as the knees straighten and the trunk tenses. It multiplies as the shoulder rotates, the upper arm swings, and ends like a snapping spring at the fingers and wrist. At high speed, force is moving over fulcrums. When this speed is combined in a throw, or a blow, or a stride, it represents the peak of speed that begins with the feet.
>
> Therefore, the ability to strike, throw, run, or deliver a blow is dependent on the condition of the feet. It must be noted here that

American feet are not accustomed to the urgency and drive of sporting events. They need specific kind of conditioning to meet the demands of athletics. They need prevention and care. American feet have to have strenuous conditioning because they are the foundation of the athlete and the building of the athlete is no stronger than the foundation which holds him up. To accomplish stamina and endurance, he goes down the path his feet take him. If his feet hurt, he hurts all over. If his feet break down, he has "shin splints." His spine is curved and he slumps. He has neckaches and headaches and in general wishes he wasn't "out for the team."

Too often, potential stars, as well as top athletes, are lost because of the condition of their feet and legs. They are lost because someone is too content to say, "You're getting too old to play" or "If you haven't got it, you haven't got it," and that's why good feet are important in athletics.

## REFERENCES

1. J. V. Cerney, *Athletic Injuries, an Encyclopedia of Causes, Effects and Treatment* (Springfield, Illinois: Charles C. Thomas, 1963), reprinted by permission of the publisher.

# 17

## Structure, Anatomy, and Movements of Foot and Ankle

$A$side from the brain, the foot is the most complicated structure in the human body. It is composed of 26 bones, over 100 ligaments, and 12 extrinsic muscles of the lower leg, whose tendons cross the ankle joint and insert into the various bones of the feet. Its articulation with the tibia of the lower leg at the ankle joint, an architecturally weak joint, determines to a great extent a correct weight-bearing line running from the leg to the foot and ground.

A brief and simplified explanation of the foot and ankle, their anatomy, and the movements of their bony parts will assist the coach, athlete, and jogger in understanding this complicated mechanism and its importance to optimum athletic performance. It will aid them in making effective use of exercises developed to increase the balanced strength and flexibility of the ankle and foot.

### TYPES OF FEET AND LONGITUDINAL ARCHES

The shape of the foot is subject to as many individual variations as is any other part of the body. These variations are the result of the development of the human foot resulting from functional demands, heredity, body type, and racial and national evolutionary characteristics.

In general, feet can be classified into three broad areas according to their morphological structure and external appearance:

1. *Bony, narrow, slender, pointed, tapering feet.* These feet tend to be longer than the average, with the narrow heel structure. This foot is common among runners. It is not an athletic foot in the powerful muscular sense.

2. *Stocky muscular feet with thick bones supported by powerful ligaments*. There is generally a broad forefoot with toes of nearly the same length that have a powerful grip.

3. *Fat feet, generally small in size with a delicate bone structure and often displaying a higher than usual instep*. The feet are flabby and flexible.

In addition to the above, there are feet with long and short heels, long and short toes, and variations in the length of the medial longitudinal arch.

The height of the arches means little, providing they function without pain and in a manner that permits the mechanics of correct weight bearing and locomotion to be carried out without the strain or breakdown of the ligaments or bone structure.

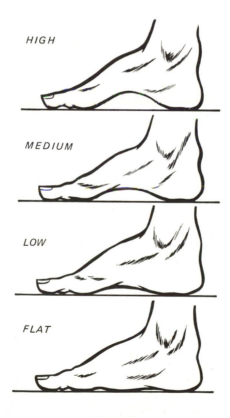

**Figure 19**
**DIFFERENT TYPES OF ARCHES**

An extremely high-arched foot (pes cavus) is the weakest and most troublesome type. The completely flattened foot (pes planus) existing from birth and (often seen in Negroes), exhibiting the normal range of foot motions, may be one of the strongest and most serviceable. A flat foot acquired in early childhood, however, is a definite abnormality.

## STRUCTURE OF THE FOOT AND ANKLE

In discussions of foot structure, four terms describing the bones and joints of the feet are used. The terms occur interchangeably with others in the literature. The calcaneus (heel) is also called the os calcis; the astragalus bone is also called the talus; the navicular bone is also called the scaphoid; the sub-astragalar joint is sometimes called the sub-astragaloid joint, as the anterior faces of the astragalus articulate with the cuboid bone on the lateral side of the foot and the scaphoid bone on the medial side of the foot.

The 26 separate bones of the foot are divided into groups (Figure 20). There are 7 tarsal bones (calcaneus, talus, navicular, cuboid, and three cuneiform); 5 metatarsal bones; and 14 phalangeal bones. The calcaneus (os calcis) and talus (astragalus) of the tarsal group make up the rearfoot; the scaphoid (navicular), cuboid, and three cuneiform bones, the midfoot; and the five metatarsal and phalangeal bones, the forefoot.

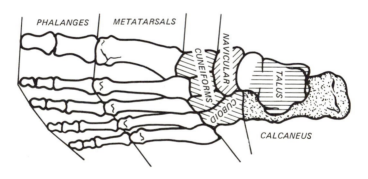

**Figure 20**
DORSAL VIEW (TOP) OF FOOT

The inner longitudinal arch consists of the calcaneus, talus, scaphoid (navicular), the three cuneiform bones, and the three medial metatarsals (Figure 21). The lateral (outer) longitudinal arch consists of the calcaneus, cuboid, and the fourth and fifth metatarsal bones (Figure 22).

A complicated system of ligaments binds and supports the bones of the foot. The most important ligament on the medial side of the

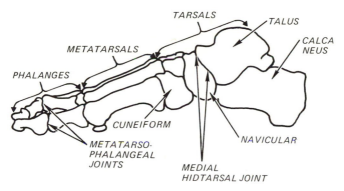

**Figure 21**
**BONES AND JOINTS OF MEDIAL LONGITUDINAL ARCH**

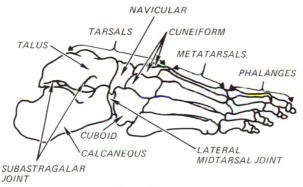

**Figure 22**
**BONES AND JOINTS OF LATERAL SIDE OF FOOT**

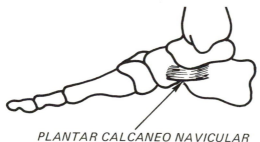

PLANTAR CALCANEO NAVICULAR
"SPRING" LIGAMENT

**Figure 23**
**MAJOR LIGAMENT SUPPORTING MEDIAL SIDE OF FOOT**

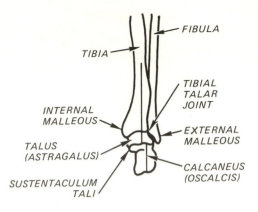

**Figure 24**
POSTERIAL VIEW OF ANKLE AND FOOT
(Note the offset weight line between leg and heel)

foot is the calcaneo-navicular (scaphoid) ligament (Figure 23), also called the spring ligament. It supports the medial mid-tarsal joint running from the sustentaculum tali on the inner side of the heel to the navicular (scaphoid) bone. It is a very heavy ligament that supports the head of the talus and is the main supporting ligament of the medial longitudinal arch. Underneath it runs the tendon of the tibialis posterior muscle which, in turn, supports the spring ligament. Lying across the foot is the transverse metatarsal arch. It is composed of a posterior arch at the posterior ends of the metatarsals and an anterior arch at the anterior ends of the metatarsals. There is a great deal of discussion in the literature about the anterior metatarsal arch. X-rays reveal that in a normal foot, in non-weight-bearing position, the first (big) toe and fifth (little) toe metatarsals are in one plane, and the second, third, and fourth metatarsals are on a higher plane, which forms a slight arch across the forefoot. Morton, however, proved that in the weight-bearing position the heads of all five metatarsal bones touch the ground.[9]

The bones of the foot are held together by ligaments, tendons of the extrinsic (calf) muscles, the intrinsic muscles of the foot, and the plantar aponeurosis on the sole of the foot.

Particular attention should be paid to the structural relationship of the calcaneus (os calcis) and the talus (astragalus) to the tibia bone of the lower leg (Figure 24).

In 1912, Osgood first called attention to the fact that the relationship of the foot structure to the leg and ankle structure is such that, uninfluenced by ligament support and muscle pulls, the normal line of weight bearing from the hips downward to the foot

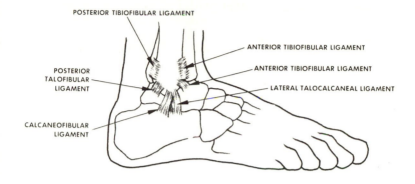

POSTERIOR TIBIOFIBULAR LIGAMENT

ANTERIOR TIBIOFIBULAR LIGAMENT

ANTERIOR TIBIOFIBULAR LIGAMENT

LATERAL TALOCALCANEAL LIGAMENT

POSTERIOR TALOFIBULAR LIGAMENT

CALCANEOFIBULAR LIGAMENT

*Figure 25*
LIGAMENTS INNER (MEDIAL) SIDE

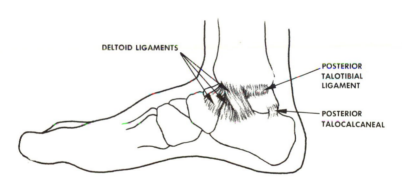

DELTOID LIGAMENTS

POSTERIOR TALOTIBIAL LIGAMENT

POSTERIOR TALOCALCANEAL

*Figure 26*
LIGAMENTS OUTER (LATERAL) SIDE

tends to fall to the inner side of the foot and to depress the medial longitudinal arch.[10]

Scholl commented on this in 1915, pointing out that in the true structural sense the heel lay to the outer side of the astragalus and there was a tendency of the heel towards insecurity and tilting inwards.[11]

Subsequently, in a series of comprehensive studies over a period of 10 years, Schwartz and Heath proved conclusively that in the normal foot there is a malalignment between the tibia (shinbone) and oscalcis (heel).[12] Their research showed that the axis of the weight-bearing line of the tibia passes through the middle of the

157

astragalus (talus). The axis of the weight-bearing line of the os calcis (heel) is displaced laterally from one to one and five-tenths centimeters (Figure 24). They concluded that the bones of the foot and lower leg present a relationship to each other which favors instability in the direction of pronation, which is the weakest position of the foot (Figure 33).

This explains why in the evolutionary process the powerful calcaneo-navicular spring ligament (Figure 23) and the even more powerful deltoid ligament (Figure 25) of the talo-tibial (ankle) joint have developed to counteract the tendency for the foot and ankle to tilt inward.

The important ligaments supporting the medial and the lateral sides of the ankle joint are illustrated in Figures 25 and 26. The ligaments on the medial side are much stronger than those on the lateral side of the joint.

Nature never intended ligaments alone to support and bind the bones together when they are subjected to long, continued stress or when the muscles controlling a joint—due to imbalance—pull the structure out of correct alignment. Malalignment puts a constant stress on ligaments, causing them eventually to stretch.

## DEFINITIONS

To understand the movements and actions of muscles and body joints covered in the next two sections, the reader should have some knowledge of the terminology used in describing these actions in the ankle-foot complex and particularly within the foot itself.

*Abduction* - Movement of the entire foot or forefoot away from midline of body (Figure 35).

*Adduction* - Movement of the entire forefoot towards midline of body (Figure 36).

*Dorsal or Superior* - Top of foot (Figure 20).

*Eversion* - A turning outward (Figure 33).

*Inversion* - A turning inward (Figure 33).

*Plantar* - Sole of foot (Figure 28).

*Pronation* - A turning downwards—eversion (Figure 34).

*Supination* - A turning upwards—inversion (Figure 34).

*Valgus* - Outer border of foot higher than inner border—eversion (Figure 37).

*Varus* - Inner border of foot higher than outer border—inversion (Figure 37).

The terms valgus or varus can apply to the entire foot, the rearfoot, or the forefoot.

Certain of these terms in relation to foot movement and position are interrelated in useage:

Inversion-adduction-supination-varus (Figure 34).

Eversion-abduction-pronation-valgus (Figure 34).

## ANATOMY OF THE FOOT AND ANKLE

The extrinsic (calf) muscle tendons support the ligaments and intrinsic muscles of the foot in the static position. Their balanced action keeps the foot, ankle, and leg in correct alignment.

With the exception of the gastrocnemius and soleus muscles of the calf that blend into the Achilles tendon, the other seven extrinsic (calf) muscle tendons cross the tibio-talar (ankle) joint (Figure 24), the sub-astragalar joint (Figure 22), and the mid-tarsal joints (Figure 21 and 22). They insert in the plantar (sole) or dorsal (top) aspects of the foot (Figures 28 and 29) ahead of the mid-tarsal joint None of them insert into the talus (Figure 20), which is the mechanical unit of the tarsus (mid-foot) bones. This shows the interdependence of all three joints in foot and ankle joint movements, as almost all the extrinsic (calf) muscles are operational through their tendons on the three joints.

It should be noted that the extrinsic (long) foot muscles provide joint motions in three planes. They are more efficient the greater the angle of the leg-foot axis and the distance between the origin and insertion of the muscle. They also have the ability to change their functions from those of invertors to those of evertors, and vice versa, according to the position of the foot. The peroneus longus muscle is a typical foot abductor. It may change its function and assist in adducting and pronating the forefoot. The dorsiflexors and plantar flexors of the foot can act as adductors or abductors, according to the varus or valgus position of the heel and midfoot.

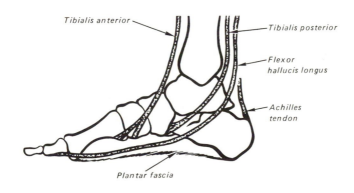

**Figure 27**

Three most important extrinsic muscle tendons supporting medial side of foot.

159

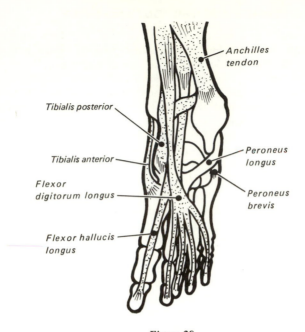

**Figure 28**
Plantar aspects of foot with insertion of intrinsic muscle tendons. Note peroneus longus that passes across sole and inserts into foot next to tibialis anterior.

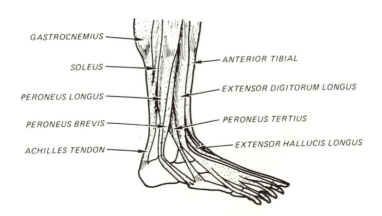

**Figure 29**
Muscles on lateral and anterior sides of ankle and foot.

## EXTRINSIC (CALF) MUSCLES AFFECTING
## FOOT MOVEMENTS AND BALANCE

*Dorsiflexion*—Prime Movers: tibialis anterior, extensor digitorum longus, peroneus tertius.

*Plantar Flexion*—Prime Movers: gastrocnemius and soleus.

*Inversion and Adduction*—Prime Movers: tibialis anterior and posterior, assisted by flexor digitorum longus and flexor hallucis longus.

*Eversion and Abduction*—Prime Movers: extensor digitorum longus, peroneus tertius, peroneus longus, peroneus brevis.

*Toe Flexion*—Prime Movers: big toe, flexor hallucis longus (four other toes), flexor digitorum longus.

*Toe Extension*—Prime Movers: big toe, extensor hallucis longus (four other toes), extensor digitorum longus.

### PLANTAR FLEXION

The gastrocnemius and soleus muscles, also called the triceps surae (Figure 30), through the Achilles tendon—their attachment to the heel—are the chief propelling force in locomotion. They provide 95 percent of the force in plantar flexion. The tibialis posterior, flexor hallucis longus, and flexor digitorum longus provide only 5 percent of the force in plantar flexion. The powerful action of the triceps surae when raising the heel off the ground tends to displace the front part of the heel downwards. This is counteracted by the intrinsic foot muscles and ligaments, assisted—if the foot is pointed straight ahead—by the flexor hallucis longus (Figure 30), tibialis posterior (Figure 30), and tibialis anterior (Figure 30).

If the Achilles tendon is shortened and the latter group of muscles and ligaments cannot counteract the pull, the added super-imposed body weight causes the navicular (scaphoid) and talus (astragalar) bones (Figure 21) to sink downwards and inwards, which stretches the spring ligament (Figure 23) and the short intrinsic plantar muscles in turn causing the medial longitudinal arch to flatten.

### DORSIFLEXION

Of the three muscles classed as prime movers for dorsiflexion of the foot, the anterior tibialis muscle (Figure 30) is the most powerful. Its strength capacity comprises 60 percent of the total work capacity of all dorsiflexor muscles. As noted in Figure 27, its tendon crosses the instep and is inserted into the foot at the base of the first metatarsal and the anterior side of the first cuneiform bone.

Its action, outside of dorsiflexion, in weight bearing is dependent on the position of the foot. If the foot is pointed straight ahead, and

161

# ANTERIOR — POSTERIOR LOWER LEG

## Anterior Lower Leg

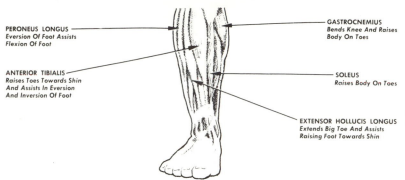

PERONEUS LONGUS
*Eversion Of Foot Assists*
*Flexion Of Foot*

ANTERIOR TIBIALIS
*Raises Toes Towards Shin*
*And Assists In Eversion*
*And Inversion Of Foot*

GASTROCNEMIUS
*Bends Knee And Raises*
*Body On Toes*

SOLEUS
*Raises Body On Toes*

EXTENSOR HOLLUCIS LONGUS
*Extends Big Toe And Assists*
*Raising Foot Towards Shin*

## Posterior Lower Leg

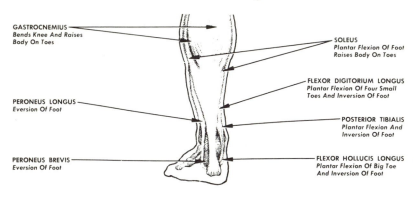

GASTROCNEMIUS
*Bends Knee And Raises*
*Body On Toes*

PERONEUS LONGUS
*Eversion Of Foot*

PERONEUS BREVIS
*Eversion Of Foot*

SOLEUS
*Plantar Flexion Of Foot*
*Raises Body On Toes*

FLEXOR DIGITORIUM LONGUS
*Plantar Flexion Of Four Small*
*Toes And Inversion Of Foot*

POSTERIOR TIBIALIS
*Plantar Flexion And*
*Inversion Of Foot*

FLEXOR HOLLUCIS LONGUS
*Plantar Flexion Of Big Toe*
*And Inversion Of Foot*

*Figure 30*

the invertor-adductor muscles are stronger, it assists them in inversion and adduction of the foot with a supination-varus posture of the foot. If the foot is pointed outwards and the evertor-abductor muscles are stronger, it assists them to increase the evertor-abductor action and the pronation (valgus) posture of the foot.

## INVERSION, ADDUCTION, SUPINATION, VARUS

The tibialis posterior muscle (and its tendon) is classed by most authorities as the major extrinsic supporting muscle of the medial

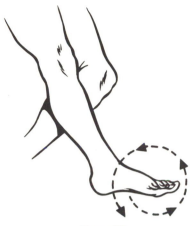

**Figure 31**
**Rotation**

longitudinal arch (Figure 27). It is also classed as the only prime mover muscle in adduction and inversion of the foot, although in that case it is assisted by the flexor hallucis longus (Figure 30) and flexor digitorum longus muscles. Its tendon is inserted into the base of the navicular (scaphoid) bone.

In contrast to this opinion, Bettman maintained that the flexor hallucis longus is the most powerful long muscle inserted into the bones of the foot.[1] He quoted Hoke, who classed this muscle as the medial longitudinal arch preserver.[4] Bettman stated that it supports the sustentaculum tali (Figure 24) bone on the inside of the heel, preventing the heel from going into eversion, and is the main support of the plantar flexors, adductors, and supinator muscles of the foot.

As can be seen in Figure 27, the tendon of the muscle is inserted into the foot at the base of the big toe. Its action in keeping the big

## MOVEMENTS OF ANKLE JOINT

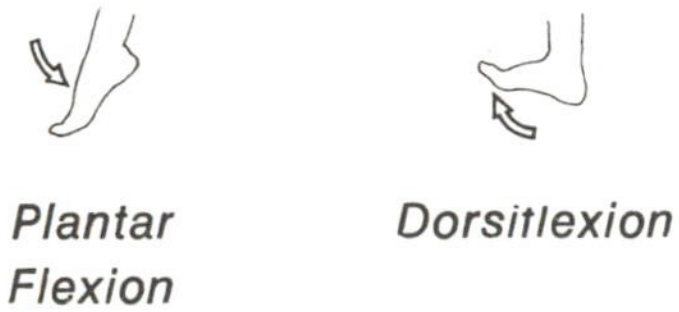

Plantar
Flexion

Dorsiflexion

**Figure 32**

163

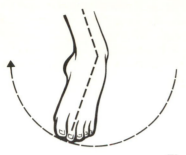
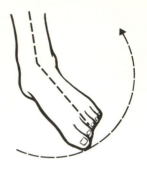

**Figure 33**

INVERSION                    EVERSION

toe on the ground makes it the major muscle of forward propulsion of the foot. However, this is true only when the foot is pointed straight ahead. Any deviation of the foot in an outward (abducted) position detracts from its efficiency in this respect.

The plantigrade (entire foot sole on ground) foot position is dependent to a great extent on the peroneus longus muscle (Figure 29), which is a prime abductor muscle of the foot. The muscle is situated on the outside of the calf. Its tendon winds around the external malleous of the fibula bone—down, under, and across the sole of the foot—inserting into the base of the first metatarsal and first cuneiform bones on the medial side of the foot next to the insertion of the anterior tibialis muscle, the prime mover in dorsiflexion of the foot.

The action of the peroneus longus muscle is to keep the inner side of the forefoot flat on the ground—but only if the foot is held in an inverted-adducted position by the tibialis posterior—and to depress the big toe. If it cannot do this, the forefoot goes into a varus (inner edge of forefoot off the ground) position as in Figure 37A. The peroneus longus muscle is assisted in depression of the big toe by the action of the abductor hallucis, an intrinsic (short) muscle of the foot.

Wiles maintained that the maintenance of the normal-arched foot and the plantigrade position of the foot depends largely on closely-balanced action of the tibialis posterior (invertor-adductor) and the peroneus longus.[14]

However, even though the foot may be in a corrective inverted-adducted position (pointed straight ahead), the peroneus longus cannot depress the big toe and the inner side of the forefoot unless the action of the anterior tibialis (dorsiflexor) is inhibited. The latter muscle dorsiflexes the big toe and raises the inner edge of the forefoot off the ground into a varus position.

In substantiation of his position, Wiles pointed out that the tibialis posterior and peroneus longus muscles are often classed as antagonist muscles, as the former is an invertor-adductor and the latter is an abductor-evertor muscle. He stated that in some cases they may be so; but for the most part, they must act as synergist (cooperative) muscles in maintaining the plantigrade position of the forefoot. He contended that the real functional antagonist to the posterior tibialis is the peroneus brevis (Figure 22), an abductor of the foot, and that the functional antagonist to the peroneus longus is the anterior tibialis.

## EVERSION, ABDUCTION, PRONATION, VALGUS

Tests by Fick,[3] Martin,[8] and Osgood[10] disclosed that the natural strength of the invertor-supinator adductor muscles is stronger than the abductor muscles—the peroneals (Figure 29).

However, the mechanical advantage of the peroneal muscles, to which is added the normal malalignment of the calcaneus-astragalus weight-bearing line—as shown by Schwartz and Heath[12]—and the effect of gravity and superimposed body weight which acts as a pronatory force offset the strength advantage of the invertor-supinator adductor muscles. If the invertor-supinator muscles weaken, the peroneals (evertor-pronators) will raise the outer border of the foot upwards into a valgus posture and depress the inner border of the foot into a position of pronation (Figures 34 and 35).

### INTRINSIC FOOT MUSCLES

There are three layers of short intrinsic foot muscles which help in adjustment of the posterior and anterior transverse arches. The normal foot becomes shorter and narrower on weight bearing, because the extrinsic (long) flexor muscles act as stirrups, or drawbridge arms, while the intrinsic (short) muscles by bowstring action stiffen the medial longitudinal arch against the thrust of gravity.

The intrinsic foot muscles serve as stabilizers for the arches of the foot and prevent the bones from spreading out. They are assisted in this binding effect by the peroneus longus muscle, whose tendon crosses the sole of the foot and inserts into the medial side of the first metatarsal (Figure 29). The short muscles also increase the flexor powers of the long foot muscles.

### LIGAMENTOUS OR MUSCULO-TENDINOUS SUPPORT OF THE ARCHES

The functions of the human foot are to provide support for the weight of the body (static weight bearing) and to provide a lever to raise the body and propel it into motion (dynamic propulsion in walking and running).

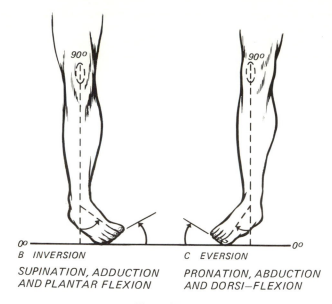

*Figure 34*
COMBINED MOVEMENTS OF FOOT

All medical and anatomical authorities have accepted the fact that the musculo-tendinous tissues of the foot and leg are the primary support of the arches and the balance of the foot during the dynamic phase of weight bearing. The ligaments play a secondary role in this function.

For the past century, however, a controversy among authorities has existed in the literature relating to the foot over the anatomy and structure of the foot as they pertain to the respective roles that muscles, tendons, and ligaments play in support of the arches during static weight bearing.

In 1935, Dudley Morton, an American anatomist, wrote: "Standing involves continuous static strain for periods of greater or lesser duration. This is the type of strain which ligamentous tissue is specifically designed to withstand."[9] His contention was that as far as the arch is concerned, static weight-bearing stance calls for ligamentous function only, while locomotion utilizes both ligamentous security and muscular protection and activity. Also, he maintained that the main function of the musculo-tendinous tissues of the leg and foot is to balance the body of the foot during static weight bearing. His primary supporter in this was British orthopedic specialist Norman Lake.[6]

Earlier, the opposing viewpoint had been set forth by Sir Robert Keith, British anatomist.[5] In 1928, he wrote:

Thirty years ago it was not uncommon to meet with surgeons who regarded "flat foot" as the collapse of a mechanical arch—one which depended on the shape of bones and the strength of supporting ligaments. I thought this conception, a vitally wrong one for men in practice, would die with the generation which held it, but in this I find myself mistaken. My young friend Dr. Dudley J. Morton holds that "the term balance as applied to the foot structure does not refer to muscle activity, but to the arrangement of the bones and ligaments which furnishes a stable base upon which body weight can be supported with the least demand for muscular exertion and propelled evenly balanced upon the lever axis."

A foot may be well-balanced or ill-balanced; but in either case, we cannot maintain the weight of our bodies poised on the soles of our feet unless every muscle of our legs and feet is in a state of reflex activity. Above all, we must reckon the two peroneal muscles and the two tibial muscles among the purely postural muscles, whose main activities are directed toward the safeguarding of the arch. With the maintenance of the normal arch, ligaments are not directly concerned. Nature never uses ligaments as prime supporters in the structure of the animal body; always, muscles are used for this purpose. Ligaments serve only as safeguards; they come into action only when the muscular defense has broken down.

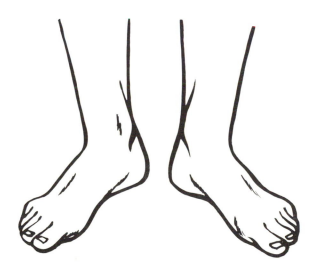

*Figure 35*
ABDUCTION DUE TO EXTERNAL LEG ROTATION

Keith cited many famous foot authorities to support his conclusion, but stressed one study in particular:[2]

...Of the proofs which have been furnished to demonstrate that the arches of the human foot are maintained by muscular action, none are so convincing or so complete as those provided by Dr. H. L. Dunn of the Medical Reserve Corps of the U.S. Army. He measured the height of the arch in the feet of soldiers under all conditions of health and load; he observed that the arch was maintained or gave way according to the state and strength of the postural muscles of the leg.

A review of later literature reveals that Keith's contention rather than Morton's is accepted by the majority of orthopedic specialists in America and Britain. In an article in *Military Surgeon*, Steindler, whose book *Kinesiology of the Human Body Under Normal and Pathological Conditions* is considered to be the classic in its field, wrote:

There are certain muscles which assist in the supporting of the arches. It is the elasticity of these muscles which first takes up the burden of the strain. Only after the muscles give way the strain comes directly on the ligaments and when they, too, give way, the arches yield and deformity begins. The anterior arch of the foot is supported by the muscles which balance the toes. Any factor which will prevent the free play of the toes, anything which will cramp the toes and force the toes back will reduce relaxation of this arch with a strain of all the ligaments which normally support it. This one consideration teaches two things. First, that in order to break through the line of defense which a normal foot displays against disability, the muscles must first be put out of commission. Second, when they are unable to do their work the ligaments next must be strained to the point of yielding. Only then the actual deformity takes place.[13]

Lewin commented:

Ligaments are not directly concerned with the maintenance of the normal arch. Nature never uses ligaments as prime supporters in the structures of the animal body; muscles are always used for this purpose. Ligaments serve only as safeguards; they come into action only when the muscular defense has broken down.[7]

Keith's conclusions are also shared by Osgood, Bettman, Wilson, Wiles, Bankart, and many others.

### JOINT MOVEMENTS OF FOOT AND ANKLE

There are three principal axes of movements in the ankle and foot. They are the tibio-talar (ankle) joint (Figure 24), the sub-talar (astragalus) joint (Figure 22), and the mid-tarsal (medial and lateral) joints (Figures 21 and 22).

The shape of the foot joints (1) enables the bones of the foot to be held in the desired position within a minimum of muscular effort,

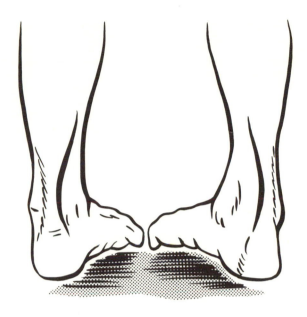

**Figure 36**
ADDUCTION DUE TO INTERNAL LEG ROTATION

and (2) gives the foot resistance to absorb the enormous stresses to which it is subjected. Movements of the ankle and foot occur both in the non-weight-bearing position and in the weight-bearing stance.

## TIBIO-TALAR (ANKLE) JOINT

In a non-weight-bearing position, the talus bone of the foot, which joins the tibia, works as a unit with the tibia due to the fact that the talus is held in a tight mortise between the internal and external malleous (Figure 24). When the foot moves against the leg in the non-weight-bearing position, it is a combination of tibio-talar (ankle) joint and sub-talar (astragalus) joint motion which curves the foot around the leg in a circling movement (Figure 31). This movement combines adduction, supination, and inversion with plantar flexion (Figure 34) and abduction, pronation, and eversion with dorsiflexion (Figure 34).

In the weight-bearing position, the talus acts as a bone of the foot. The tibio-talar (ankle) joint has freedom of motion in one plane only—plantar flexion and dorsiflexion (Figure 32).

With the patella of the knee facing straight ahead, the axis of the ankle joint runs obliquely from outward and backward to forward and inward, which corresponds to the normal outward rotation of the lower end of the tibia. Due to this normal outward tibial torsion, the foot at the ankle joint is normally rotated outwards in relation to the knee joint. Because of this obliquity in the ankle joint axis in an upright standing position, the foot moves in the ankle joint upward and medially in dorsiflexion and downward and laterally in plantar flexion.

## SUB-TALAR (ASTRAGALUS) AND MID-TARSAL JOINTS

In the weight-bearing stance, movements of the foot occur simultaneously in the sub-talar joint (Figure 22) and the medial mid-tarsal joint (Figure 21).

The sub-talar joint normally has one degree of freedom of motion in the weight-bearing position about an axis which runs obliquely from outward, backward, and downward to inward, forward, and upward. The outward movement involves inversion, supination, adduction, and plantar flexion (Figure 34). The inward movement involves everson, pronation, abduction, and dorsiflexion (Figure 34).

There is little movement possible in the calcaneo-cuboid mid-tarsal joint (Figure 22) on the lateral side of the foot. In contrast, the talus-scaphoid (navicular) joint (Figure 21) on the medial side is a ball and socket joint that permits a wide range of rotatory and gliding movements.

The importance of the medial tarsal joints lies in their ability to take care of compensatory movements in the foot. They enable the forefoot to hold firmly to the ground in a plantigrade position even though the back part of the foot is in an eversion-pronation position or an inversion-supination position (Figure 34). They also permit a slight abduction and adduction in the forefoot while the rear foot remains in vertical alignment. This permits a slight rotation to an inversion (varus) position (Figure 37B) or an eversion (valgus) position (Figure 37A) in the forefoot.

All foot joints ahead of the mid-tarsal joints permit only a very slight movement. However, the joints between the scaphoid (navicular), first cuneiform, and first mid-tarsal bones on the medial side of the foot (Figure 21) do allow a fair amount of rotary movement in the sagittal plane (flexion and extension of big toe).

Abduction (Figure 35) or adduction (Figure 36) of the entire normal foot is the result of rotation of the legs at the knee joint or hip joints or due to tibial torsion.

## CRITERIA OF NORMAL AND STRONG FEET

Before considering the more common types of faults and defects found among runners, hurdlers, and joggers, we should consider the established criteria for normal strong feet:

1. A normal weight-bearing line, with the heel centrally located

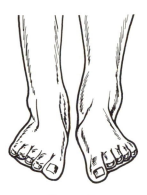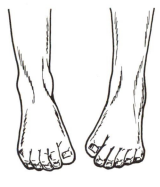

Figure 37A
VALGUS
(Pronation of Forefoot)

Figure 37B
VARUS
(Supination of Forefoot)

under the leg.

2. A normal range of active motion at the ankle joint and in the posterior tarsal joints of the foot; straight and flexible toes with no tissue contractures.

3. Bones of the foot bound together by strong ligamentous bands and properly placed and well-articulated with one another.

4. Good muscle tone and balanced muscle strength of the extrinsic leg muscles whose tendons insert into the bones of the foot to support the medial longitudinal arch and properly balance the leg on the foot.

5. Strong ligamentous and fascial bindings and well-developed small intrinsic muscles to maintain the bones and toes in straight alignment and to support the so-called anterior metatarsal arch.

6. Proper heel-toe motion in walking and running and maintenance of the foot in a relatively straight ahead position.

7. Absence of any pain or tiredness in the feet.

To meet these criteria, the foot and lower leg must be in proper balance. Foot balance is dependent on two factors, i.e., structural and postural stability.

*Structural stability* is dependent on the proper arrangement of the bones and the ligaments that bind them together, assisted by the intrinsic plantar muscles and the tendons of the lower leg muscles inserted into the bones of the foot.

*Postural stability* is dependent on the tone and strength of the extrinsic leg muscles and their tendons which cross the ankle joint and insert into the bones of the foot to maintain the balanced posture of the leg on the foot, as well as the tone and strength of the intrinsic plantar muscles.

The above two factors are interdependent. Any loss of structural stability affects postural stability, and any loss of postural stability

171

affects the position of the lower leg on the foot and results in an unequal distribution of weight stresses over the foot.

REFERENCES

1. Bettman, Ernst H., "The Human Foot," *Archives of Physical Therapy,* January 1944.
2. Dunn, H. L., "The Statistics of the Human Arch When Subjected to Body Weight," *Military Surgeon,* June 1933.
3. Fick, R., "Anatomie und Mechanik der Gelenke," Teil III, *Spezielle Gelenk und Muskelmechanik,* Fischer, Jena, 1911.
4. Hoke, M., "An Operation for the Correction of Extremely Relaxed Flat Feet," *Journal of Bone and Joint Surgery,* 13, 773, 1931.
5. Keith, Sir Arthur, "The History of the Human Foot and Its Bearing on Orthopedic Practice," *Journal of Bone and Joint Surgery,* 2, 1928.
6. Lake, Norman C., *The Foot* (London: Bailliere, Tindall and Cox, 1952).
7. Lewin, Phillip, *The Foot and Ankle* (Philadelphia: Lea and Febiger, 1959).
8. Martin, E. G., "Tests of Muscular Efficiency," *Physiological Review,* Vol. 1, 1923.
9. Morton, Dudley J., *The Human Foot* (New York: Columbia University Press, 1935).
10. Osgood, Robert B., "Pathologic and Symptomatic Weight Bearing: A Consideration of the Prevention and Cure of Foot Strain," *American Journal of Orthopedic Surgery,* February 1912.
11. Scholl, William M., *The Human Foot* (Chicago: Foot Specialist Publishing Co., 1915).
12. Schwartz, R. Plato and Heath, Arthur L., "Some Factors Which Influence the Balance of the Foot in Walking," *Journal of Bone and Joint Surgery,* April 1933.
13. Steindler, Arthur, "Anatomical and Physiological Conditions of the Feet," *Military Surgeon,* Vol. 86, 1940.
14. Wiles, Phillip, "Flat Feet," *Lancet,* November 17, 1934.

# 18

## Foot Faults and Defects

After reviewing statistics on foot problems compiled by numerous researchers, in addition to his own findings, Dudley Morton commented that, with the sole exception of tooth decay, foot disorders are the most common form of physical impairment among civilized peoples.[18] Kuhns stated that disturbances in the function of the foot are among the most frequent and most disabling of all ills that befall civilized man.[14] Eighty percent of all adult persons are said to suffer from some form of foot disorder.[4] Fifty-eight percent of growing children have been found to suffer from weakness or other disability of the feet.[3]

A massive study of 20,000 children up to 12 years of age by podiatrists in the Washington, D.C. area between 1968 and 1970 disclosed that 37 percent of the children had orthopedic foot disorders and 16 percent displayed gait problems resulting from foot disorders.[23] This project was sponsored by the U.S. Public Health Service, and was the first study of a large group of young children conducted in the United States since the famous Chelsea Study of 50 years ago. It is important for two reasons: (1) It is well-established that most hidden faults and defects of the feet in young children rarely cause pain or discomfort. (2) Unless there are obvious visual abnormalities, foot problems during the early years of life rarely reach the offices of podiatrists or orthopedic specialists.

When the above statistics are combined with the tremendous stresses imposed by modern training methods, it is easily understandable why there is a constant increase in overuse syndrome injuries affecting the feet and lower extremities of athletes in all sports, but particularly in middle and longer distance runners. The figures also add tremendous weight to Cerney's statement that 80 percent of American athletes display symptoms of weak feet.

Though not subjected to the training stresses imposed on competitive runners, physical fitness joggers—after years of inactivity sitting at desks and riding in automobiles—have allowed the muscles, tendons, and ligaments of their feet to deteriorate. To a lesser degree, they are faced with the same problems as the younger competitive runners.

Before we proceed further in this discussion, a clarification of terms used in describing structural (bone) and musculotendinous problems of the foot and ankle is in order. In the literature, they are many times used interchangeably to describe the same conditon.

## DEFINITIONS

*Fault* - A malposition or incorrect alignment of the foot that subjects the foot or ankle to abnormal weight-bearing stress. The fault has not affected the structural alignment of the foot bones. It can be corrected by the voluntary action or will of the person through posture training, exercise, and—where required—assistance with orthotic appliances.

*Anomaly or Architectural Defect* - A marked deviation, imperfection, or absence from the normal standards of alignment of the foot structure. A fault becomes a defect when it finally affects the structure of the foot. A defect cannot be corrected by the will or voluntary effort of the person.

*Deformity* - A visible distortion or general disfiguration of the foot, involving both the bony and musculo-tendinous-ligamentous structures of the foot.

## PREDISPOSING FACTORS

Numerous causes of foot faults, weak feet, and foot disabilities have been advanced by orthopedic specialists in foot disorders and chiropodists, now known as podiatrists, over the past 150 years. Those causes that could not under any circumstances have been prevented by the person affected will not be considered here. They include disabilities or deformities resulting from inheritance, disease, or congenital causes—such as improper development during intra-uterine life.

The remaining causes can be divided into two basic categories: (1) Those that may or may not be within the control of the person affected. Parents, teachers, pediatricians, and general medicine specialists also play a large part in prevention and correction of these. (2) Those that can be classed as "hidden factors." The prospective athlete or jogger is completely unaware of their presence and, with a few exceptions, writers of athletic injury texts, team physicians, coaches, and trainers are completely unaware of their widespread existence among the general population. Where they do possess such knowledge, they attribute little or no importance to them as predisposing causes of foot problems.

The emphasis in this text is being placed on the "hidden factors," and the first category listed above is discussed only in passing. The causes included therein have been adequately covered by numerous texts and in a multiplicity of articles. The most universally accepted one is poorly fitting or poorly constructed shoes. Among others are physical weakness and fatigue in childhood; disease requiring prolonged periods of bed rest or inactivity; long-term or sudden obesity; malnutrition; walking on hard surfaces with bare feet; occupational standing in relatively static positions for long periods of time; wearing high-heeled shoes; poor sitting and sleeping habits during infancy and early childhood; long continued crossing of legs, crouching, squatting, or kneeling; and slender (gracile) small-boned feet.

*N.B.:*

> In any consideration of athletic injuries, two potential complicating factors should be kept in mind. One is the tendency of athletes who incur minor strains or sprains to work or run off the injury or to change their walking or running gait to avoid pain. In either case, the continued activity leads to far more serious problems. Another is the possibility that the athlete may disregard the advice of the trainer or attending doctor and fail to engage in the proper rehabilitation prior to returning to training or competition.

Among the more basic predisposing causes classed as "hidden factors" are muscle imbalance, antereo-posterior posture and lateral pelvic tilt, short leg, leg rotation, faulty leg alignment, tibial torsion, outward foot rotation in walking or running, and architectural anomalies or defects of the foot or lower leg.

## MUSCLE IMBALANCE

In 1855, during his classic investigations of muscle function, Duchenne reached the conclusion that faulty weight bearing and foot strain were more commonly caused by a faulty balance between the group of muscles that inverted the foot and elevated the arches, and the group whose contraction tended to evert the foot and depress the arches.[7] Bick, in his *Source Book of Orthopedics*,[2] credits Delpich,[6] who at that time was the dean of French orthopedic surgery, with making a similar observation. Thus the myogenetic (muscle) etiology of static foot deformity dominated the thinking of French students of the late 19th and early 20th centuries.

In 1908, Osgood and his associates conducted tests on 123 pair of feet, using a *chatillon* spring balance measuring device.[20] He noted that the study was motivated by the belief that lack of muscle balance was of great importance in the development of foot strain and that the establishment of a proper balance was a great factor in the cure of weak feet.

Osgood classified the 123 pair of feet into four groupings:

*Normal* - feet practically free from pronation and with no evidence of objective or subjective foot weakness.

*Symptomless Pronated*- feet which, while manifesting no symptoms or only those of vague tiredness, showed faulty weight-bearing lines and seemed to have the potential for trouble.

*Weak or Strained* - flexible but markedly pronated feet, showing definitive symptoms of tiredness and foot discomfort.

*Acute Flat Feet* - fairly flexible feet, showing signs of acute strain, swollen, congested, tender, and very painful.

Osgood's testing reflected the average ratio of strength as follows:

*Normal* - (22): adductors 10, abductors 8.2.

*Symptomless Pronated* - (23): adductors 10, abductors 10.5.

*Weak or Strained* - (46): adductors 10, abductors 10.8.

*Acute Flat* - (32): adductors 10, abductors 12.2.

From this study he concluded that in the normal foot the adductor group is composed of muscles having a stronger combined pull than the abductor group. This latter group, however, favored as it is in the position of weight bearing by the planes of the joint surfaces, may—because it over-balances the adductor group—become comparitively the stronger and favor foot strain. Conversely, he concluded that the weaker the adductors, the more likely the foot structures are to be strained, and—other things being equal—the more severe the subjective symptoms will probably be.

Antereo-Posterior Posture and Lateral Pelvic Tilt

In 1934, Wiles coined a new phrase, "postural pes valgus," to describe the loss of the medial longitudinal arch due to a complicated rotation in which the forefoot is everted, pronated, and abducted, as distinguished from the term "functional flat foot," generally used to describe the majority of non-congenital flat feet.[31] He maintained the condition began early in life due to weak anti-gravity muscles and poor postural habits (see Chapter 9, Figure 7).

Wiles went on to state:

...general bodily posture can also have a direct influence on the posture of the feet. The person with lumbar lordosis and forward tilting of the pelvis is a good example. Here the center of gravity of the body is carried slightly forward in front of the acetabula (hip sockets) and stabilization is obtained by internally rotating the femora (thigh bones). This in turn causes in-toeing which may be corrected either by external rotation of the knee or by eversion (pronation) and abduction of the feet. The former is not comfortable as a permanent posture, so the latter, or valgus foot, position is assumed. This shows the danger of trying to force a child who in-toes to turn out his feet. There may be a perfectly good postural reason for the in-toeing and the two defects must be corrected together.

Subsequently, in a series of articles describing the same condition, Graham used the term "weak foot."[8] He maintained that the weak foot was the earliest anatomical abnormality in a commonly recurring syndrome of foot malposture that produced a whole series of clinical symptoms. He named the total syndrome "sub-talar dystrochoides," which described the numerous progressive changes in the bones, muscles, tendons, and ligaments of the foot whose starting point was poor antereo-posterior body posture.

Atkins described the effects of lateral pelvic tilt, whatever its cause, on the posture of the foot (see Chapter 12, Figure 9).[1] He pointed out that with a lateral tilt there is a relative degree of adduction (internal rotation) of the thigh on the side of the high ilium (see Chapter 9, Figure 3B), and a relative abduction (external rotation) of the thigh on the lower side of the pelvic tilt. The abducted thigh on the lower side forces that leg and knee into extension and the opposite leg on the high side into flexion.

Commenting further, he stated:

> Incident to these changes in the thigh arrangement there are evidences other than those mentioned at the knee. They are seen in comparing the two legs. The relatively abducted one is seen in some external rotation, that is, the foot "toes out" more than the other. The ankle is less freely movable than its opposite. History reveals that the more freely movable one turns easily. A similar comparative finding will be seen in the feet. The abducted one shows a lightened and tender plantar fascia, restricted joint movements, callouses, and corns; whereas its opposite evidences less severe symptoms of failure. The distortions of weight bearing outlined should be coupled with the normal predisposition to foot failure seen in the bony arrangements in the ankle.

Referring to an article by Schwartz and Heath,[23] he continued:

> Such a predisposition is seen in the medial offset of the midline of the tibia in relation to that of the talus (Schwartz and Heath). Together, these factors produce—or tend to produce—pronation of the ankle and consequent malalignment of the talo-calcaneal arrangement.

### SHORT LEG

Whether a short leg is due to a lateral pelvic tilt, muscle imbalance in the hips, arrested structural development, unilateral knock-knee, or flat foot, the entire short leg will almost always rotate outwards in an abducted (toed-outwards) foot position. Klein, whose studies on the effect of lateral asymmetry as a predisposing factor in knee injuries are monumental, did extensive work on the short leg syndrome.[13] He commented:

> ...in observing gait patterns of people with lateral asymmetry, abnormalities may be noted in the movement of the leg, ankle, and foot. Common observations are the "toeing outward" of the foot on the short leg side, an ankle pronation as the foot is place on the ground, as well as a valgus knee position as the leg is carried forward. On the opposite side, the knee and the foot will be carried straight forward toward the foot's contact with the ground. These observations will be fairly consistent.

> It may be surmised there is a neurological basis for this action in that, as the short leg swings forward, the toe will automatically point outward to balance the abnormal lateral sway of the body when the foot is shifted to the short leg side. A slight foot supination, ankle pronation, and valgus knee commonly accompany this body action.

## LEG ROTATION

In 1908, Lowman began a study, which contained over a period of 12 years, on the effects of leg rotation on malposture of the foot. His first paper, published in 1912, summarized the results of his initial four-year study of 300 patients—50 percent of them under the age of 18—suffering from valgus-pronated foot postures.[17] Lowman stated that his study was based on the problem of postural strains and muscle balance which a number of authorities had been pointing to at that period of time. He pointed out that the common condition of valgus at the ankle spoken of as "pronation," "knock-ankle," "in-ankle," etc. (excluding congenital causes or disease), is caused most frequently by bad statics or paralysis; but he studied only the former cause as it related to postural strain and muscle balance.

Lowman first looked into the effects of orthotic appliances (arch supports) on the position of the foot, especially in those with pronated feet. Many of the patients would obtain relief of their symptoms for a time, but the valgus-pronated posture of the foot was not corrected.

Next he studied the effects of treatment by foot and leg exercises. Here he found that after persistent and careful work the muscles would be in good tone, pain would be less, cramps in the feet eased, etc., but the valgus-pronated foot position persisted, although in some cases it was considerably modified.

Finally he studied the occurrence of pain, cramps, tired feeling, etc., in the back, hips, legs, and pains in the knee of which so many of his patients complained. Treatment of these patients with orthotic appliances and foot and leg exercises left only a few relieved of these symptoms.

Lowman also found that among the 300 patients observed, nearly everyone showed a condition of inward rotation of the leg. This deviation from normal weight-bearing line of the leg caused this line to fall on the medial side of the foot. This condition of exaggerated internal rotation was more pronounced in those cases that walked in a "weak-footed" or "toed-out" position.

His work reflected that in each of the 300 persons who were given an external leg rotation exercise to correct internal leg rotation, along with the assistance of orthotic appliances and foot exercises, the valgus position of the feet was eventually eliminated and so were related pains and cramps in the feet, legs, hips, and low back.

## FAULTY LEG ALIGNMENT

Caldwell and his associates showed that almost every normal child passes through a physiological cycle in regard to alignment of the lower extremities:[5]

1. Child is born with moderate bowlegs.
2. On standing or walking, he assumes a wide base for balance with feet toed outwards.
3. This is usually corrected by development of a knock-knee deviation, although thigh and tibia bowing may still be present.
4. Child then toes inward as he walks, in an attempt to correct the knock-knees, and the thigh rotates internally at the hips, with the lateral side of the knee facing more to the front.
5. With the internally rotated leg fixed firmly on the ground, as child takes each step forward, the forward thrust of weight through the knees tends to straighten out the knock-knees. Also, the inner border of the foot is raised by toeing-in, and the medial longitudinal arch is developed and formed.
6. In the normal cycle, after the knock-knees are corrected and the arch is formed, child tends to toe straight ahead or slightly outwards.

This cycle can be broken by obesity, malnourishment, congenital anomalies, structural defects in the feet or legs, and internal or external rotator muscle contracture at the hips. It has been well established that either obesity or malnutrition is a predisposing cause of postural deviations, and that congenital anomalies and structural defects are beyond the control of the person so affected. This discussion will therefore concern itself with rotator muscle contracture, which is directly related to Lowman's findings on leg rotation.

External rotator contracture of the hip, with exaggerated external rotation of the leg, is relatively rare except in those children who when they first stand rotate their feet and legs in a widely toed-out position to maintain balance and then fail to toe in as they go through the knock-knee cycle.

Internal rotator contracture of the hip and internal rotation of the leg may develop in children whose tendency to toe inward exceeds the normal. There is a greater tendency, however, for children who may not excessively turn their feet inward during their developmental growth stage to develop a permanent internal rotation of the entire leg due to factors discussed earlier.

As Wiles pointed out, some children displaying excessive inward toeing will toe their feet outwards to compensate for the toeing in. This can lead to the development of the comparatively rare external tibial torsion and also holds the knees in the knock-kneed position.

If the legs remain in internal rotation during the growth stage, with the feet abducted outwards, the weight line will drop to the medial side of the foot—leading to a pronated valgus foot and ankle.

If development is arrested in the bowlegged position, the child may develop an internal tibial torsion and hyperextended knees.

## TIBIAL TORSION

Internal tibial torsion directly affects the talus in its relationship to the heel and mid-tarsal bones. It rotates the talus downward and inwards and is the beginning point for eventual pronation-valgus position of the feet.

## OUTWARD FOOT ROTATION IN WALKING AND RUNNING

Beginning in 1887, Royal Whitman undertook concentrated studies of flat feet in human beings.[30] He presented many papers on this subject before medical groups. As orthopedic historian Bick has pointed out, his writings on the subject, later incorporated into his textbook on orthopedic surgery, still remain among the finest of their kind.

Whitman's main contribution to the field of orthopedic foot disability lay in distinguishing between (1) the true flat foot of congenital origin, which is generally rare in human beings and an hereditary anomaly that rarely if ever produces symptoms of pain and disability; and (2) pseudo-flat foot (which he named "weak foot"), in which the foot is initially everted and painful but still flexible, and later becomes a more or less rigid acquired functional flat foot.

In 1907, he summarized his 20-year study, the results of which supported his hypothesis as to the major causes of weak foot that advanced to acquired functional flat foot:

From this standpoint, the popular term flat foot is so misleading and inadequate that it has been discarded for one that calls attention primarily to impaired ability, rather than to deformity, which is in most cases, the result of disordered function. To illustrate, one recognizes two contrasting postures of the foot, that of activity and that of inactivity. The first is exemplified by the runner, in whom the foot points directly forward so that a line projected from the center of the limb would fall over the second toe. In this attitude the weight is balanced on the center of the foot by muscular effort. The contrasting posture is that in which the individual stands at ease, the foot serving as a support, the muscles inactive, and the strain falling upon the ligaments.

Whitman commented that it would be impossible to enumerate all the factors near and remote that may predispose to the weak foot, or hasten the progression of deformity. He listed as one of the major classes of predisposing factors "improper attitudes that subject the foot to mechanical disadvantage in the performance of its function," and went on to state:

...the most common of these is outward rotation of the limbs in walking. Outward rotation of limbs, "toeing-out," must not be confounded, as it usually is, with abduction or eversion of the feet which characterize all grades of deformity. In the first, the hip joints are concerned; in the second, the medio-tarsal and sub-astragaloid joints. Outward rotation of the limbs is the attitude peculiar to civilized people...(and also)...by placing the feet at a mechanical disadvantage, by checking alternation of posture, and thus by disuse weakening the muscles is one of the most important of the predisposing causes of the weak foot.

It should be noted that at the time he wrote, the military posture of extremely toed-out feet was an outgrowth of a general posture developed by the German Army of the 19th century, one that dominated both military and physical education authorities' concept of good posture for many years.

In summarizing his descriptive sketch of this disability, Whitman stated:

Habitual outward rotation of the feet combined with slight abduction is characteristic of the predisposing or early stage of weak foot, while marked abduction, with outward, and with even inward rotation of the limbs, characterizes advanced deformity, the apparent degree of out-toeing being the same in each instance. The statement may be made that all weak feet, in the sense in which the term is used here, are abducted feet. All flat feet are abducted feet, but all abducted feet are not flat feet.

Whitman's findings were substantiated 40 years later by Hartley in his study of flat feet among soldiers in the United States Army.[10] In commenting on the effect of the position of the foot in standing and walking on the longitudinal arches, Hartley stated:

The position of attention requires the heels to be placed together with a 45-degree angle between the feet. This means that each hip joint must be externally rotated almost 22.5 degrees. In this position a great deal of strain is placed on the longitudinal arches. Ideally, this position should be held only for short periods. Since the command, "Forward March!" is always given from the position of attention and the soldier is required to step off in cadense, the tendency of troops is to walk with the lower extremities in external rotation. This gets to be a habit which is projected into ordinary walking and commonly observed among trained soldiers.

In a series of photographs to prove his conclusions, Hartley found the effects of bad mechanics (toeing outwards) on the arch could be so severe that a normal foot could be made to resemble a case of pes planus (flat foot) simply by a change of weight bearing position. He concluded: "The photographs serve to support the thesis that incorrect walking on a normal foot can actually produce a flat foot and that correct walking (toeing straight ahead) in a case of pes planus can cause the foot to more closely resemble the normal."

The advice usually given to runners with respect to running efficiency and injury prevention has been to run with the feet pointing straight ahead. An interesting cinematographical study of runners was recently conducted by the biomechanics laboratory of Dalhouise University in Canada.[12] Nine trained runners—three sprinters, three middle distance, and three distance runners—together with four untrained runners served as subjects for the study. Of three factors analyzed, one—the angle of abduction (toeing out) and adduction (toeing in) of the foot at the instant of first contact—pertains to this discussion. The results of that analysis were as follows:

A toed-out or abducted position of the foot was predominant throughout the study in most of the subjects. Greater abduction

## THE POSITION OF THE FEET IN WALKING

CORRECT POSITION    INCORRECT POSITIONS

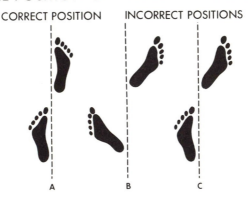

A                B                C

*Figure 38*
**Correct and incorrect angle of foot position in walking and running.**

182

occurred in the untrained runners and decreased progressively from the distance runners through to the sprinters. Generally, the trained runners had less than 10 degrees of abduction at all speeds, with sprinters and middle distance groups having less than 5 degrees abduction. There was a tendency toward asymmetry in all subjects on this variable. The right foot generally exhibited more abduction than the left.

Travers, writing about injury due to faulty style, commented that any deviation from correct style will upset the balance of muscle action and will therefore predispose to injury.[28] Among the deviations listed were two that applied to runners: splay foot (toeing out) gait and scissor gait (similar to the splay foot gait in its mechanics).

## ANOMALIES OR DEFECTS OF FOOT AND LOWER LEG

It was pointed out in the previous chapter that good foot posture and foot balance were dependent on structural and postural stability. Any factor which decreases structural stability will make postural stability more difficult to maintain. It will increase the work required of the foot and leg muscles and subject the foot to chronic strain, creating a predisposition toward eventual structural breakdown of the foot.

Defective architecture due to anomalies or defects in bones of the foot or lower leg is a major factor in decreasing structural stability. This may be due to hereditary, congenital, or developmental causes. Among such anomalies or defects are the following: hypermobility of the first metatarsal; shortness of the first metatarsal; posteriorly located sesamoid bones; metatarsal varus primus; accessory scaphoid or prehallux; faulty development of the calcaneus (heel) or talus (astragalus); obliquity of ankle joints; and pes cavus (hollow or claw foot).

Dudley Morton should be given the credit for emphasizing the first three defects mentioned in the preceding paragraph. From his intensive research and testing, Morton proved that in weight bearing the five metatarsal bones of the forefoot all bear weight, instead of the first and fifth only, as previously claimed by other authorities. On this basis, he maintained that the forefoot is the prime factor in a balanced posture of the foot.[18] Of the five metatarsals, the first has been shown by his research to be of the greatest functional importance in locomotion, bearing twice as much weight as any of the other four.

1. *Dorsal Hypermobility of the First Metatarsal Segment:* Dorsal hypermobility of this type is due to relaxation of the ligaments binding the first metatarsal with its digit and the medial cuneiform bone (see Figure 40). This allows an unusual amount of mobility in

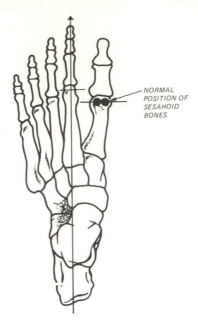

*Figure 39*
MORTON'S TOE

the joints between the scaphoid and the medial and middle cuneiform bones. When the heads of the other metatarsals, which are not relaxed, come in contact with the bearing surface, the first metatarsal continues to flex dorsally due to its mobility. This causes the foot to roll inward and pronate, which causes the ligaments on the medial side of the foot to become strained and stretched.

Morton identified three degrees of pronation: first, second, and third. In *first degree pronation,* hypermobility is slight, ground contact is quickly gained, and movement is arrested. *Second degree pronation* is the stage when the vertical weight line has moved to the medial side of the foot until the line projects forward through the head of the first metatarsal. According to Morton, the medial margin of structural stability is now eliminated, and only the muscles and the ligaments on the inner side of the ankle and foot remain on the inner side of the ankle. The pronated posture of the feet now begins to alter the position of the joint surface beneath the talus, depressing its inner margin (see Chapter 17, Figure 37A). *Third degree pronation* presents two distinct types, i.e., the rigid and the flexible flat foot. Morton contended that rigid flat foot results from progressive degrees of pronation over a period of time, while flexible flat foot is traceable to an unusual degree of ligament laxity in early childhood.

In *Human Locomotion and Body Form,*[19] Morton and Fuller wrote:

Statistics from various surveys indicate that hardly more than 10 percent of feet have perfect posture. A mild amount of pronation (first degree) is found in about 45 percent of feet and may be regarded as within the normal range of variation insofar as posture and functional performance is concerned. It is as common among athletes and sprinters as in other groups. Greater fault in posture (second degree pronation) covers another large group of about 40 percent, with the remaining 5 percent accounting for severely pronated feet and other serious deformities.

In an earlier work, Morton had pointed out that the progressive course of longitudinal arch disorder clearly stamped second degree pronation as the critical stage in progressive breakdown of foot structure.[18]

2. *Shortness of the First Metatarsal Bone:* Morton saw a short metatarsal as impairing the effectiveness of the first metatarsal segment chiefly in locomotion, because the more advanced position of the head of the second metatarsal causes the latter to act alone as the fulcrum of the foot's leverage.[18] The second metatarsal bone, because of the concentration of weight stresses, hypertrophies and becomes thicker and more robust (see Figure 40). Also, the foot must roll inward in order that the head of the first metatarsal may come in contact with the weight-bearing surface. This results in a greater or lesser degree of pronation of the foot, depending upon the amount of shortness of the first metatarsal.

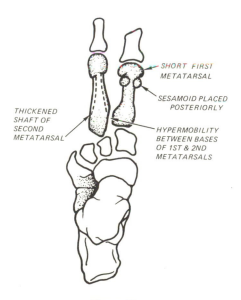

THICKENED SHAFT OF SECOND METATARSAL

SHORT FIRST METATARSAL

SESAMOID PLACED POSTERIORLY

HYPERMOBILITY BETWEEN BASES OF 1ST & 2ND METATARSALS

**Figure 40**
**Morton's Syndrome**

185

Up until recently, it was often maintained that 50 percent of the population displayed evidences of a short first metatarsal, sometimes to the extent of one centimeter. George Sheehan, however, in a 1974 article in *Runner's World*,[25] noted the finding of Dr. Richard Schuster, a New York podiatrist, that 80 percent of 1,000 patients demonstrated evidences of a short first metatarsal.[22]

Morton claimed that the short first metatarsal is hereditary in nature, and most authorities tend to agree with him. However, it is interesting to note the viewpoint of Doctor John Hiss, a prominent orthopedic foot specialist in the 1930's, who believed otherwise.[11] Hiss maintained that a short first metatarsal is a compensatory developmental anomaly resulting from eversion and abduction of the feet during developmental growth, and also that the amount of shortening correlates closely with the degree of eversion and abduction. He commented that even if it were a congenital deformity, the slowness of bone growth during development would give the feet sufficient time to adapt to the condition and thereby develop sufficient function for human activity.

The famous law of Julius Wolff, formulated in 1892, that living bone adapts its structure to changes in mechanical load lends weight to Hiss's opinion. The modern version of this law is: "The form of the bone being given, the bone elements place or displace themselves in the direction of the functional pressure and increase or decrease their mass to reflect the amount of functional pressure."

It is well-known that an everted-abducted foot makes the first metatarsal relatively inoperative as a factor in forward propulsion. The stresses being placed on the second metatarsal naturally develop an increase in mass, while the first metatarsal—receiving relatively little pressure—would fail to develop normally in terms of mass.

3. *Posteriorly Located Sesamoid Bones:* These two small bones, situated normally at the head of the first metatarsal (see Figure 39), provide protection to the flexor hallucis longus tendon, the muscle of forward propulsion when the foot is pointed straight ahead. Morton stated:

> Of similar effect as shortness of the first metatarsal, a third factor has been identified in a rearward position of the two small sesamoid bones that normally underlie the head of that bone. Since these sesamoids represent the contact points of the first metatarsal with the ground, whenever they are located more proximally towards the neck of that bone and posterior to the head of the second metatarsal they create a potential shortage of the former and affect the mechanism of the foot accordingly.[18]

He added that rearward-placed sesamoids are usually regarded as a contributory factor, rather than a primary factor, in foot disturbances.

186

Morton concluded by stating that hypermobility of the first metatarsal, shortness of the first metatarsal bone, and posteriorly located sesamoid bones may exist singly, but usually occur in combination. Due to this fact, several writers have classed the triad of defects and the resulting symptoms as "Morton's Syndrome" (Figure 40).

4. *Metatarsus Varus Primus:* In this condition, the first metatarsal projects medially (inward) beginning at the joint between the base of the first metatarsal and medial cuneiform bone (Figure 40), at an acute angle. There is a wide interspace between the first and second metatarsals at the toes. Almost invariably, this defect is associated with laxness or hypermobility of the first metatarsal.

The deviation of the first metatarsal deprives the medial longitudinal arch of definite stabilizing support. The hypermobility is similar to that discussed by Morton, as the first metatarsal bone does not properly contact the ground surface due to its lack of rigidity. The lack of stability on the inner side of the foot causes the foot to roll inward and downward under the stress of weight bearing, which leads to eventual pronation of the foot.

5. *Accessory Scaphoid or Prehallux:* Lewin stated that this is the most common anomaly found in cases of flat foot.[16] The prehallux is an accessory bone attached to the inner border of the scaphoid (see Chapter 17, Figure 21). The posterior tibialis tendon in the normal foot is inserted into the internal cuneiform and first metatarsal (see Chapter 17, Figure 27). When a prehallux is present, the tendon attaches to the prehallux instead. The tendon then pulls backward and inward, instead of upward as it would in the normal foot. The long lever arm of the prehallux turning inward forces the tendon and its muscle to a greater length of contraction in order to produce a given amount of lift at the center of the arch. The effort to lift the arch or adduct the foot is quickly stopped by nearness of the prehallux to the internal malleous (see Chapter 17, Figure 24). The crowding of the tissues between the prehallux and internal malleous causes pain, which is relieved by abduction or pronation of the foot.

6. *Faulty Development of the Calcaneus (Heel) and Talus (Astragalus):* Harris and Beath, in examination of 3,000 Canadian recruits, found many cases of what they termed "hypermobile flat feet with short Achilles tendon," due to developmental faults in the calcaneus and talus.[9] They concluded from their study that a common type of severe flat foot deformity in childhood and young adult life was due to abnormalities of the tarsal bones, which result in instability of the talus, manifested when weight is superimposed on the foot. The chief lesion was inadequate support of the head of the talus by the calcaneus. Dorsiflexion of the foot was greatly limited, but an increased range of mobility at the sub-talar and

mid-tarsal joints existed (Chapter 17, Figure 21).

7. *Obliquity of the Ankle Joints:* In this condition, the lower articular surfaces of the tibiae fail to develop evenly. It slopes a little medially instead of being parallel with the ground. When non-weight-bearing, the soles of the feet are in a slight varus position (facing each other). However, when bearing weight, the soles of the feet are restored to the horizontal position by eversion into the valgus position (Figure 44). While some cases are the result of faulty development, others are due to a severe in-curving of the tibiae (tibial varum).

8. *Pes Cavus (Hollow or Claw Foot):* Frank Weinstein used the term "pes cavus syndrome" to describe the characteristic signs of the pes cavus.[29] This terminology can be used to identify all degrees of high-arched foot, from the extremely high arch—a deformity—to the moderate and mild types of high arch.

The extremely high arch, not found among athletes, is considered to be a congenital deformity. It results from a structural defect in which there is a drooping of the forefoot due to a malalignment of the tarsal bones, not an actual raising of the longitudinal arches.

Many causes other than congenital ones have been advanced to explain the development of the acquired moderate and mild types of high-arched foot. Among them are: postural defects; high-heeled shoes; overdevelopment of the calf muscles; habitual posture assumed by the foot to compensate for a short leg; the kneeling position in early childhood; prolonged illness in bed with the feet held in a plantar-flexed position; muscular imbalance between the calf muscles and intrinsic foot muscles; dysfunction of the foot muscles; and pathological nervous diseases.

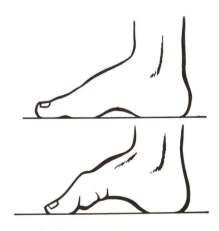

*Figure 41*
PES CAVUS TYPE OF FOOT

In *Mild Cavus* (mild high arch), the foot is still flexible. It appears to have a high arch when non-weight-bearing; but the claw foot disappears when it is weight-bearing. There is a limited dorsiflexion of the foot and a rearfoot varus position of approximately five degrees.

In *Moderate Cavus* (moderate high arch), the foot displays clawed toes when dangling (Figure 41), but they do not entirely disappear when it is weight-bearing. The foot is less flexible. The arch flattens only mildly in a full weight-bearing state. There is a greater degree of limited dorsiflexion and a tightness and firmness of the intrinsic foot muscles. The rearfoot varus position of five degrees cannot be everted or pronated beyond the perpendicular to the valgus position.

Three conditions are common to the moderate and mild degrees of pes cavus: (A) a limitation of foot dorsiflexion due to a shortened Achilles tendon or calf muscles; (B) some degree of rearfoot varus (Figure 47); and (C) various degrees of clawing of the toes.

## ANATOMICAL FACTORS

Morton maintained that shortened calf muscles are one extrinsic condition which may be either an important direct or a contributing factor in functional disorders of the foot.[18] The shortness reduces the normal range of dorsiflexion of the foot. He claimed that, though sometimes congenital in origin, it is most commonly acquired by women through constant wearing of high-heeled shoes, or may be developed through a protracted period of illness in bed. Schuster, a podiatrist long experienced in dealing with the foot problems of athletes, claimed that approximately 70 percent of athletes and non-athletes alike are unable to dorsiflex the foot beyond a right angle when the sub-talar joint (see Chapter 17, Figure 32) is held in a neutral position.[21]

Runners, like all other athletes, display a high degree of muscular imbalance in the lower leg due to the excessive use of the calf muscles which from early childhood onward normally are over five times as strong as the antagonist shin muscles. This muscular imbalance is a major factor in producing foot disorders. The shortened calf muscles or tendon stretch the weaker intrinsic foot muscles on the sole of the foot, which eventually weakens them and renders them unable to support the ligamentous structure binding the foot bones together.

The reduced dorsiflexion capacity of the foot due to a short Achilles tendon or calf muscles throws the burden of weight bearing largely upon the forefoot. The concentration of weight on the forefoot and the pull exerted by the short tendon or calf muscles on the heel tend to roll the heel inwards into a valgus position (see Figure 46). The two forces also tilt the subastragalar joint (see Chapter 17, Figure 21) downward and inward, which depresses the

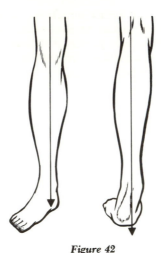

*Figure 42*

Pronated foot, note inward deviation of ankle and valgus position of heel.

medial longitudinal arch into a pronated foot position and eventually leads to acquired functional flat foot.

An additional anatomical factor in foot disorders is relaxation of ligaments. It may be a part of a general relaxation which is often found in the slender small-boned individual with a gracile (slender) foot. The relaxation may be congenital in origin, or due to long periods of illness in bed or inactivity, obesity, an occupation requiring long periods of standing, high-heeled shoes, or the short calf-stretched plantar muscle and ligament imbalance discussed previously. If the relaxation affects only the ligaments binding the tarsal bones together, it generally affects only the medial longitudinal arch and the first metatarsal bones spread apart and the true type of "splay foot" develops.

## FOOT FAULTS COMMON TO RUNNERS, HURDLERS, AND JOGGERS

Excluding the two most common structural defects, short and/or hypermobile first metatarsal (Figures 39-40), the two most common foot faults found among the general population and among athletes are minor degrees of foot pronation (Figure 42) and abducted toed-out foot postures (Figure 43). In addition to these, according to Schuster, the most common faults or defects found among runners and joggers are equinus influences (short heel cord or calf muscles); forefoot varus (Figure 45); reduced sub-talar motion; rearfoot (sub-talar) varus (Figure 47); rearfoot (sub-talar) valgus (Figure 46); and gracile (slender small-boned) feet.[21]

Schuster pointed out that minor structural deviations or faults in the feet of athletes may become painful problems due to constant pounding; whereas the ordinary individual with the same kind of foot abnormalities would experience no problems from them.[21]

## FOOT PRONATION

As the reader will recall, Morton and Fuller stated that 45 percent of the population, including athletes, display symptoms of first degree pronation. This is manifested in a very slight degree of a valgus heel (Figure 46), valgus forefoot (Figure 44), and downward displacement of the talus (astragalus).

Steindler pointed out that as the pronation enters the second degree stage the forefoot will attempt to maintain contact with the ground, despite the fact that the rearfoot has gone further into the pronatory or valgus position.[26] The mid-tarsal joint has three axes of joint movement. One of these axes, motion around the longitudinal axis, is expressed in the pronatory and supinatory torsion motion which the forefoot executes against the rearfoot. Said Steindler: "The torsion of the posterior foot is followed by a detorsion of the anterior foot."

The compensatory torsional action of the forefoot occurs only during the dynamic phases of walking and running. In the static standing position, the forefoot may display a very slight varus posture (Figure 45).

## ABDUCTED TOED-OUT FOOT POSTURE

Anything beyond a 15-degree deviation of each foot (30 degrees for both) from the midline of the body in a standing position, or five degrees of each foot in running, may be considered a definite reflection of poor foot posture (Figure 43).

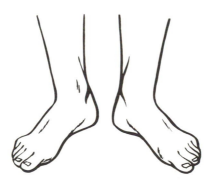

*Figure 43*
ABDUCTED (TOED-OUT) FOOT POSITION

191

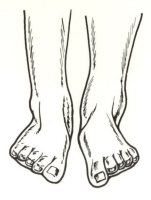

**Figure 44**

FOREFOOT VALGUS

Heel bone is normal, but the forefoot has a pronounced inward tilt.
Requires a twisting motion of forefoot to meet the ground.

## EQUINUS INFLUENCES
## (SHORT HEEL CORD OR CALF MUSCLES)

Schuster commented that 10 degrees of dorsiflexion at the ankle
when the heel is held neutral is ideal for both walking and
running.[21]   About 80 percent of his runner patients were incapable
of dorsiflexing beyond a right angle. Laird suggested tight medial
hamstrings as a cause of equinus foot posture and sometimes of
rearfoot varus (Figure 47) posture.[15] The hamstrings may be truly
short on a congenital basis; or the muscle may be short as an
accommodation phenomenon and, as such, considered in a state of
contracture; or the muscle may be considered short because of more

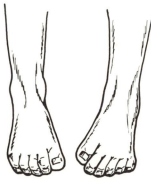

**Figure 45**

FOREFOOT VARUS

Heel bone is normal, but the forefoot has a pronounced outward tilt.
Requires a twisting motion of forefoot to meet the ground.

rapid bone growth than muscle growth, which has left a discrepancy in length. The condition causes an internal rotation of the leg prior to heel contact.

## FOREFOOT VARUS

Schuster considered it noteworthy that almost every runner he and his associates treated on a mechanical basis showed a moderate to severe forefoot varus (Figure 45). It occurred with much higher frequency among runners than among their other podiatric patients. The usual cause was congenital, i.e., retention of some fetal characteristics. He termed it the most serious potential foot problem in runners.

There are two other factors that must be considered in cases of forefoot varus:

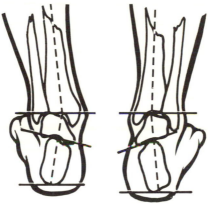

*Figure 46*
REAR FOOT VALGUS HEEL

Also known as sub-talar valgus. Heel bone is out of alignment with rest of lower leg.

1. Most children, when they first stand, display a certain degree of foot pronation and a toed-out position in order to balance themselves. If they remain in this pronated abducted foot position for any great length of time, the forefoot will go into the compensatory-supinatory position, as Steindler pointed out. As they begin to toe more straight ahead, and to wear shoes with heels, they tend to correct most of the rearfoot valgus posture. If the pronation is still quite pronounced, inserts on the medial (inner) side of the shoe will be recommended. However, as Steindler noted, medial wedges only, for the entire foot, throw the forefoot into a varus position because the former pronated foot posture has already developed the detorsion of the forefoot. For this reason, he recommended that medial inserts should be used to correct the valgus heel, but lateral inserts should be used on the forefoot. If this

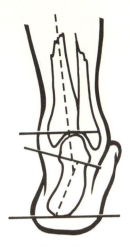

**Figure 47**
REAR FOOT VARUM HEEL

This is also known as sub-talar varus. Heel bone is out of alignment with rest of lower leg.

is not done, a permanent forefoot varus foot posture will result.

2. In the writer's opinion, forefoot varus can also result from muscle imbalance between the tibialis anterior muscle of the lower leg and the much weaker peroneus longus muscle (see Chapter 17, Figure 29). The reader will recall Wiles' contribution to the explanation of pronated and poor foot posture, discussed in Chaper 11. It is well-established that the shin muscles, while relatively weak as compared to the calf muscles, are powerful decelerating muscles as the foot strikes the ground during walking, running, and jogging. They automatically become much stronger than their primary antagonist muscles in respect to the functions of the muscles controlling the plantigrade (flat on ground) position of the forefoot. As Wiles pointed out, the primary responsibility of the peroneus longus in maintaining the plantigrade forefoot posture is to hold the first metatarsal on the ground. If its basic antagonist muscle, the anterior tibialis, is much stronger, it cannot carry out this function and the forefoot goes into a varus position.

The peroneus longus muscle is rarely given specific exercises to strengthen it, and ice skating is the only athletic activity that builds a high level of strength in this muscle.

## REDUCED SUB-TALAR MOTION

Schuster commented that another problem of runners not usually found in general practice has to do with the sub-talar joint (see

Chapter 17, Figure 22). He pointed out that the average sub-talar range of motion is about 30 degrees—20 degrees inversion and 10 degrees eversion. He found runners with smaller ranges of subtalar motion—12, 15, or 17 degrees instead of the usual 30—who complained of pain in the groin and upper thighs. He went on to state that the narrow sub-talar range does not permit adequate eversion-abduction of the foot at the contact phase of the stride, and that as yet a successful way of handling this problem has not been found.

Fahey found reduced sub-talar motion in ballet dancers and others who were affected with the "retarded leg" syndrome and resultant faulty foot posture of the short leg.

Excluding any structural defects of the sub-talar joint, deviations in lower leg alignment (such as tibial varum), varying degrees of the high-arched foot (pes cavus), and pronation, the basic cause of a reduced sub-talar motion is muscle imbalance and reduced flexibility due to the muscle imbalance. The muscle imbalance involves the adductor-invertor and the abductor-evertor muscles that control the lateral stability of the ankle and the movements of the foot on the lower leg.

## REARFOOT (SUB-TALAR) VARUS

Schuster maintained that rearfoot varus is an important factor in the foot problems of runners but, in his experience, low on the list of situations that contribute to arch strain. He suggested that this may be due to the fact that many runners make minimal or no heel contact, and pass through the heel contact phase of running much too quickly for it to be significant (see Figure 47).

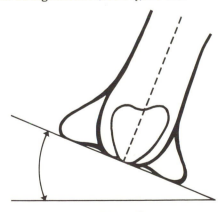

*Figure 48*
Tibial Varum
**Entire lower leg of right foot is out of line.**

On the other hand, Sabotnick, a podiatrist specializing in the foot problems of runners, maintained in describing foot types and overuse injuries that among distance runners, rearfoot varus appears commonly or is apt to develop.[27] In his opinion, it usually arises from athletic training.

Rearfoot varus may also be caused by faulty development of the calcaneus and talus (Harris and Beath);[9] obliquity of the ankle joints (Wiles);[31] severe tibial varum (bowing of lower leg); short Achilles tendon and high-arched foot; and muscular imbalance of the muscles controlling the lateral stability of the ankle joint. Subotnick commented that the rearfoot varus feet are moderately flexible, but tend to have a mildly limited total range of motion of the sub-talar joint. These feet may display a range of motion of 15 to 17 degrees of supination (inversion) with 4 to 5 degrees of pronation (eversion).

## REARFOOT (SUB-TALAR) VALGUS

This condition is invariably associated with the various degrees of pronated foot. In the case of a runner, hurdler, or jogger, it is a most serious type of foot fault (Figure 47).

## GRACILE (SLENDER SMALL-BONED) FEET

According to Schuster, gracile feet is not a common problem, although it does exist, causing frustrating foot strains, and it is not one of the easiest problems to treat. As a result of heredity, the foot is not structurally able to withstand the stress of the intensive training required of those participating in the distance runs.

## REFERENCES

1. Atkins, Charles E., "Pelvic Imbalances as Causative Factors in Foot Disturbances," *Clinical Osteopathy,* July 1938.
2. Bick, Edgar M., *Source Book of Orthopedics* (Baltimore: William & Wilkins Co., 1948).
3. Bivings, L., "Classification of Weak Feet in Children and a Method of Analyzing Foot Prints and Heel Prints," *American Journal* (Disabilities for Children), 49, 1935, 1164.
4. Bruce, J., "Management of Flatfoot," *Practioner,* 142:299, 1939.
5. Caldwell, Guy A; Shorkey, R. L.; and Duncan, T. L.; "Treatment of Mild Knock Knees and Pronated Feet in Childhood," *New Orleans Medical Journal,* 104:304, 1952.
6. Delpich, J. M., *L'Orthomorphie,* Paris, 1829.
7. Duchenne, Guillaume, B. A. *Physiologie des Mouvements,* Paris, 1855.

8. Graham, James, "Complications of the Weak Foot (Subtalar Dystrochoides)," *American Journal of Surgery*, November 1938.
9. Harris, R. I., and Beath, T., *Army foot Survey* (Ottawa: National Research Council of Canada, 1947).
10. Hartley, Joe L., "Gait and the Soldier: Importance of Gait in the Prevention and Cure of Foot Strain and in the Treatment of Symptomatic Flat Foot," *Military Surgeon,* February 1945.
11. Hiss, John Martin, *Functional Foot Disorders* (Los Angeles: University Publishing Co., 1937).
12. Hopkins, Ronald F., and Holt, L. E., "Foot Plant and Stride Length," *Modern Athlete and Coach* (Australia), July 1974.
13. Klein, Karl K., "Developmental Asymmetry of the Weight Bearing Skeleton and Its Implication on Knee Injury," *20th Annual Meeting A.C.S.M.*, Seattle, May 7, 1973.
14. Kuhns, John G., "Physical Therapy in Disabilities of the Foot," *The Physiotherapy Review,* Vol. 21, No. 3.
15. Laird, Patrick, "Examination of Gait," *Second Annual Sports Medicine Seminar,* California School of Podiatric Medicine, San Francisco, April 27-28, 1974. ("The Overuse Syndrome of the Foot and Leg, Part II.")
16. Lewin, Philip, *The Foot and Ankle* (Philadelphia: Lea & Febiger, 1959).
17. Lowman, Charles L., "Relation of Thigh and Leg Muscles to Malpostures of the Feet," *Boston Medical and Surgical Journal,* January 18, 1912.
18. Morton, Dudley J., "Foot Disorders in General Practice," *Journal of the American Medical Association*, October 2, 1937.
19. Morton, Dudley J., and Fuller, Dudley Dean, *Human Locomotion and Body Form* (Baltimore: William & Wilkins Co., 1952). Reprinted by permission of the publisher.
20. Osgood, Robert B., "The Comparative Strength of the Adductor and Abductor Groups in the Feet," *American Journal of Orthopedic Surgery,* January 1908.
21. Schuster, Richard O., "Overuse Syndrome: Arch Strains, Heel Pains, Shin Splints," *Annual Sports Medicine Seminar,* California School of Podiatric Medicine, April 28-29, 1973.
22. Schuster, Richard O., "Podiatry and the Athlete," *Journal of the American Podiatry Association*, Vol. 62, No. 12, December 1972.
23. Schwartz, R., and Heath, Arthur, "Some Factors Which Influence the Balance of the Foot in Walking," *Journal of Bone and Joint Surgery*, April 1933.
24. Shapiro, Jerome, "Podiatry and Public Health, a 7-Year Experience in the District of Columbia," *American Journal of Public Health*, October 1973.

25. Sheehan, George, "Morton's Foot: the Big Crippler," *Runner's World*, August 1974.

26. Steindler, A., "The Supinator, Compensatory Torsion of the Forefoot in Pes Valgus," *Journal of Bone and Joint Surgery*, Vol. 2, 272, 1929.

27. Subotnick, Steven R., "Foot Types and Overuse Injuries," *Second Annual Sports Medicine Seminar*, California Schools of Podiatric Medicine, April 27-28, 1974.

28. Travers, P. R., "Injuries Due to Faulty Style," *Track Technique*, No. 11.

29. Weinstein, Frank, *Principles and Practice of Podiatry* (Philadelphia: Lea & Febiger, 1968).

30. Whitman, Royal, "A Consideration of the Causes and Characteristics of the Weak Foot," *Medical Record*, August 31, 1907.

31. Wiles, Philip, "Flat Feet," *Lancet*, November 17, 1934.

# 19

## Effects of Foot Faults, Defects, and Faulty Foot Positions

The terms pronated, everted, and valgus have been used in the orthopedic literature to describe a foot fault in which the inner border of the foot is lowered towards the floor in various stages until it actually touches the floor, at which point it is termed an acquired functional flat foot—as opposed to the congenital flat foot. In many cases, "abduction" is the term used to describe the out-toeing or duck-foot position (see Chapter 18, Figure 43). True abduction, however, refers to the outward movement of the forefoot at the mid-tarsal joints during the progressive stages of the acquired functional flat foot.

In 1907, Royal Whitman wrote:

Twenty years ago when I first became interested in the weak foot as representing more particularly the less advanced type of deformity commonly called flat foot, practically nothing was known of it, at least nothing relative to what is now considered as its importance. It may be fairly stated I think, that the importance of the weak foot, the most common and the most disabling of all the postural deformities, was unsuspected.[29]

In defining the causes of weak feet, Whitman maintained that improper attitudes subject the foot to a mechanical disadvantage in the performance of its function. The most common of these attitudes is outward rotation of the limbs in walking. Outward rotation of the limbs "toeing out" must not be confused, as it usually is, with abduction or eversion of the feet, which characterizes all grades of deformity.

Subsequently, in his textbook on orthopedics, Whitman used the terms splay foot, pronated foot, and the flat foot as synonyms for weak foot.

Lewin stated that "the concept of the 'weak foot,' flaccid in its early stages and rigid in advanced cases, has almost entirely superseded the older concept of flat foot."[12]

Thirty years after Whitman, Graham commented that classification of congenital structural anomalies and the numerous traumas and infections of the feet presented no difficulty.[5] However, the great majority of humans with foot complaints could not be placed in the above classifications, as their symptoms were manifestations of abnormalities in the weight-bearing function, both static and dynamic, and in this respect there was utter confusion. He went on to state:

> The field of surgery will not be defined clearly until the dominant disorder of weight-bearing weak foot, pronated foot, fallen arches, flat foot had been identified, properly named, and considered as a disease entity with definite etiology and symptomatology, nor until such sequels of this condition as rigid foot, arthritis, muscle spasm, callous, etc., are viewed clearly as complications of this common disorder and not as clinical entities in themselves.

Graham, combining the internal thigh rotation concept of Lowman in 1912 with the postural pes valgus (flat foot) concept of Wiles in 1934 due to forward pelvic tilt, pointed out that the starting point of the weak foot was a relative valgus (pronated) foot position forced by an improper reception of superstructure body weight, reflected in a forward tilt of the pelvis, internal rotation of the thighs, and femoral-tibial internal rotation of the astragalus (talus) bone of the foot. He wrote that the complications resulting from a weak foot were the progressive steps of structural destruction: (1) heel eversion; (2) forefoot extension and separation of the metatarsal bones; (3) development of first metatarsal (big toe) hypermobility; (4) splay foot; (5) pronation of the foot; and (6) compensatory supination of the forefoot into a varus position.

Some writers have termed the first stage of weak foot as "strain foot," and as the impending stage of eventual acquired functional flat foot.

## EFFECTS OF CHRONIC STRAIN FOOT

The reader will recall that Morton and Fuller stated that 45 percent of the population displayed evidence of first degree pronation. This does not interfere with function, and clinical symptoms will not appear except in those individuals highly overweight, on their feet most of the day, or engaged in repetitive foot strike during training and competing in athletics. With first degree pronation, the ligaments on the medial side of the foot, the plantar ligaments, and plantar fascia begin to stretch.

The outstanding difference between strain foot and weak foot is that in the former condition no evidence of abnormality is seen in the foot when it is in a standing position.

Symptoms are reflected first by a feeling of fatigue and the inability to stand without constantly shifting the weight first to one foot and then to the other. Gradually, the feet become definitely painful, the pain being noticed chiefly during the day when the athlete is standing or walking, or during the evening after a severe work-out. The symptoms are manifested in a fairly steady pain under the medial longitudinal arch and a burning sensation along the sole of the foot due to the stretching of the plantar fascia.

## EFFECTS OF WEAK FOOT (SECOND DEGREE PRONATION)

Morton and Fuller reported that in addition to the 45 percent of the population displaying evidence of first degree pronation, another 45 percent were affected by various degrees of second degree pronation. Also, Morton claimed that the progressive course of medial longitudinal arch disorder clearly stamped second degree pronation as the critical stage in the progressive breakdown of the foot structure.[15]

The early symptoms of weak foot are manifested by pain and the beginning of loss of spring in the feet. The pain and tenderness are found along the medial side of the foot, including the bones, muscles, and ligaments. The latter two structures begin to stretch. The further they stretch, the greater the lengthening of the inner border of the feet due to separation of the heel bone from the scaphoid bone (see Chapter 17, Figure 21), which stretches the spring ligament (see Chapter 17, Figure 23) between the two bones. The heel begins to evert, and from the rear view the Achilles tendon is curved downward and outward (see Chapter 18, Figure 42).

As the progress of weak foot continues, the feet begin to swell, especially in front of the internal and external malleous (see Chapter 17, Figure 24). The foot lists to the inner side. The weight-bearing line, which normally drops from the middle of the kneecap to a point between the first and second toes, begins to move to the center of the big toe, and eventually moves to the medial side of the great toe.

The first stage of second degree pronation is limitation of the ordinary movements of the foot, particularly adduction (inward). Later, there may be an actual shortening of the abductor muscles and of the other tissues on the outer aspect of the feet. The limitation is in great part due to muscle spasm resulting from the chronic strain the foot is continually subjected to during the day.

Graham pointed out that weak feet lead to shortening of muscles on the lateral side and stretching of muscles on the inner side of the feet, stretching of the plantar fascia, increased muscular spasm with eventual development of degenerative foot disease—osteo-arthritis and rigid flat feet.[5]

Tucker provided an excellent description of the pronated (valgus) foot and its effect on the active athlete.[26] He wrote:

> In *active alerted posture* at the ankle joint and foot level, the weight should be carried on the outer side of the foot and the toes should grip the ground. In this way, ankle and foot should form a tense bow which allows for spring and resistance.
>
> The opposite of this is a flat valgus foot, with the strain on the longitudinal arch and the anterior transverse arch. Both arches are flattened and this foot is likened to the bow in which the strings are loose and there is lack of resilience and no recoil as in the *active alerted posture* position. The ankle is in danger of being sprained because there is not that balanced tension in the muscles of the ankle and foot which allows for firm fixation of the foot on the ground. If there is slight unevenness of the ground, the ankle will tend to rick over, spraining the lateral ligaments and the structures on the outer side of the ankle, as well as compressing the structures on the inner side. The flat valgus position of the foot also tends to produce acute foot sprains involving the tibialis anticus and posticus and tendons and the spring ligament, with symptoms of pain and swelling in relation to the tarsal scaphoid. If this strain is allowed to persist, the anterior transverse arch (forefoot) may become so flattened that persistent strain produces a stress fracture of one of the metatarsal shafts. Stress fractures of the metatarsal, fibula, or tibia can be seen to be due to a whipping movement as the result of muscle imbalance.
>
> Also, in the everted valgus position of the foot, strain is transferred to the fibula and typical stress fractures may take place about 6" from the lower end of this bone. Stress fractures can also occur in the tibia.
>
> If the transverse arch (forefoot) has been strained for some time, Morton's metatarsalgia with enlargement of one of the digital nerves may occur. This is often associated with bursitis between the metatarsal heads. Chronic foot strain also affects the circulation and tends to produce varicosity of the veins of the foot. If a sudden movement at the take-off occurs with the foot flat, the calf muscles, particularly the muscles making up the tendo-Achilles, are taken off guard, and a shock strain is produced with either the production of tendonitis, a tear of the calf muscles, or even a rupture of the tendo-Achilles.
>
> The flat-footed valgus ankle with knees braced back also produces strain on the structures on the medial side of the knee, and this will start a trend of symptoms leading to a chronic strain of the medial collateral ligament and may even involve the medial meniscus. In walking with flat valgus feet there is a cross drag on the patella and the ligament patellae and this in time can be an important factor in producing patello-femoral chondromalacia.

The flat valgus foot producing a strain of the foot and the knee will also produce a shearing strain on the hip, so that there is a tendency for the head of the femur to sublux out of the acetabulum. This can often account for strain on both the medial and lateral aspects of the hip joint, particularly causing strain on the adductors on the medial aspect and the gluteal muscles on the lateral posterior aspects. I consider that in time this flat-footed condition of the foot can be an important factor in the production of osteo-arthritis of the hip joints.

Subotnick maintained that the pronated foot leads to overuse symptoms of the posterior tibial tendon with generalized tendonitis, myositis, shin splints, and chondromalacia.[25] If a forefoot varus (Chapter 18, Figure 45) is also present, the results will be foot strain, plantar fasciitis, plantar calcaneal spurs, and bursitis.

Sheehan commented that pronated feet are the major cause of "Dutch Elm Disease" (chondromalacia) among runners.[20] He stated that when the arch flattens with pronation, it transfers a torque of six to seven degrees to the knee. The patella moves to the side, instead of sliding up and down on the groove. The underside of the patella rubs on the knob (condyle) of the thigh bone.

Hiss pointed out that the internal lateral ligaments of the knee (Chapter 15, Figure 18) are attached to the internal semilunar cartilage.[7] The pronated everted foot will in many cases pull this cartilage into a position of extreme tension, resulting in the typical symptoms and pathology of a dislocated internal semi-lunar cartilage.

Spastic weak foot, sometimes named spastic flat foot, in which the forefoot is held in pronounced abduction and eversion, is caused by a spasmodic convulsive contraction of the lateral leg and ankle muscle. While the spasm lasts, it resembles a rigid flat foot with marked pronation. This type of weak foot is most frequently found in young adult males of the robust muscular type and in adolescents, due to long-continued standing, walking, or running in which the feet are markedly abducted (outward) in the forefoot due to the progressive stages of pronation or from continually toeing outward.

As a result of these faults, the muscles on the anterior surface of the leg which adduct the foot (inward) tire. They begin to relax and are unable to counteract the pull of the muscles which abduct and dorsiflex the foot—the extensor longus digitorum and the peroneals. The latter become irritated by the continued contraction and react in spasm.

## THE PRONATION SYNDROME AND LOW BACK PAIN

Though orthopedic physicians early in this century emphasized the interrelationship between faulty foot posture and faulty upper body posture, two orthopedic physicians of the 30's and 40's, one of whom concentrated solely on foot problems, emphasized in their writings that pronated everted feet were a direct cause of low back pain and sciatica.

Walker pointed out that Hiss, who directed the Hiss Foot Clinic in Los Angeles, found that of 150,000 patients he had treated, half had backaches.[27] Of these 75,000 cases, nearly 40,000 originated in foot problems. Hiss, in his textbook, stated that in his experience, 75 percent of the backaches disappeared when the feet were corrected and correct posture was re-established.[7]

Lowman, who 35 years earlier had called attention to related foot and posture problems, subsequently wrote:

> Since a faulty foundation produces added stress on all the joints above, such conditions as legache, backache, neuritis, sciatica, varicose veins, and many other widespread reflex conditions can be caused or contributed to by this means.[13]

It was Jones, an orthopedic surgeon, who developed his "pronation syndrome" theory, claiming that a variety of symptoms in addition to those of low back pain could be caused by an exceedingly common type of faulty foot posture; namely, pronation or internal rotation of the feet.[9] Jones made this observation after a four-year study involving more than 200 cases of low back pain and 26 cases of sciatica. He commented that pronation of the foot caused the entire leg to rotate inward, resulting in a forward pelvic tilt. He pointed out that pronation *per se* has been found to be present to some degree in the vast majority of people. This statement agrees with Morton and Fuller's observations previously cited above and in Chapter 18.

Jones maintained that from the diagnostic standpoint, the presence of the pronation syndrome should be suspected when confronted by one or all of four cardinal symptoms: generalized fatigue, dull legaches of various distributions; low back pain of various patterns; and sciatic neuritis or sciatica.

The faulty weight lines due to the pronation syndrome first produce secondary inflammatory changes and pain in any area, whether it be the foot, ankle, knee, thighs, or spine. In the beginning, these are largely peri-arthritic (tissues around a joint); although, when long continued, the intrinsic joint structures are finally affected.

Jones successfully cured the low back problems of the 200 patients. Of the 26 sciatica patients—five of whom had previously been told by neurosurgeons that their symptoms were due to inter-vertebral disk protrusion—all 26 were treated satisfactorily, with only one being classed as a complete failure. Jones accomplished this by correcting the pronation of the feet with orthotic appliances and good shoes. Lowman had accomplished much the same thing 40 years earlier (see Chapter 15) by correcting the internal leg rotation at the hip joints.

In 1947, at the National Convention of the American Medical Association, Jones summarized his postural symptom complex before a committee concerned with the various neuralgias. Commenting that pronation gives rise to a series of related anatomical distortions from the foot upward that combine to produce elongating tensions which can affect the central nervous system in varying degrees, he pointed out that long-continued malalignments could produce non-infectious inflammation of: (1) nerves (neuritis); (2) arteries and veins (arteritis and phlebitis); (3) muscles (myositis); (4) fascia (fibrositis); (5) ligaments (periarthritis); and (6) joints (arthritis).

## EFFECTS OF STRUCTURAL FOOT DEFECTS

The structural defects of the short first metatarsal (big toe) and dorsal hypermobility (excessive) of the first metatarsal and of the posteriorly located sesamoid bones at the base of the big toe are generally grouped together under the term "Morton's Syndrome."

Morton commented that uneven distribution of weight is associated with all three of the structural factors.[14] The superficial symptoms are reflected in a burning sensation in the soles of the feet, followed by a callous formation under the heads of the second and third toes. The strain on the basal joints sets up a traumatic arthritis, which involves irritability or inflammation of the medial plantar nerve—whose branches flow out to the various toes—resulting in various types of metatarsalgic pain.

The second source of symptoms, according to Morton, is loss of the medial stability of the foot, usually due to dorsal hypermobility and leading to pronation, with muscle exhaustion and spasm and pain from strained ligaments along the inner border and arch of the foot.[14]

After the establishment of the inflammatory condition, symptoms and change of a secondary nature appear. Signs of nerve involvement are expressed in pain extending up the legs and thighs to the back, while localized areas of sharp pain or numbness and tingling develop in the feet.

If the destructive process in the feet continues, the tarsal bones become altered in shape and the foot is gradually depressed into a fixed and rigid flat foot deformity (third degree pronation). In the metatarsal area, progressive claw toe deformity is the most characteristic change.

In Chapter 18, Morton is noted as having pointed out that a short first metatarsal causes the shaft of the second metatarsal to hypertrophy (thicken). Slocum, in commenting on the overuse syndromes of the lower leg and foot, found a similar condition in runners who have trained in track over a period of years, one which appears to occur whether or not the first metatarsal is short.[24] He attributed this to the strong repetitive thrust at take-off. He also commented that there appears to be a widening between the bases of the first and second metatarsals and their associated cuneiform bones which accompanies the second metatarsal hypertrophy, which he attributed to the fact that the feet of most good runners are extremely flexible in the forepart of the foot—far more so than those of the general population.

It should be noted that Morton maintained that the increased flexibility of the first metatarsal (dorsal hypermobility) was due to slack ligaments that placed a larger burden of weight stress on the second metatarsal, causing it to hypertrophy.

Sheehan wrote that Morton's Foot (short big toe) occurs in about 33 percent of the population; though Schuster found, in a patient population of 1,000 which he studied, an 80 percent incidence of short first toe. Sheehan stated: "I recently surveyed all the available X-rays and orthopedic texts in the local hospital, and discovered that every stress fracture (metatarsals) pictured in these books had occurred in a Morton's Foot!"[21] Slocum commented that stress fractures are more easily incurred if mechanical defects of the foot are present, such as the short big toe, splay foot, or hallux valgus.[24] However, he pointed out that in his experience, stress fractures of the second, third, and fourth metatarsals have not been encountered with a hypertrophied second metatarsal. Schuster noted: "Most runners with metatarsal problems have either a short first metatarsal (Morton's Syndrome) and/or a varus forefoot."[19]

The fact that in the presence of repetitive foot strikes a round-shouldered head forward position and an increased pelvic tilt which throws the weight line of the body forward onto the ball (metatarsals) of the foot become a predisposing cause of metatarsal stress fractures should not be overlooked. The same is true of pes cavus (high arched foot).

Sheehan claimed that numerous disorders of the foot and knee are due to the short first metatarsal:[22] stress fractures of the metatarsals; plantar fascitis; heel spurs; arch pain; Achilles tendonitis; stress fracture of the fibula; posterior tibial tendonitis; and knee pain due to pronation of the foot.

## EFFECTS OF TOED-OUT FOOT POSITION

Habitual outward rotation of the feet combined with slight abduction, pronation, or forefoot valgus results in the following: a loss of spring in the feet; discomfort and pain manifested in a sensation of weakness; tiredness and strain along the inner border of the feet and beneath the medial longitudinal arch; and, sometimes, pain in the heels. The pain may extend to the calves, knees, and lower back during long periods of standing. Over a period of time, the flexor hallucis longus and posterior tibialis tendons begin to stretch. The power of foot adduction (inward) is lessened, while the abductor muscles (peroneals) on the lateral side of the foot and ankle begin to contract. This contraction can lead to eventual muscle spasm, and in young people to spastic flat foot (previously described) after periods of unusual activity.

In running, the line of drive goes across the metatarsal bones instead of straight ahead. The tremendous stress on the metatarsals can lead to fractures of these bones. Tendonitis can develop from the constant and unusual tension of the muscle tendons mentioned in the paragraphs above. In the writer's opinion, the toed-out foot position is a major predisposing cause of very troublesome "shin splints," one of the more common overuse syndromes that affect running athletes and joggers.

### EFFECTS OF PES CAVUS (HIGH-ARCHED FOOT)

In the mild type of pes cavus, the feet are predisposed to calcaneal (heel) bruises, plantar fascia, and medial longitudinal arch strains.

A moderate pes cavus condition places unusual stress on the metatarsal heads as they strike the floor or track. The metatarsal bones are highly disposed toward metatarsal arch strains, plantar fascia strains, and stress fractures. Subotnick stated that this foot is subject to callouses on the ball of the foot and frequent sprain of the ankles; has poor shock-absorbing qualities, with the shock being transferred to the ankles, knees, and back—with attendant problems.[25] Also, there is bony limitation of dorsiflexion at the ankle joint, and talar exostosis (bone growths) are not uncommon. He maintained that a severe pes cavus deformity or a very high-arched foot (Chapter 18, Figure 41) is unsuitable for the rigors of athletic competition and requires surgical correction before it can sustain them.

### EFFECTS OF LOWER LEG ANATOMICAL AND STRUCTURAL FACTORS

A congenital or acquired short Achilles tendon or short gastrocnemius-soleus calf muscles can aggravate any other foot fault an athlete or jogger may have. Newel affirmed that these conditions force the feet to function for the most part fully pronated, with a valgus heel strike throughout the stance and foot strike stages, which leads to many symptoms, e.g., low back pain, hyperextended knees, chondromalacia of the patella, shin splints, medial longitudinal arch discomfort, heel spurs, early hallux valgus (big toe bending inward toward second toe), etc.[16]

The short heel cord is highly susceptible to Achilles tendon strain, tendonitis, tendosynovitis, and bursitis. Because the runner or jogger is forced to run more on his toes, unusual stresses are placed on the forefoot. In the distance runs and in jogging, the short heel cord may lead to metatarsal stress fractures and arch strains, and in shorter runs to plantar fascia or longitudinal arch strain.

Tibial varum (bowleg) causes the heel to remain in a permanent varus position (Chapter 18, Figures 45 and 48). Foot strike causes the heel to pronate (Chapter 18, Figure 42). A normal degree of pronation is four degrees. If the pronation (valgus) exceeds this range, pains in the foot and knee occur. Bowleg also leads to medial longitudinal arch strain, runner's knee (chondromalacia), Achilles tendon problems, and heel spurs. Over a period of time, it can bring about irritation of the posterior tibialis tendon, with resulting tendonitis and/or shin splints.

## EFFECTS OF FOOT FAULTS COMMON AMONG RUNNERS AND JOGGERS

According to Schuster, "A four-year experience treating runners has indicated beyond a doubt that the runner differs considerably from the non-runner in the occurrence of mechanical foot problems."[19] The faults covered previously in this chapter tend to occur more often in runners and joggers. Podiatrists specializing in the foot problems of these groups, however, have become aware of several faults particularly common among their patients. These include forefoot varus, rearfoot varus, narrow sub-talar range, gracile (slender small-boned) feet, and shin splints.

## FOREFOOT VARUS

Schuster stated: "In our experience this is the major cause of metatarsal neuritis, stress fractures, fascia strain, vague but annoying forefoot symptoms and incidentally, knee pains. (About half of our 'runner' practice has knee pains that we feel are directly related to forefoot varus.)"[19]

Subotnick pointed out that athletes with forefoot varus are prone to postural fatigue that causes pains in the arches and back of the legs.[25] In addition, the turning inward of the foot causes an internal rotation of the thigh which may result in knee, hip, or low back pain.

Pagliano maintained that forefoot varus is a major predisposing factor in Achilles tendon strains, tendonitis, and eventual tendon rupture.[17] In an unstable foot, the pronatory effect is often carried out to extremes, and the heel is everted past its normal limits (Chapter 18, Figure 42). The Achilles tendon that is attached to the heel also experiences this extreme eversion force and undergoes severe tension and stretching. He stated that forefoot varus produces an extremely unstable type of foot. There is excessive pronation of the foot and excessive eversion of the calcaneus (Chapter 18, Figure 42), causing undue strain on the Achilles tendon. Instead of the tendon being stretched the normal few degrees, it is being stretched through an extra five to eight degrees. If this motion is repeated several hundred times, a rupture or tear is bound to occur. There are many other foot conditions which cause this pronatory force, but in Pagliano's opinion the forefoot varus appears to be the most common.

## REARFOOT VARUS

Subotnick described this type of foot as moderately flexible, but tending to have a mildly limited total range of motion at the sub-talar joint (Chapter 17, Figure 21).[25] This frequently permits a partially compensated rearfoot varus, which results in excessive strain upon the ankle and knee joints. Besides the usual runner's bumps (heel), chondromalacia of the patella, shin splints, plantar strains, spurs, and bursa, there is an increased tendency toward hamstring pulls and soft tissue problems around the buttocks and hips. Subotnick found that rearfoot varus is more common, or even more apt to develop, in distance runners.

## NARROW SUB-TALAR RANGE

Schuster wrote that in his experience narrow sub-talar joint range has been the second most common cause of arch strain and other related problems of runners.[19] When there is a narrow subtaler range, the rearfoot complex does not have the full capacity to act as a kind of universal joint. Because of this limitation, the foot cannot freely adapt to variations in the terrain unless it stresses other foot joints, thereby leading to arch strain. Also, the reduction of adduction (inward) and abduction (outward) seems often to be compensated for in the hip, which in turn brings on signs of strain in the groin.

## GRACILE (SLENDER SMALL-BONED) FOOT

As mentioned earlier, Schuster classified this type of foot problem as difficult to treat and indicated that it can be the cause of frustrating foot strains.[19] When the slender heel occurs in this type of foot, the heel is an unstable heel and easily subject to ankle sprains.

## SHIN SPLINTS

Shin splints, or shin soreness as it is sometimes named, is one of the most common overuse syndromes peculiar to athletes in all the running sports and, at the same time, the most controversial issue in the field of athletic injuries with respect to its cause, diagnosis, and treatment.

Leach commented that shin splints have been reported to account for 10.6 percent of all distance running injuries.[11] In his opinion, however, the injury is much more common than the *Runner's World* survey that was the source of that figure may have revealed.

The controversy over the primary causes of the lesion and the anatomical or structural factors involved was resolved to some extent in 1966. After a survey of several hundred physicians, trainers, and physical educators, an American Medical Association sub-committee on Medical Aspects of Sports arrived at a standardized definition of shin splints. Its report stated in part: "Diagnosis should be limited to musculo-tendinous inflammations, excluding fracture or ischemic disorder."

This definition limits the condition to pain and discomfort in the tibial (shin) area of the lower leg due to the anatomy of the leg. The source of the inflammation must lie at the origin, belly, or musculo-tendinous junction of the plantar flexor or dorsiflexor foot muscles.

1. *Anatomy*—Of the 12 muscles of the lower leg, 7 have their origins in either of the posterior, lateral, or anterior side of the tibia and/or fibula and the interroseus membrane that lies between the tibia and fibula bones. All seven, through their tendons, insert into the bones of the foot. Four—tibialis posterior, flexor digitorum longus, flexor hallucis, and soleus—are involved in plantar flexion (Chapter 17, Figure 30), and arise from the posterior and medial sides of the tibia and/or fibula. Three—tibialis anterior, extensor digitorum longus, and extensor hallucis longus—are involved in dorsiflexion (Chapter 17, Figure 30), and arise from the lateral and/or anterior sides of the fibula or tibia.

2. *Site of Injury (Lesion)*—Authorities writing on the subject of shin splints are divided in their opinions as to the specific anatomical structure that is the site of the lesion and the direct cause of inflammation and subsequent pain.

Slocum pointed out the specific muscles of the leg may be more involved in one sport than another, and in this sense the lesion is occupational in that certain types of athletic activities require the use of selected muscles.[23] For example, he has found that in track, the lesion is most commonly located in the lower third of the leg along the medial border of the tibia in the region of the posterior tibialis.

In contrast, Hobbs, after 15 years' experience in treating shin soreness among Australian football and rugby players, stated that in his opinion the lesion was centered in the flexor digitorum muscle on the medial side of the tibia.[8]

Leach reviewed 31 sources of literature on the shin splint

syndrome, and the authorities he cited named one or more of the following anatomical structures as the site of the lesion: tibialis posterior; anterior tibialis; interroseus membrane; the soleus and flexor digitorum longus; and the extensor hallucis longus and extensor digitorum longus.[11]

3. *Cause of Shin Splints*—A review of the literature relating to the shin splint syndrome discloses that over 30 predisposing factors to it have been noted by various authorities. Only two will be covered in this discussion: weak or strained feet and walking and running in the toed-out position.

Cerney listed weak or strained longitudinal arches and pes cavus (high-arched foot) as predisposing factors.[1] Drake listed pre-existing foot or arch problems as one of five causes of the syndrome.[3] Flood and Naubert pointed out that some athletes with inherent weakness, such as poor arch structure or poor running mechanics, are more susceptible to it than others.[4] Dolan and Holladay commented that in seeking causes for the syndrome, most trainers look for a sprained or weak longitudinal arch.[2]

Hirata, in discussing the shin splint syndrome, said that in every case of shin splints treated by him the condition was directly related to running "duck-footed."[6] Slocum said that during the foot dorsiflexion stage in running (foot strike) the plantar flexor muscles may be stretched beyond their normal working range due to a shortened excursion caused by flat feet or toeing-out gait.[19] Juvenal wrote: "In looking for a common denominator, we found that every athlete with shin splints shared one thing in common with every other; to a greater or lesser extent, they ran or walked "duck-footed" (toed-out).[10]

## EFFECTS OF FAULTY FOOT POSITIONS ON PERFORMANCE

Three faulty positions of the feet that directly affect the performance of a competitive runner or jogger are: pronated or weak feet, pes cavus (high-arched foot), and toeing out.

### Pronated or Weak Feet

The gripping action of the toe flexors and the pulling action of the anterior tibialis muscle are lost through the stretching of the muscles and ligaments on the medial side of the foot. The loss of spring from the stretched plantar flexors affects the push-off force from behind and the traction of the forefoot on the ground in front.

### Pes Cavus (High-Arched Foot)

The forefoot thrust tends to be outward instead of straight ahead. The associated short Achilles tendon prevents a forceful thrust and take-off. With a shortening of the plantar flexors and extensor

211

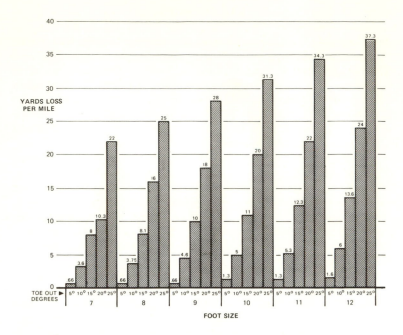

*Figure 49*
RUNNER'S LOSS OF DISTANCE WHEN TOEING-OUT

Computation of loss of distance over a mile based on the angle of deviation from the straight ahead foot position for each foot size.

muscles, there is a loss of spring in the feet.

## Toeing-Out

Many authorities have commented on a runner's loss of distance on each stride and over a course of one mile when toeing-out is involved. Robison, *et al.* pointed out that with 20-degree outward toeing, the forefoot would be about one-half inch outward from the straight ahead position.[18] Figuring a six-foot stride (880 foot strikes per mile), a runner would lose 12 yards in distance during a mile run. It should be pointed out, however, that these authorities did not indicate the size of the runner's foot—an item that should be taken into account, since each foot size deviates outward at a greater or lesser angle. Using a strike figure of 1,000 foot strikes per mile (which Subotnick, Sheehan, and Schuster considered the usual number), this writer asked an engineer friend to compute the loss of distance over a mile and the angle of deviation from the straight ahead foot position for each size foot. The results of his computations are reflected in Figure 49.

# REFERENCES

1. Cerney, J. V., *Athletic Injuries* (Smithfield, Illinois: Charles C. Thomas, 1963).
2. Dolan, Joseph P., and Holladay, Lloyd J., *Treatment and Prevention of Athletic Injuries* (Danville, Illinois: The Interstate Printers and Publishers, 1967).
3. Drake, E. C., "Shin Splints from the Trainer's Point of View," Presented at *The 8th National Conference on the Medical Aspects of Sport,* Las Vegas, November 27, 1966.
4. Flood, Jim, and Naubert, Jerry, "Shin Splints," *Scholastic Coach,* December 1967.
5. Graham, James, "Complications of the Weak Foot," *American Journal of Surgery,* November 1938.
6. Hirata, Isao, *The Doctor and the Athlete* (Philadelphia: J.B. Lippincott co., 1968).
7. Hiss, John M., *Functional Foot Disorders* (Los Angeles: University Publishing Co., 1937).
8. Hobbs, Kevin, "Shin Soreness," *Australian Journal of Sports Medicine,* May-June 1972.
9. Jones, Laurence, "Low Back Pain: A Different Cause and Treatment," *Industrial Medicine,* Vol. 16, No. 2, February 1947.
10. Juvenal, James P., "Shin Splints and Duck Feet," *Scholastic Coach,* December 1973.
11. Leach, Bill, "Shin Splints," *Track and Field Quarterly Review,* Vol. 74, No. 2, June 1974.
12. Lewin, Philip, "The Foot and Ankle," *Minnesota Medicine,* November 1938.
13. Lowman, C. L., "Feet and Body Mechanics," *Journal of Health and Education,* March 1940.
14. Morton, Dudley J., "Foot Disorders in General Practice," *Journal of the American Medical Association,* October 2, 1937.
15. Morton, Dudley J., *The Human Foot* (New York: Columbia University Press, 1935).
16. Newel, Stanley G., "Prolonged Pronation of the Foot," *2nd Annual Sports Medicine Seminar,* California School of Podiatric Medicine, San Francisco, April 27-28, 1974.
17. Pagliano, John, "Achilles Tendon Strain," an unpublished paper.
18. Robison, Clarence E.; Jensen, Clayne R.; James, Sherald W.; and Hirschi, Willard M.; *Modern Techniques of Track and Field* (Philadelphia: Lea & Febiger, 1974).
19. Schuster, Richard O., "Overuse Syndrome: Arch Strains, Heel Pains, Shin Splints, *Annual Sports Medicine Seminar,* California School of Podiatric Medicine, San Francisco, April 28-29, 1973.

20. Sheehan, George, "The Dutch Elm Disease of Long Distance Runners," *Medical Times*, Vol. 100, April 1972.

21. Sheehan, George, "Morton's Foot: The Big Crippler," *Runner's World*, August 1974.

22. Sheehan, George, "Structural Troubles," *The Complete Runner (Mountain View, California: World Publications, 1974)*.

23. Slocum, Donald B., "The Shin Splint Syndrome," *American Journal of Surgery*, December 1967.

24. Slocum, Donald B., "Overuse Syndromes of the Lower Leg and Foot in Athletes," *Instructural Course Lectures,* Vol. 17, 1960 (St. Louis: C. V. Mosby, 1960).

25. Subotnick, Steven I., "Foot Types and Overuse Injuries," *2nd Annual Sports Medicine Seminar,* California School of Podiatric Medicine, San Francisco, April 27-28, 1974.

26. Tucker, W. E., "Postural Training in Athletes," Lecture presented at Royal Northern Hospital, England, 1974.

27. Walker, Morton, *Your Guide to Foot Health* (Chicago: Follet Publishing Co., 1964).

28. Whitman, Royal, "A Consideration of the Causes and Characteristics of the Weak Foot," *Medical Record*, August 31, 1907.

# 20

## The Injury Prone Athlete

In addition to the three predisposing musculo-skeletal hidden factors of injuries and overuse syndromes so far discussed, there is a fourth hidden predisposing factor—the injury prone personality. This personality is encountered in all areas of life, including the field of athletics.

The athlete, like his fellow human beings, is subject to the everyday pressures, stresses, and tensions of living—conflicts in inter-personal relationships, the search for economic security in a highly competitive world. He, too, needs to have his personal needs, wants, and hopes fulfilled.

In fact, the performer faces as a matter of course extremes of pressure and stress far beyond the norm, particularly if his motivation to succeed and excel is a strong one.

The openly straightforward quest of the successful athlete for public recognition and approval demands overwhelming motivation and subjects him to equally tremendous psychological wear and tear—to which he must adapt. In competition, the athlete's total ego is at the mercy of the critical judgments of others. Only an indomitable determination to excel enables him to risk it again and again. Such formidable forces are not born of an uncomplicated psyche.

When an athlete whose physical qualifications for successful competition are apparent chokes up during an important contest, or is constantly plagued with chronic minor injuries that prevent him from participating, or fails in some other way to perform to the level of his potential, the cause lies more often than not in emotional or motivational conflicts.

A psycho-diagnosis by Antonelli of 418 Italian athletes selected to participate in the Tokyo Olympics disclosed the following psycho-pathological phenomena: 3 (0.6%) dysthymically psychotic; 70 (19%) emotionally immature; 87 (20%) hypermotivated and anxious; 106 (26%) insecure; 26 (7%) constitutionally depressed; and 26 (7%) lacking resistance to frustration. Antonelli commented that more than a third of the athletes presented attitudes or phenomena which merited psychological guidance, especially during the long prepara-tory phase.[2]

In commenting on the same diagnostic evaluation, Pollini pointed out that the athlete's relationship to society was altered in 59 cases (16%) owing to unsociability; in another 59 (16%) owing to introversion; in 6 cases (1.4%) as a result of inadaptability; and in 1 case because of a tendency to indiscipline. The self-evaluation picture was found to be even more disturbed: 110 athletes (27%) were ambitious; 33 (9%) were narcissistic; and 106 (26%) were insecure. Pollini noted that among those who were hypermotivated and anxiety prone, track and field athletes predominated. They were 87 in number and accounted for 20% of the group.[1]

In 1966, a year after Antonelli announced the results of his study, Ogilvie pointed out that, in general, highly successful athletes of international caliber will be driven by most of the following personality traits: emotional stability; psychological endurance; tough-mindedness; self-assertiveness; self-control; and conscien-tiousness. They will possess basically trusting natures, and be homogenous with respect to need for achievement, desire for recognition, aggressiveness, and a highly-organized lifestyle.[13]

In spite of this very positive picture, however, the greater the athletic challenge, the higher the probability that even those athletes with international talent will begin to manifest negative psycho-physiological reactions. This was reflected in the increase in psychosomatic complaints reported by the U.S. medical team at the 1968 Olympic Games in Mexico City. Vanek, the team psychologist for the Czech team, reported that slightly over ten percent of these superior athletes were what "might be termed problem athletes."

## PATTERNS OF EMOTIONAL RESPONSE

Emotions are responses to stimuli received from the external world through the sensory organs. Their control and expression are centered in the brain.

There are three types of emotional response to the stimuli: (1) the *perceptual aspect* located in the upper brain, that involves the recognition of a situation as being threatening, pleasurable, fearful, surprising, humorous, etc.; (2) the *sensory aspect* located in the upper brain, which is the feeling tone associated with specific emotions of rage, anger, fear, pleasure, pain, etc.; and (3) the

216

*physiological aspect* centered in the lower brain, which reflects the automatic changes in the respiratory, circulatory, glandular, muscular, and other body systems. Cannon pointed out that from a physiological standpoint, emotions are a reactive pattern with characteristics that depict those of a simple reflex pattern.[4]

## EMOTIONS AND PHYSIOLOGICAL CHANGES

The involuntary nervous system under the control and direction of the lower brain responds to stimuli with an emotional context in a *prompt, uniform, and stereotyped manner*. In the lower brain there are centers for the expression of emotions and for the maintenance of the basic functions of the body concerned with survival of the organism, such as circulation, maintenance of body heat, circulation of body fluids, combustion of sugar, etc.

Cannon demonstrated clearly that when rage, fear, or other intense emotional states are expressed, there is an automatic, stereotyped response to them by the various body systems.[4]

Under such conditions, the gastro-intestinal body functions are inhibited, and the flow of salivary, gastric, and pancreatic juices may even come to a complete stop. Contrastingly, the functions of the cardiovascular system are sharply increased, resulting in altered coaguability of the blood, an increase in number of red blood corpuscles and in blood sugar, and higher levels of fat lipids and serum cholesterol in the bloodstream. In addition, the genito-urinary system undergoes an acceleration manifested by emptying of the bladder. Thus the lower brain and involuntary nervous system put the organism on a "war footing," and prepare it for "fight or flight." Simultaneously, the muscular system of the body tenses in anticipation of the coming physical action.

## CHRONIC EFFECTS OF EMOTIONS ON BODY FUNCTIONS

If emotional tension and emotional excitement are prolonged, the physical changes accompanying them become chronic in nature; or, if the body cannot adapt to it, the continued stress will lead to the development of organic symptoms and disease. Such disease resulting from prolonged overactivity of the involuntary nervous system under constant stress is termed psycho-physiological, psycho-somatic, or psychogenic disorder.

Set forth below are a few of the diseases that chronic emotional stress can cause to eventually affect various body systems:

*Musculo-Skeletal*: Arthritis, tension headaches, backache, muscle cramps, psychogenic rheumatism.

*Respiratory*: Asthma, common colds, hay fever, sinusitis, recurring bronchitis.

*Cardiovascular*: Hypertension, migraine headache, excessive heart beat, vascular spasm, anginal syndrome.

*Glandular*: Hyperthyroidism, diabetes, obesity.

*Dermatological*: Hives, allergic eczema.

*Gastro-Intestinal*: Colitis, peptic ulcer, constipation, gastritis, hyperacidity, heartburn, diarrhea.

*Genito-Urinary*: Impotence, frigidity, menstrual disorders, false pregnancy, infertility, painful urination, enuresis (bed wetting).

*Neurological*: Neurasthenia, anxiety reaction, body image disturbances.

*Sensory*: Disorders of smell, hearing, taste.

## STRESS DISORDERS

A great deal has been written of late on the topic of stress and the athlete. In origin, athletic stress may be biological, psychological, or both.

*Biological stresses* call upon the physical defenses of the body to adapt or eventually break down. Among these stresses are: (1) acute and chronic disease; (2) malnutrition; (3) excessive noise; (4) all kinds of handicaps and defects; (5) extreme heat or cold; (6) starvation; (7) poisoning; (8) injury; and (9) drugs.

*Psychological stresses* impact upon their victim's ego defenses by (1) threatening his sense of security, his confidence, and/or his will power; (2) producing feelings of anger, fear, grief, guilt, failure, disappointment, and/or tension; (3) depriving him of satisfaction of basic human needs and/or the opportunity to grow, develop, and fulfill his human potential.

*Social and cultural stresses* stem from (1) family and peer relationships; (2) school situations; (3) the opposite sex; (4) feelings about race, nationality, and/or national honor; and (5) coaches, trainers, teammates, and/or alumni. Pressures upon an athlete to perform well, and/or fear on his part that he will let down his supporters will generate anxiety and tension in varying degrees.

Anxiety and emotional tension are always accompanied by various degrees of muscle tension which fatigues muscles and renders them vulnerable to strain.

In some instances, a person will be simultaneously subjected to both biological and psychological stress. This occurs in athletics, combat, and natural catastrophe, as well as in extended illness, severe injury, and chronic fatigue arising from overwork, tension, or psychological conflict.

Even high-grade athletes of international caliber fall victim to stress, brought on by tensions and emotional conflicts to which the body or mind cannot adapt. Hanley surveyed the disease patterns of athletes at games in Rome (1960); Tokyo (1964); Winnipeg (1968); Mexico (1968); and Sapporo (1972).[7] He found that infections accounted for the largest number of clinic visits, with upper

218

respiratory tract, gastro-intestinal tract, and skin infections leading the list. Hanley stated that several physicians gained the impression that athletes seem to have more infections than non-athletes of the same age group; and that those who are trained down to the finest edge, such as endurance type athletes, are more susceptible than the rest. He speculated that this is probably due to the existence of a chronic fatigue factor in intensive training.

Hanley also found that chronic conditions (e.g., ulcers and diabetes), allergies, and emotional problems accounted for three of the seven categories of disease patterns.

In commenting on emotional problems, he pointed out that the motivating force which drives world-class athletes to compete in spite of disabilities is a strong one. This stands out clearly when a world-class athlete loses his motivation, that is, decides he is not willing to pay the price. He does not realize at first that this decision is under way. It usually appears several times in the consciousness of the athlete, and is rejected or repressed by him before he finally admits he has "had it." In some cases, this emotional conflict occurs just prior to a major competitive effort. All through his training for it, the athlete may have been experiencing nagging doubt about wanting to continue and, as the "moment of truth" draws near, his emotions become difficult to control.

Hanley related the case of a 34-year-old athlete involved in a sport where there was a real possibility of serious injury. This excellent athlete had experienced a series of injuries ranging from minor to moderately severe during the previous four months, which had left him actually terrified; but he continued to practice daily and to compete, because "it was expected." However, he experienced increasing tenseness, irritability, and insomnia. After a couple of tearful discussions, the athlete agreed that medical justification existed for his withdrawing from competition.

Patti pointed out that when an athlete is irrationally trained because of wrong timing, too few rest periods, improper technique or method, or when he is overtrained, i.e., has reached his best form but is attempting to obtain even better, he can develop—apart from harmful physical overfatigue—a condition of profound psycho-pathological depression.[15] When this happens, serious personality changes are observed, along with phenomena of anxiety, dejection, lack of confidence, and inferiorty.

Irrational training or overtraining may be due to a psychological factor on the part of the athlete, such as fear of failure; or it could be the result of faulty leadership by a coach or trainer who has wrongly interpreted the athlete's physical and psychological peak level (optimum readiness for competition).

Whether they are due to biological, psychological, social, cultural, or environmental factors (altitude, temperature, living conditions), the effect of stressor agents on athletes is manifested in various physiological symptoms. Indeed, training and competition are in themselves stressor agents. If others accompany them, mild physiological symptoms will develop. In the past, these symptoms have been identified with a condition of "staleness," resulting from overtraining. Today, they are recognized as warning signs that the body is failing to adapt to the increased stress and the athlete may be heading for a physiological or psychological breakdown.

Among the symptoms of impending physiological breakdown are: (1) sore throat; (2) excessive nervousness, depression, irritability, headaches, inability to relax, and insomnia; (3) constant fatigue; (4) persistent soreness and stiffness of the body's muscular system; (5) stomach pains; (6) loss of appetite and weight; (7) diarrhea or constipation; (8) various skin eruptions; (9) swelling and aching of the lymph glands; (10) lack of interest in life or exciting activities; and (11) increased muscular tension.

## PSYCHOLOGICAL PREDISPOSING FACTORS

Psychologists and psychiatrists specializing in the psychology of sports agree that there are characteristic types of personality patterns or psycho-neurotic disorders identified with the problem of injury prone athletes. Such injury prone individuals, due to acquired or unconscious motivational drives, enter the field of athletic competition accompanied by these patterns of behavior or disorders that can affect performance or act as predisposing factors to injuries and overuse syndromes.

These personality behavior patterns and psycho-neurotic disorders develop in the same manner: (1) Distorted relationships or damaging experiences arise in childhood within the family structure. (2) The child adopts certain personality patterns to attain personal security, or adopts faulty behavior patterns which will lessen his capacity for adjustment when faced with conflicts, problems, and inter-personal relationships later in life. (3) Because he cannot cope successfully or attain personal security, the child feels anxious and threatened. (4) To ward off anxiety and gain personal security, he reverts to infantile behavior and develops characteristic personality patterns. (5) In time, these patterns develop into rigid unconscious neurotic patterns of adaptive reactions to life.

Originally, personality trait disturbances and psycho-neurotic disorders arise from the small child's desire to satisfy his basic needs and acquire personal security, in contrast to his being frustrated in satisfying his needs and fearful of losing his personal security.

Subsequently, many factors may contribute to the development in the child of a faulty adaptation to the basic conflict. Among these are: (1) reactions to rejecting or dominating parents; (2) direct conditioning experiences in the home; (3) imitation of parental behavior; (4) jealousy of other children in the family; (5) feelings of failure and lack of self-acceptance stemming from unrealistic aspirations; (6) disturbing emotional experiences in childhood; (7) failures in inter-personal relationships with peers; (8) overprotective parents who smother the child and interfere with his development as an individual; (9) personality immaturity that leads to ego-centrism; (10) feelings of guilt, despair, and emptiness that leave the child without the courage to shape his own existence, causing him to yield instead to a shadow life of group conformity; and (11) an environment which threatens a child's self-image and sense of worth.

The following specific types of personality disturbances share a common denominator of immaturity, inability to maintain emotional stability, and failure to withstand minor stress. Their possessors revert to ineffectual childish behavior when subjected to stress or emotional conflict.

*Passive-Aggressive:* Various forms of emotional dependence accompanied by hidden or open resentment; expressed in predominantly passive dependence, passive aggressive, or active aggressive types of behavior.

*Compulsive*: Rigidity, inhibition, perfectionism, overconscientiousness, and inability to relax.

*Hysterical*: Self-centeredness, proneness to emotional outbursts and theatrical behavior to attact attention and dominate others.

*Obsessive*: Worry over trifles, imposition of severe standards on self and others, excessive orderliness and caution.

*Emotionally Unstable*: General excitability, inability to control emotional reactions, low stress tolerance, poorly controlled temper, lack of judgment under pressure.

*Immature*: Little control over emotions, inability to tolerate stress or frustration, reversion to infantile tactics and behavior when opposed.

Psycho-neurotic disorders are characterized by disturbing emotional symptoms and the use of exaggerated defense mechanisms in order to cope with underlying emotional conflicts and the anxiety they produce. There are six major types of reactive patterns: (1) conversion reaction; (2) dissociative reaction; (3) depressive reaction; (4) phobic reaction; (5) obsessive-compulsive reaction; and (6) anxiety reaction.

Ogilvie, who has tested some 40,000 athletes for psychological and motivational traits, pointed out that the athletes who realize their potential present a picture of extremely mature, symptom-free, non-neurotic young men.[14] Seventy percent of the athletes tested conformed to this positive picture. The other thirty percent may achieve greatness energized by motivational forces based upon satisfaction of neurotic needs, but their performances will be highly variable. On any one day, or on any one occasion, such an athlete may be a winner or end up last in the contest.

Ogilvie and Tutko, commenting on the effect of deep unconscious emotional conflicts as causes of neurosis, noted that the two most frequently found neurotic reactive patterns among track men are obsessive compulsiveness and anxiety depression.[11]

In an *obsessive-compulsive* reaction, the individual unconsciously seeks to ward off dangerous impulses by becoming preoccupied with persistent irrational thoughts and actions which are symbolically related to these impulses. He shows outward symptoms of obsessive thoughts or compulsive acts.

In an *anxiety-depressive* reaction, the individual gives in to defeat, failure, or other setbacks because when he tries to face his problems directly he is overwhelmed by anxiety. He shows outward symptoms of despair, discouragement, and resignation.

## THE INJURY PRONE PERSONALITY

As indicated earlier, certain emotional traits, personality traits, and behavior patterns mark the injury prone person, regardless of his field of activity or endeavor. Yost, writing about industrial workers, stated:

> Studies have listed personality traits which lead to accidents. Some of these traits are aggressiveness, anger, attention getting, being easily offended, competitiveness with inability to lose, excitability, feelings of inferiority or superiority, frequent conflict with authority, frustration, guilt feelings, and unconscious need for self-punishment.[20]

Dunbar, in his 1947 study of accident prone industrial workers, found they displayed traits of impulsiveness, concentration on daily pleasure with little interest in long-term goals, and extreme resentment of authority.[5] Most had evidenced neurotic traits in childhood, such as bed wetting; sleep walking or talking; constant use of minor illness to escape responsibilities or punishment; and persistent lying, stealing, and truancy. Later in life, these tendencies disappeared and were replaced by the accident habit. He went on to point out that the personality patterns of accident prone persons tend to match those of the juvenile delinquent and adult criminal. Their early childhood history is one of poor adjustment to authority in home or school, usually accompanied by a story of outright or subtle parental rejection.

Montanini, *et al.*, in 1965, maintained that there is a different psychogenous pattern distinguishing the amateur from the professional accident prone athlete.[9] The accident prone amateur athlete will exhibit hostility toward superiors (resulting from unsolved family problems going back to childhood); impulsiveness; a disorderly tendency to adventure and evasion; superficiality; bursts of aggression; anti-conformism; moods tending toward depression; and fickleness in feelings and attitudes. The accident prone professional athlete, on the other hand, will exhibit psychogenetic mechanisms more akin to those of workers in general, i.e., feelings of embarrassment, inferiority, or superiority as regards the work done; difficulties in inter-personal relations with fellow workers, etc.

They contend that, in general, accident prone athletes have a very rigid super-id (conscience and guilt), and nurture an unconscious hostility toward the sport they practice. Only by having an accident (thereby punishing themselves) can their guilt feelings be placated.

In writings by Ryan[17] and Seaton,[18] the injury prone athlete has also been characterized as easily distracted; emotionally unstable; sometimes extremely aggressive and intolerant of others demonstrating an attitude of superiority; and exhibiting patterns of repressed anger, strong feelings of inferiority, and a desire to be the center of attention.

Beisser, in the book *The Madness in Sports*,[3] and Goff, in a paper on "The Injury Prone Athlete,"[6] have affirmed that an athletic injury may be used by the athlete to escape—from an intolerable situation or from pressure to perform well that has become too great.

It is well-established in psychosomatic literature that when anxiety has been building up for a long time, due to its victim's inability to solve an emotional conflict, a clinical syndrome called conversion reaction (hysteria) may develop, with attendant psychosomatic symptoms. With the appearance of the physical symptoms, the anxiety disappears. They remove the individual from the anxiety situation, gain him sympathy and the attention of others, and many times fulfill the needs that initially generated the anxiety.

One general practitioner in England documented several cases of athletes suffering from minor injuries who were actually trying to escape from unpleasant emotional decisions and the anxiety that accompanied them by means of the conversion reaction syndrome.[1] One of these involved a female athlete, pre-eminent in her sport, who had been suffering from a chronic leg injury for a long period of time. She had earlier developed a pseudo father-daughter relationship with her coach—a close friend of her deceased father. The coach had high hopes for her and expected her to do well.

As it turned out, she had become engaged to be married. By developing the leg injury, she was able to take time away from practice to spend with her fiance without disappointing her coach. The injury also provided an excuse for not performing well due to the lack of practice. Subsequently, she married and the leg injury disappeared.

Slatton has written of the pressures of society (peer groups) that force the athlete to opt for injury rather than continued participation.[19] Group pressure raises the level of aspiration and sometimes contributes to an overestimation of one's abilities. Tension results, the athlete is afraid of group disapproval should he fail, and injury gives him a socially acceptable "out."

Motivations are based on biological needs and human wants. Wants are in turn based on psychological and social drives. Ogilvie identified *conscious* motivational factors that may be associated with athletes.[14] They include: (1) affiliative need or need to "belong;" (2) desire for social approval; (3) status motives; (4) security motives; and (5) the achievement motive.

The most complex motives, however, are buried in the *unconscious*. They are disguised by such psychological mechanisms as rationalization, regression, repression, and sublimation. According to Maslow's and Mittlemann's *Principles of Abnormal Psychology*, unconscious motives usually involve the avoidance of pain, danger, or emotional hurt, or the protection of self-esteem or security.[8]

Ogilvie and Tutko pioneered the research on the personal traits of the successful athlete and the psychological traits and adaptive behavior patterns of the problem athlete.[11] The injury prone athlete is in the latter category. Their classic *Problem Athletes and How to Handle Them* should be required reading for every coach, trainer, and medical specialist dealing with athletes, regardless of the level of competition involved, and it has served as the primary source for the following discussion.

Ogilvie and Tutko grouped injury prone athletes into three major categories: the bonafide injury prone athlete, the psychologically injured prone athlete, and the malingering athlete.

### BONAFIDE INJURY PRONE ATHLETE

This type of injury prone athlete is unduly critical of himself. His standards are beyond his reach, and his failure to come up to them constitutes self-punishment. Others in this category are often frightened of their underlying hostile or aggressive tendencies. To injure someone makes their hostility very real to them. Self-punishment is not the only unconscious motivation applicable to this group, however. In many instances, the incurring of injury serves to punish others, often parents, against whom they cannot openly express hostility for fear of disapproval or loss of love.

The athlete who has been pushed into sports which he does not like by an athletically frustrated father may hate the father for it and yet be afraid to quit and risk being disapproved of or rejected by that father. This type of injury prone athlete is the offspring of particularly hard and overbearing parents, whose demands on their children have been extreme. In such a family, where the value of getting to the top by rugged individualistic means is over-

224

emphasized, rewards are hard to come by. Success brings only temporary expression of affection. The athlete can feel accepted only if he works himself relentlessly, especially if there are other children in the family. Any type of failure of his part is subtly or overtly criticized as falling short of the accomplishments of other athletes or even of his brothers and sisters.

## PSYCHOLOGICALLY INJURY PRONE ATHLETE

There is no more perplexing athlete than one who continually complains of injury or pain when no medical evidence can be found to support his claim. This type of athlete experiences a high degree of anxiety and apprehension, and his defense against this may take the form of the conversion hysteria syndrome discussed earlier in this chapter.

The general clinical picture of the psychologically injury prone athlete is one of an anxiety prone, very dependent, almost infantile person, attempting by athletics to satisfy his dependency needs. To be injured is to succeed in this, since it means others must take care of him. These athletes are not without a touch of showmanship. They limp just a little more than necessary and in such a fashion that they immediately attract attention. All of their reactions to injury extend beyond the normal.

Most psychologically injury prone athletes are just average in ability. By being injured, they gain more of the attention and sense of importance their dependent personalities crave than they could through use of their talents. They also feel threatened by those whose ability is superior to their own and live in constant fear of being replaced, which to them would equal rejection or abandonment.

Hence injury serves this athlete in two-fold fashion. It enables him to avoid the responsibility of really testing (and thereby exposing) the limits of his potential, and it calls forth the attention and sympathy he desperately needs in order to be reassured that others do care about him.

A psychologically injury prone athlete will emerge from a family in which the parents are rejective and non-giving. Their standards for love and acceptance are high, usually just out of his reach, so that he must continually do a little more to achieve either. The rejection, however, is subtly extended; he cannot be loved even in winning. Such parents are too much concerned about their children. They are continually looking after them. Although they reject them, they also keep a close rein on them. Often the child's health is a major worry, and at the slightest indication of illness the parents become deeply involved. (Some parents interpret this concern as an indication of love for the child.) Children thus learn to use sickness or injury as a means of escaping from punishment and, at the same time, gaining attention. For them, that attention has to substitute for acceptance.

*N.B.*: Pain tolerance and pain threshold must be considered when discussing the injury prone athlete. Over-protective and apprehensive parents generally make their children's health a major issue. If an insecure child finds he can gain undue attention and sympathy and escape from responsibility through very minor illness, he will develop a low threshold of pain. As athletes, these persons are constant visitors to the training room complaining of minor aches and pains. Studies have shown that the superior athlete has a greater tolerance and higher threshold of pain than the average athlete. He can train more vigorously, continue longer in competition, and require less treatment after an injury.

## MALINGERING ATHLETE

The most complete reason for feigning an injury is to avoid athletic practice, and there are several varieties of athlete given to doing so:

1. *Veteran athletes*, who feel they know all there is to be known and that any future practice will be of little if any benefit to them.

2. *Hypochondriacal athletes*, who feign injury because they feel they actually will be injured in practice.

3. *Vindictive athletes*, aware of their value to the team and intent on "getting even with" or "paying back" a coach.

4. *Untalented athletes*, aware of their shortcomings and afraid that if they expose them they will be dropped from the team or group—to which they want very much to belong.

5. *Disinterested athletes*, naturally talented but negative toward the sport; pressured into it, or in search of other rewards. For these athletes, quitting is difficult—either because they are unable to resist the pressures put upon them if they do so, or because they feel they owe the sport and the people supporting them a sort of debt. They are willing to participate in active competition; but practice is more than they can stomach.

Again, these different types of malingering athletes come from similar family backgrounds, wherein as children they used lies to escape from responsibilities, to avoid being held accountable for their actions, to obtain sympathy, and to gain attention. Such a background usually involves overly protective parents. The child is never confronted with the reality of a situation, and he is able to control, manipulate, and even be excused or rewarded for lying. The parents continue to defend him or rationalize his behavior, despite the fact that the child is obviously in error.

## PASSIVITY VERSUS AGGRESSION

Moore stressed the conflict between passivity and aggression as a basic predisposing factor in the development of the injury prone athlete.[10] He maintained that each growing child must learn how to achieve an uneasy compromise between his urges to be actively aggressive motor-wise and his wishes to be pleasing to his parents. He also contended that the expression of aggression in today's world has been blurred by the roles men and women play in the home. The father may like ball games and playing golf; but he is also expected to wash dishes, make the beds, and help with household chores. He does not appear as powerful as the mother. As a result, the young boy is less certain as to what is acceptable male aggressive behavior and he becomes confused.

In a typical middle class culture, parents desire their children to be "well-adjusted," that is, "well-controlled." The young boy soon learns that uncontrolled aggressive behavior brings him not gain, but pain—as he is punished through withdrawal by his parents of their love and approval, or by stern criticism from his teachers, and probable loss of comradeship with his peers. The equation becomes clear to him: To express aggression means to receive aggression in return—sometimes greater than he can tolerate or defend himself against.

The young boy incorporates this disapproval; if he is too aggressive, he develops feelings of guilt and anxiety, and ultimately even the contemplation of aggression brings on a sense of uneasiness. At this point, he can be labeled "civilized" and "well-adjusted."

Moore pointed out, however, that society contains two situations where aggression is not only permitted, but encouraged and rewarded—war and sports.

In World War II, the psychiatric disabilities among infantrymen resulting from conflict within them between passivity and aggression almost overwhelmed our medical facilities. Infantrymen who had been trained to impartially, impersonally, and in cold blood kill enemy troops refused to fire their guns, even in self-defense, and waited passively in their fox holes. Even in training camps, psychiatric breakdown occurred in men who could not even tolerate the aggression demanded of them in bayonet drill against straw dummies.

Participation in sport, on the other hand, is voluntary and aggression there is rewarded. As noted earlier, the young boy faces a dilemma, particularly during adolescence, in defining his masculine and sexual roles.[10] The athlete has always, in the past, been idolized as a symbol of masculinity. What better way could there be, then, for a boy to assert his own masculinity than by becoming an athlete? However, it may happen that neither a boy's talent nor his underlying aggressiveness is sufficient to meet the requirements of the chosen sport or to enable him to fulfill his human potential within it.

Moore described two types of athlete in whom proneness to injury is due to an underlying conflict between passivity and aggressiveness. In one type, the young athlete wants to prove himself by being more aggressive than his ability allows him to be; so he must extricate himself by injury before he is defeated—thus avoiding any final proof of what he feels others will perceive to be his unmanliness. In the second type, a boy with great athletic potential cannot allow himself to manifest it because evidence of the aggressive component of this talent would cause a decrease in his passivity-demanding parents' love for him. Here, too, injury is the ideal way out.

In his studies of successful athletes, Ogilvie determined that a very high degree of aggressiveness is a key trait among them.[12] The achieving athlete must be aggressive to the point of confronting other players and opponents with his need not only to compete with them, but to walk right over them. In discussing this trait, Ogilvie quoted golfers Arnold Palmer and Gary Player, who told him: "In order to win in this game you have to retain the killer instinct." Each of these men, according to Ogilvie, had discovered that winning demands an aggressive, dominating, and extroverted spirit.

He agreed with Moore that the injury prone personality is developed early in life out of a background of inter-personal relationships and attitudes within the family. As an adult, the possessor of this personality will instinctively react with feelings of guilt whenever he is called upon to express any form of aggression, and in sports he will psychologically retreat from competition, either by incurring injury or losing the contest.

## REFERENCES

1. Anonymous, "Some Psychological Factors in Sports Medicine," *Coaching Newsletter,* May-August 1964.
2. Antonelli, F., "Psychopathology and Psychotherapy in the Sporting Phenomenon," *International Congress of Sports Psychology,* Rome, April 1965.
3. Beisser, Arnold R., *The Madness in Sports* (New York: Appleton-Century Crofts, 1967).
4. Cannon, Walter B., "The Mechanism of Emotional Disturbances of Bodily Functions," *New England Journal of Medicine,* June 14, 1928.
5. Dunbar, Flanders, *Mind and Body: Psychosomatic Medicine* (New York: Random House, 1947).
6. Goff, Robert, "The Injury Prone Athlete," Paper presented to the *6th Annual Illinois Swimming Association Clinic.*

7. Hanley, Daniel F., "Health Problems at the Olympic Games," *Journal of the American Medical Association,* August 28, 1972.

8. Maslow, A. H., and Mittlemann, B., *Principles of Abnormal Psychology* (New York: Harper and Brothers, 1951).

9. Montanini, R.; Mastruzzo, A.; and Zucchi, V.; "Psychological and Psychopathological Aspects of Sporting Accidents," *International Congress of Sports Psychology,* Rome, April 1965.

10. Moore, Robert A., "Psychological Factors in Athletic Injuries," *Journal of the Michigan State Medical Society,* December 1960.

11. Ogilvie, Bruce C., and Tutko, Thomas A., *Problem Athletes and How to Handle Them* (London: Pelham Books, 1966).

12. Ogilvie, Bruce C., "Build a Winning Psychology," *Golf Digest,* November 1966.

13. Ogilvie, Bruce C., "Psychosocial Variables That Influence Attitudes Toward Injury," *Sports Psychology Bulletin,* March 1971.

14. Ogilvie, Bruce C., "Future Contribution of Motivational Research in Track," *Track Technique,* September 1963.

15. Patti, M., "Psychopathological Effects of Irrational Training and Overtraining," *International Congress of Sports Psychology,* Rome, April 1965.

16. Pollini, L. M., "Frequency of Psychopathological Elements in 418 Italian Athletes Selected for the Olympic Games," *International Congress of Sports Psychology,* Rome, April 1965.

17. Ryan, Allan J., "Prevention of Sports Injury: A Problem Solving Approach," *Journal of Health, Physical Education and Recreation,* April 1971.

18. Seaton, Don C., *Safety in Sports* (New York: Prentice-Hall, Inc., 1948).

19. Slatton, Bonnie, "The Injury Prone Athlete," *Athletic Training* March 1975.

20. Yost, Charles P., "Total Fitness and Prevention of Accidents," *Journal of Health, Physical Education and Recreation,* March 1967.

## RECOMMENDED READING

*Problem Athletes and How to Handle Them*

by

Bruce Ogilvie and Thomas Tutko

This book is a classic. It can be purchased direct from the author, Dr. Bruce Ogilvie, at San Jose State University, San Jose, California, or from *Track and Field News*, P.O. Box 296, Los Altos, California, or *Runner's World*, P.O. Box 366, Mountain View, California.

# Part Three

## The How of Prevention and Correction

# 21

# Exercises in
# Prevention and Correction

In discussing what role exercise plays in preventing or correcting muscle imbalance and postural and foot faults, the reader should keep three important points in mind:

1. As pointed out in Chapter 6, every person begins life with a high degree of muscle imbalance and there is no such thing as a perfectly complete muscle balance in the human body. If the human born with a predominant flexor strength, in comparison to extensor strength, fails to develop a comparable relative strength of the anti-gravity extensor muscles, the result is postural and foot faults and predisposition to strains, sprains, and overuse syndromes.

2. Exercise *per se* is not a complete answer to correcting postural or foot faults that results from congenital structural defects, diseases, traumatic injuries, or arthritis or from long-standing postural or foot faults that have altered the structural skeleton of the upper body, legs, or feet.

3. With respect to the factors being discussed, more emphasis will be placed on correction and rehabilitation than on prevention. Statistical studies over the past 60 years bear out the veracity of this statement.

In Chapter 6, several studies of children and adults which showed the high degree of muscular imbalance evidenced in the general population and among athletes were summarized. As to postural faults, the Chelsea study found that over 80 percent of 1,708 children and adolescents between 5 and 18 years of age exhibited poor or bad posture.[12, 18] A Harvard University survey of 746 adults disclosed that 80.3 percent displayed poor or bad posture.[2] Cook's testing of 1,393 students disclosed that only 25 percent exhibited a normal spinal curvature.[5] Cerney's statement that 80 percent of

233

American athletes have weak feet gains support from the findings of numerous foot specialists during the past 60 years, i.e., that 80 to 85 percent of the general population in industrialized societies have weak feet.[3]

The statistics and estimates quoted above and in previous chapters include various degrees of mild, moderate, and serious deviation from a normal body alignment and a relative inequality in balance of flexors and extensor muscles.

## CORRECTION
### Posture

It has been well established among orthopedic, osteopathic, physical medicine, and corrective physical education authorities that exercise, in addition to postural reflex training and elimination of any psychological or nutritional problems, plays a highly important role in the correction of postural faults.

Corrective exercises applied by Phelps and Kiputh to 3,503 college students with mild, moderate, and severe postural faults produced the following results:[18] Forward head and shoulders—41% completely corrected, 27% improved; forward shoulders—84% completely corrected, 4% improved; kyphosis—44% completely corrected, 23% improved; lordosis—36% completely corrected, 35% improved; moderate scoliosis—49% completely corrected, 27% improved; severe scoliosis—21% completely corrected, 27% improved.

Cook compiled complete records on 500 Yale college students over a two-year period, which, through testing, he had classified by specific postural faults graded in severity from one to four.[5] They were given 15 weeks of corrective postural exercise. Commenting on the results, Cook pointed out that he and his co-workers saw complete correction of 212 cases and partial correction of 145 cases out of a total of 428 cases of forward head and neck, and complete correction of 101 cases and partial correction of 94 cases of lateral curves varying from one-quarter to one inch out of a total of 280 cases of scoliosis. With respect to various faults in the antereoposterior plane, they were able to completely correct 66 cases and partially correct 116 cases of kypholordosis (total round back—see Chapter 10, Figure 7) out of a total of 274 cases, and to completely correct 53 cases and partially correct 8 cases of kyphosis (round upper back) out of a total of 103 cases.

Cook noted that in his experience with the group the correction of total round back (kypholordosis) was the most difficult to achieve. In England, some 10 years later, Wiles made the same observation on correcting the total round back.[21] He stated that the difficulty was due to the lack of normal mobility in the upper lumbar and lower dorsal regions of the spine.

All postural authorities maintain that serious acquired postural faults or those due to congenital factors that have affected the skeletal structure and alignment of the spine can be corrected only by surgery, casts, and various types of corsets. Exercise, however, plays an important role in the rehabilitation process.

## Leg Alignment

Internal or external rotation at the hip joints that creates internal rotation of the thighs and a pronated foot, or outward rotation of the entire leg with toed-out foot position, can be corrected by exercise and changes in foot position during walking. Excessive degrees of knock-knee or bowlegs can be corrected up to three or four years of age by exercise and braces. Kite demonstrated how excessive internal tibial torsion and pigeon-toes or excessive external tibial torsion and toeing out can be corrected up to two or three years of age by manipulative exercises performed on the child by the mother.[11] Hyperextended knees can be corrected by exercise only if due to obesity or muscular imbalance, not if the condition is one of compensation for bowleg or internal tibial torsion. If the quadriceps is stronger than the hamstrings, the goal is to strengthen the latter group of muscles; if the reverse is true, the goal is to strengthen the quadriceps.

## Foot Faults

Studies concerning the effect of exercise on correction of foot faults appear infrequently in the literature. However, over the last 70 years, several hundred articles and books on orthopedics, osteopathics, physical medicine, physical education, and surgical and general medicine have dealt exclusively with problems related to the foot, including faults, congenital defects, and anomalies. Of the many researched by the writer—including works by 59 orthopedic specialists, 5 surgeons, 5 chiropodists (now known as podiatrists), 13 corrective physical education specialists, and 1 anatomist—all recommended foot exercises as an integral part of prevention, correction, and rehabilitation of weak feet, strained feet, pronated feet, abducted toed-out feet, and non-rigid minor grades of acquired functional flat foot.

Since the start of this century, the approach to the correction and treatment of foot faults has included: (1) properly fitted shoes; (2) exercises; (3) manipulation; (4) deep heat; (5) contrast hot and cold foot baths; (6) proper use of the foot in walking; (7) flexible casts and taping; (8) massage; (9) retraining of postural reflexes; (10) custom-made shoe inserts or arch supports (orthotics); and (11) surgery.

Ignoring most of these methods, particularly exercise and manipulation, today's podiatrists specializing in the treatment of foot problems among runners depend almost exclusively on the use of orthotics in correcting foot faults and foot plant problems during running. This fact is substantiated by the editors of *Runner's World* magazine in their publication *The Athlete's Feet.*[8]

It should be noted that three specialists—Wiles,[22] Lowman,[15] and Graham[10]—who emphasized in their writings that poor pelvic posture associated with the internal rotation of the thighs was a major factor in developing the pronated foot also maintained that the treatment and correction of the common foot faults of pronation and/or abduction could not be successful unless there was at the same time correction of upper body faults.

## CORRECTIVE EXERCISE

This writer is strongly in favor of exercise as a contribution to the prevention, treatment, and correction of muscular imbalance and foot postural faults, and the following discussion serves to support that position.

Pollock conducted an experiment on public school children among whom were 30 with weak foot and arch strain, 38 with beginning stages of flat foot, and 29 with advanced type of flat foot.[19] They were given 28 periods of corrective exercises over a seven-week period, which also included prescription of proper shoes, massage, and contrast foot baths. The results of this experiment showed that in 75 percent of 97 children some sort of improvement took place.

Funk divided a group of 30 high school students aged 14 to 16 and displaying various degrees of foot eversion (25-degree toeing out) and/or pronation, into two groups of 15 each.[9] Experimental and control tests on vertical jump reach and 100-yard run and a rope skip trial of 100 feet were given all 30 boys. The experimental group was given four resistance foot exercises and its members were encouraged to walk on the outside of their feet, with an exaggerated inversion of the feet, during the day. The experiment covered a period of five weeks (25 days). Funk's findings revealed that "despite the relatively short time of exercise administered, more than one inch was added to the vertical jump reach and the time of the 100-yard dash was reduced four-tenths of a second."

Vorobiev, the Russian track and field team physician, commenting on the problems of pronation and metatarsal arch problems among runners, joggers, jumpers, race walkers, and throwers, recommended specialized exercises to increase the functional capabilities of the foot both in prevention and in treatment of these problems.[20] He also provided one of the best explanations why today's podiatrists and sports medicine physicians emphasize orthotics and other mechanical means of treatment rather than exercise:

> In comparison with the hand, the foot is not so flexible and that is why exercises for its development are not very dynamic, do not have

emotional appeal and quickly become boring. The number of exercises directed primarily towards developing the muscles of the foot is relatively small. The effect of these exercises takes place after two to three months of regular daily practice. But not everyone has enough patience to do these exercises day after day. Some sportsmen lose faith in these exercises and give up doing them.

Osgood, commenting in 1942 on his 30 years' experience in correcting the pronated foot due to muscle imbalance through exercise, made a like observation.

> Most patients still expect a pill to cure these ills; almost as many pin their faith to an injection. A small number are willing to be massaged and exercised if the physical therapist does most of the work.[17]

Lewin, in describing the treatment for pronated valgus foot found in adolescents with long, slender, rapidly-growing feet or who are overweight noted that the objectives of the treatment are to teach proper walking, to increase the power of the supporting structures, to increase the local circulation, to support the weakened structures, to produce supination, and to correct the associated pathology, such as knock-knee, bowlegs, etc.[13] He stated that the methods of attaining these objectives included prescribing proper shoes, exercises, massage, contrast foot baths, felt pads, plaster of paris casts, and surgery. He further stated that exercises are the most important factor in the treatment of all forms of pronated flat foot other than those involving rigid flat foot or congenitally short Achilles tendons (which require surgery).

Bettman, quoting the definition of orthopedics given by Dr. Andry in 1741, i.e., "the art of preventing or correcting deformities in childhood," claimed this applies especially to the feet, as the foot is the victim of degenerating shoe styles, which mark it as the most neglected organ of the human body—in spite of the fact that next to the brain it is the most distinguishing feature of the human race.[1] Further, he maintained that "the resulting mechanical and muscular disorders can be corrected by proper exercises, the wearing of plates being restricted to a minimum. The exercise treatment applies to all weak feet due to a pronation valgus position of the heel." (See Chapter 18, Figure 46).

In treating chronic foot strain of the postural type, McMillar recommended manipulation followed by active exercises.[16] In treatment of flat foot, he first altered shoes or shoe inserts, but insisted that exercises were the most important factor in treatment of this condition because they improved mobility and strength.

Graham pointed out that success in the treatment of weak foot due to poor posture depends upon the intelligent employment by the doctor and the patient of five separate but simultaneous lines of attack: (1) maintenance of correct posture; (2) proper use of feet in walking; (3) exercise for the re-education of foot and leg muscles; (4) properly constructed shoes that fit correctly; and (5) a temporary crutch in the form of an arch support.[10]

Commenting on arch supports, Graham stated:

The arch support is the factor of least importance in the uncomplicated weak foot; in the complicated weak foot, it plays a very important role. Great caution must be exercised with the support. It is a temporary measure and it should be used only after the patient fully appreciates that the arch support will not cure his condition and that it is the factor of least importance in the treatment. Its value of aiding easily exhausted muscles and in giving the patient the feel of correct foot posture is overshadowed and invalidated when the patient thinks the support is the cure.

Diveley, in commenting on the correction of foot imbalance, stated:

Supports, shoes, braces, and strapping may hold the foot in the corrected position and relieve pain and discomfort, but such measures must be considered only as passive agents. One must add to these measures others of an active character, which are the true and natural supports of both the longitudinal and transverse arches. This building up can be accomplished only by exercises carefully planned and consistently executed.[6]

In discussing treatment of the painful foot, Drew wrote:

Certain mechanical aids (orthotics) to treatment have been described, but they should be considered as being of an interim nature only. Their value lies in protecting and adjusting the foot pending its more complete rehabilitation by physical medicine. Physiotherapy as applied to the treatment of the painful foot includes manipulation, application of heat, and exercises.[7]

Wiles, in discussing the treatment of postural pes valgus (various degrees of pronation), distinguished four types of cases, two of which are important to this discussion: (1) those due to forward pelvic tilt and internal rotation of the legs, and (2) those—the great majority—in which the faulty posture of the foot is due to muscular failure.[21] In the latter group, Wiles maintained, exercises strengthen muscles, but they are not the right approach to the acquisition of a new habitual posture. The person must develop new postural reflex habits. He pointed out that the function of exercises is mainly to teach the patient to move into the new foot posture and to give him conscious control over the movements involved, and he devised exercises to accomplish this objective. As to arch supports, Wiles noted that it has been shown that it is anatomically impossible for supports alone to correct the fault. The most they can accomplish is to give some help to a patient who can produce a voluntary correction. The object is to teach the muscles to maintain a new posture, and any mechanical aid is likely to interfere with the acquisition of the new muscle balance.

In commenting on the chronic foot strain of valgus feet, Wiles pointed out two methods of treatment. One of these is palliative, and it aims at preventing full movement of joints so that strain falls on the "adhesion." Arch supports are used for this purpose and they provide temporary relief. The other method of treatment is curative. The "adhesions" are ruptured by manipulation and prevented from reforming by subsequent massage and exercises.

The authors cited in the above discussion are men who have devoted a great part of their careers as orthopedic physicians to specializing in foot problems among the general population.

For a final corroboration of his contention that exercise is necessary in the correction of foot faults, the writer requested Dr. J. V. Cerney, a present-day doctor of podiatry and a doctor of physical medicine with long experience in the handling of athletic injuries, to evaluate a chapter on orthotics in the *Runner's World* publication *The Athlete's Feet*.[8] Cerney selected three items for comment:[4]

1. "This type of appliance (orthotics) offers functional control."

*Cerney's Opinion:* In athletics, and in motion, such an appliance controls nothing. It can only guide. It can only gently persuade the foot into postural balance that aids athletic mobility. It is true that they (orthotics) do not weaken the feet. They provide a temporary crutch until such time as physical therapy and exercising reestablish the duties of muscles, tendons, and ligaments that establish the capability of the foot to do its job. It is true they do reduce "overuse." So would a crutch. So does getting the boy off his feet. But what does this solve?

2. "The use of orthotics is to normalize abnormal feet."

*Cerney's Opinion:* At no time can feet be normalized. Especially by arch supports, prosthetics, etc. Orthotics only assist in finding an environment conductive to establishing comfort and producing a more stable postural balance. An exercise program may help to do this. Physical therapy may assist. Nutritional controls help. Taping helps. Surgery establishes new weight-bearing points. But orthotics normalizing abnormal feet? Never in a million years.

3. "Does the athlete become dependent on orthotics?"

*Cerney's Opinion:* Yes, he does. He does so only when the doctor has failed to correct the reasons for mechanical dysfunction in the first place. In other words, muscles, ligaments, tendons, and possible congenital bone defects create many difficulties in athletics. Orthotics, in this case, become an unwholesome crutch. They are an admission of failure. They are "something to do" when you can't solve the problem. Using such a device in athletics should always be a temporary adjunct until the real job gets done.

## PREVENTION

All authorities in the athletic world believe that a high level of athletic fitness (strength, flexibility, endurance, and agility), along with proper application of skills, is the best protection against incurring injuries. However, general athletic fitness does nothing to stop the further progress of muscular imbalance or postural and foot faults that may be only minor in degree but will surely progress further if they are not corrected or eliminated at the start of an athlete's career.

Zohar, in commenting on preventive conditioning for athletes in relation to muscular imbalance, stated:

> When an engineer designs a structure, he calculates the maximum anticipated stress, then adds a safety factor to cover unexpected contingencies. In most athletic training programs, the safety factor is either missing or insufficient. Remember the old saying about a chain being only as strong as its weakest link? The approach to the athlete's body is being ignored in the conventional conditioning program. The coach fails to detect and strengthen the weak links. He fails to condition the athlete's muscles equitably, to see that not a single muscle weakness remains uncorrected, as one poorly conditioned muscle can cause an injury. What is needed is a different kind of conditioning—preventive conditioning—which isolates the weaknesses, corrects them, and builds into the body a high safety factor against abnormal forces...To provide maximum muscle protection against injuries to any part of the leg, it is necessary to individually condition every muscle group in both legs to levels far beyond the normal requirements of the sport.[23]

Lowman, the pioneer in relating postural and foot faults to athletic performance, pointed out that an inventory of any elementary or junior high school will reveal postural deviations in from 60 to 80 percent of students, the exact percentage depending on the skill of the examiners.[1] The principal deviations will be found in the feet, legs, and shoulder girdles. However, 40 to 50 percent of students will exhibit a lateral tilt of the pelvis or short leg. He wrote as follows:

> Since the body machine is subject to the same biomechanical laws as an inanimate machine, we may think of the bony structure as the shafts or working parts, the joints (where these parts articulate) as the bearings, and the muscular system as the motors that make the machines go. We are all familiar enough with automobiles to understand what is meant by "wear and tear." But teachers of physical education and coaches often think in terms of muscle action or motors rather than of joints or bearings. This wear and tear element is definitely proportionate to the alignment of shafts and bearings. Hence structural deviations of skeletal parts, as evidenced by postural faults, indicate muscular insufficiency in the anti-gravity muscles, and faulty

neuromuscular habits, as well as hereditary factors and environmental stresses which act on the malaligned body machine.

Lowman went on to point out that in making the analogy to an inanimate machine, there is one notable difference—growth. Structural growth takes place in the epiphyses or growth centers (the growth plates at the end of the long bones), and the ossifying centers in the irregular bones. These centers appear at various ages. Growth cartilages at adolescence are under maximum stimulation and are very sensitive to stress and trauma. Their vulnerability is increased when height or weight (or both) are disproportionate to physiological age and when asymmetries of alignment in body segments exist:

> When, in the presence of rapid growth, postural faults also exist, the addition of further stress from athletic activities increases the possibility of injury to these growth cartilages as well as to the joint components (ligaments, lining, cartilage, and muscle attachments).

This observation also applies to overuse syndromes. The reader will recall that the statistics of injury and overuse syndromes presented in Chapter 4 disclosed that the largest number of runners suffering from chondromalacia of the kneecap were in the 14- to 16-year-old age group.

Lowman commented that the occurrence of acute traumatic episodes, such as fractures, dislocations, sprains, strains, muscle and ligament tears, is not the major issue. It is the minute day-after-day trauma to the growing skeleton that should be taken into account:

> Frequent results of this wear and tear that physicians and orthopedic specialists rate in the post-school years are early signs of arthritic changes in and about the joints, slipping or displacement of femoral epiphyses, osteo-chondritic sequele in spine, upper tibial growth plate (Osgood-Schlatter) syndrome, neuritis and muscle soreness in the shoulder girdle area, sciatic and low back symptoms, and leg aches and cramps.

No other athletes subject the joints of the feet, ankles, knees, and pelvis to the continual repetitive stresses that middle and long distance runners or the physical fitness joggers do; and it should be noted that the jogger uses a shorter stride, with a greater up and down movement than the competitive runner and also performs more on hard pavements and roads.

## OBJECTIVES OF PREVENTIVE AND CORRECTIVE EXERCISE PROGRAMS

The basic objectives of a preventive program, as it relates to the further development of muscular imbalance and postural and foot faults, are two-fold:

1. Develop a balanced and strong musculature around the most vulnerable body joints.

2. Increase the range of movement of body joints where required, and insure that correct body alignment of the structural skeleton is maintained.

The basic objectives of a corrective exercise program are to eliminate the wide degree of muscular imbalance around body joints, and to correct where possible the skeletal misalignment through exercise, training of postural reflexes, and correction of poor foot positions in walking and running.

To truly accomplish these objectives, the coach and the trainer will undoubtedly require the assistance of various specialists— orthopedic physicians, osteopathic physicians, physical medicine physicians, podiatrists, physical therapists, and corrective physical education specialists.

## CONCLUSION

It is doubtful whether any young prospective athlete, when first entering the athletic world, will fail to display a high degree of muscle imbalance in one or more muscle groups or fail to show evidence of one or more minor postural deviations. The coach and trainer can easily correct muscular imbalance or lack of flexibility with properly selected strength development and flexibility exercises. This depends on adequate testing and screening and on the absence of serious postural or foot faults.

Because hidden congenital defects or anomalies cannot be determined by visual observation only, it is this writer's firm conviction that X-rays should be taken of every young athlete's spine, pelvis, legs, and feet.

Any athlete displaying even minor postural or foot faults should be sent to an orthopedic physician who is posture oriented, or to a podiatrist who is posture and sports oriented, for examination. To prescribe corrective exercise in these cases without a complete medical examination is to do a great disservice to a young boy or girl. Any reader who is not convinced of this should read Lowman's and Young's book *Postural Fitness*.[15] In it they cite many cases of improperly used exercises that seriously damaged the skeletal and anatomical structures of the adolescent boys and girls involved.

## REFERENCES

1. Bettman, Ernest H., "The Human Foot—New Functional Exercises," *Archives of Physical Therapy,* January 1944.
2. Brown, L. T., "A Combined Medical and Postural Examination of

746 Young Adults," *American Journal of Orthopedic Surgery,*
Vol. 15, No. 11, November 19, 1917.

3. Cerney, J. V., *Athletic Injuries* (Springfield, Ill.: Charles C.
Thomas, 1963).

4. _____, in a personal communication of January 20, 1975.

5. Cook, Robert J., "Results of Exercise for the Correction of
Postural Faults," *New York Medical Journal and Medical Record,*
February 9, 1923.

6. Diveley, Rex, "Foot Imbalance," *Journal of the American Medical
Association,* November 17, 1934.

7. Drew, J. F., "The Painful Foot," *Medical Journal of Australia,*
February 23, 1957.

8. Editors, *Runner's World, The Athlete's Feet* (Mountain View,
California: World Publications, 1974).

9. Funk, Hermann, "Foot Eversion and Pronation," unpublished
Master's thesis, U.C.L.A., 1967.

10. Graham, James, "Weak Foot—Pathogenesis and Treatment,"
*American Journal of Surgery,* Vol. 35, No. 3, March 1937.

11. Kite, J. H., "Exercises in Foot Disabilities," *Therapeutic
Exercise,* Sidney Light, ed. (Baltimore: Waverly Press, 1965).

12. Klein, Armin, and Thomas, Leah C., "Posture and Physical
Fitness," *Body Mechanics and Practice* (New York: The Century
Co., 1932).

13. Lewin, Philip, "Flat Foot in Infants and in Children," *American
Journal of Diseases of Children,* Vol. 31, May 1926.

14. Lowman, Charles, "The Relation of Postural States to
Competitive Sports," *The Physical Educator,* October 1952.

15. Lowman, Charles and Young, Carl H., *Postural Fitness,*
(Philadelphia: Lea and Febiger, 1960).

16. McMillar, T., "The Treatment of Minor Foot Disabilities,"
*Edinburgh Medical Journal,* Vol. 45, May 1938.

17. Osgood, Robert B., "An Important Etiologic Factor in So-
called Foot Strain," *The New England Journal of Medicine,*
April 2, 1942.

18. Phelps, Winthrop M., and Kiputh, Robert, *The Diagnosis and
Treatment of Postural Defects,* (Springfield, Ill.: Charles C.
Thomas, 1932).

19. Pollock, Meyer M., "The Road to Healthy Feet," *Journal of
Health, Physical Education and Recreation,* April 1930.

20. Vorobiev, G., "The Foot and Running," *Yessis Review of
Soviet Physical Education and Sports,* Vol. 8, No. 1, March 1973.

21. Wiles, Philip, "Postural Deformities of the Antereo-Posterior
Curves of the Spine," *The Lancet,* April 17, 1937.

22. _____ , "Flat Feet," *The Lancet,* November 17, 1934.

23. Zohar, Joseph, "Preventative Conditioning for Maximum Safety
and Performance," *Scholastic Coach,* May, 1973.

# 22

## Manipulation in Prevention Correction, and Rehabilitation

T he ancient art of manipulation as applied to the musculo-skeletal structures of the body has been expressed in many forms, including non-movement massage and traction and movements of mobilization, manipulation therapy, or surgery (non-operative). The manipulation discussed in this chapter is that applied by a second party, as distinguished from self-administered manipulation, such as self-massage, hanging traction from a bar, or voluntary mobilization (stretching).

Manipulation in all its forms has a wide range of applications in the preventive, corrective, and therapeutic contexts as related to athletic training, postural and foot fault correction, and the treatment of athletic injuries. The selection of various manipulative methods must be based on an accurate diagnosis of the goals to be attained and the problems to be overcome. An incorrect choice of manipulation as a result of misdiagnosis can lead to predisposition to injury in the athlete. Not only is proper use of manipulative techniques entirely dependent upon a correct diagnosis of the problem, but correct diagnosis is in turn dependent on a funda-mental knowledge of anatomy, physiology, and pathological changes in body joints and their surrounding tissues. Nor should manipula-tion be administered without knowledge and understanding on the part of the manipulator of the techniques of manipulative therapy.

### MASSAGE

Massage has been defined as a systematic manipulation of the soft tissues of the body. It is one of the world's oldest forms of manipulation, and has been used both in the everyday world and the world of athletics to accomplish two different ends. *Stimulating massage* is aimed at creating a psychological sense of well-being and relaxation. *Therapeutic massage* serves to initiate and promote the healing process in injured body tissue.

Therapeutic massage causes the small capillaries to dilate, resulting in a drainage of fluid that has accumulated at the site of the injury. It stimulates cell metabolism, eliminates toxins, increases lymphatic and venous circulation, and relieves pain. Theoretically, as the fluid departs, the possibility of protein breakdown and resultant fibrosis diminishes.[7] Massage prevents stagnation of the circulation in a joint surrounded by edema (swelling). It deters the formation of adhesions, assists in breaking up those that have formed, eliminates fibrosis in muscle tissue, and assists in the restoration of lost function in muscles and joints.

Lewin, in discussing the application of massage to the treatment of knee injuries, pointed out that this technique can be used to treat sprains, strains, fractures, dislocations, and stiff knees.[14] He cautioned, however, that massage should never be applied directly to the kneecap—only to the tissues above and below the joint.

The primary massage technique used in treatment of injuries is the deep stroking compression (Swedish type) of the soft tissues. For the most effective results, the stroking motions should be directed toward the heart.

## TRACTION

Traction can be applied manually or by the use of mechanical apparatus. In a preventative context, it is used to maintain the normal range of extensibility in the connective tissues of the body—hanging from a bar to stretch shoulder ligaments, for example. When used in a corrective context, its purpose is to stretch contracted and shortened connective tissues (ligaments and muscle fascia) resulting from muscular imbalance, immobility, or postural faults that restrict the normal range of joint motion.

In a therapeutic context, traction is used to relieve abnormal compression forces on the intra-auricular surfaces of body joints (such as the inter-vertebral disks of the spine) or to maintain during the healing process the normal alignment of bones that have been fractured or to establish normal bone alignment prior to the application of casts. In manipulative therapy, traction and counter-traction are applied to the joint to separate the intra-auricular joint surfaces while manipulation of the joint is performed.

## MOBILIZATION

The term "mobilization" is interchangeable with the term "manipulation." The former is used in athletics and physical education, the latter in the medical world.

Mobilization can be developed through four types of exercise: active, resistive, passive, and assistive. *Active* and *resistive* exercises are employed by the athlete himself and use flexibility (stretching exercises and strength development exercises) to maintain or improve the normal range of joint motion. *Passive* and *assistive* exercises are performed with the help of a medical specialist, therapist, or trainer. They are employed in corrective and therapeutic contexts and involve partial movement or actual stretching techniques of a general nature. Since mobilization techniques are closely associated with manipulative therapy techniques, their value and uses will be discussed below.

## MANIPULATIVE THERAPY OR SURGERY

Manipulative therapy or manipulative surgery has been defined as the correction of deformity and the restoration through non-operative means of the functions of joints, bones, muscles, tendons, and ligaments damaged by injury or disease. It is one of the oldest forms of therapy and stems from the ancient practice of "bone setting."

Bick credited Wharton Hood, a London physician, with being the first (in 1871) to publicize the so-called "secrets" of the manipulative therapy of the English "bone setters."[2] In four articles published earlier in *The Lancet*, Hood related his introduction to the art by a "bone setter" named Hutton.[9] For four years, he observed, studied, and learned the technique of manipulation under Hutton's direction.

In a summary of his experience, Hood pointed out how Hutton had successfully treated: (1) stiffness and pain of joints following fractures; (2) sprains of recent origin or old standing which had been treated by rigidly enforced rest; (3) joints that had been kept at rest voluntarily for avoidance of pain after an injury; (4) rheumatic and gouty joints; (5) displacement of cartilages; (6) subluxation (partial slippage) of foot bones; and (7) displaced tendons. Hutton excluded the use of manipulation in the treatment of true ankylosis (consolidation or union) of joints, active articular (joint) disease, and recent fractures, the wisdom of which exceptions has been verified by subsequent medical observations. Indeed, this selectivity on Hutton's part represented remarkably careful diagnosis for a layman and non-medical practitioner.

Hood pointed out that Hutton handled 1,000 cases a year in his practice, most of whom had been previously treated one or more times, without experiencing relief, by general medical practitioners and orthopedic physicians. Hutton's successes were in those cases in which there was some restraint of movement, due either to an injury or to the rest consequent upon an injury or to both together, that painfully checked joint movement, but was immediately overcome by joint manipulation.

In 1874, Dr. Andrew Still, a physician dissatisfied with many of the medical practices of that time, established in America the science of osteopathic manipulation. He was subsequently joined by a Scotch physician, Dr. William Smith (in 1892), and the two established at Kirksville, Missouri the first osteopathic college in this country. Whether Still was influenced by the writings of Wharton Hood is not known. Osteopathic medicine, however, is the only profession in the wide field of medical practice today in which training in the use of manipulative techniques is required for a degree.

In research going back over 100 years, this writer found numerous references in medical and orthopedic journals to the use of manipulation in the treatment of musculo-skeletal disorders. In the late 19th century and in this century up to 1940, numerous comments were made on this subject by orthopedic surgeons, particularly in England. Among them, it is interesting to note the statements of a relatively small number of orthopedic surgeons on the failure of members of their profession to employ this technique in various disorders of the musculo-skeletal systems of the body.

In 1931, Sir Robert Jones, in a lecture on the problem of the stiff joint, prepared in honor of Sir William Mitchell Banks, stated that in one of Banks' last letters to him the writer had deplored the fact that bone setters were making inroads on the reputation of the medical profession and asked "When shall be wake up?"[11] Commenting on manipulative surgery or bone setting, Jones stated:

I shall now deal in some detail with the subject of forcible manipulation, which is a branch of surgery that from time immemorial has been neglected by our profession, and as a direct consequence much of it has fallen into the hands of the unqualified practitioner. Let there be no mistake; this has seriously undermined the public confidence, which has on occasion amounted to open hostility. If we honestly face the facts, this attitude should cause us no surprise. No excuse will avail us when a stiff joint, which has been treated for many months by various surgeons and practitioners without effect, rapidly regains its mobility and function at the hands of an irregular practitioner. We should be self-critical, and ask why we missed such an opportunity ourselves. The problem is not solved by pointing out mistakes made by the unqualified—the question at issue is their success. Reputations are not made in any walks of life simply by failures. Failures are common to us all, and it is a far wiser and more dignified attitude on our part to improve our armamentarium than dwell upon the mistakes made by others. With few exceptions, a stiff joint is based on a clearly defined pathological basis, and a large proportion of cases cured by the manipulator represents a failure on the part of our profession. It is not a pleasant thought, but it is true.

Several authorities who have written about the use of manipulation in the handling of musculo-skeletal disorders have expressed their views as to the positive role of manipulation in the rehabilitation of patients suffering from various disorders. Douthwaite used manipulation to treat various musculo-skeletal disorders, such as chronic cervical fibrositis, chronic lumbago, shoulder peri-arthritis, osteo-arthritis (but only with associated fibrositis), and sciatic neuritis not caused by a herniated intervertebral disk.[6] Tucker and Armstrong used it to treat acute foot strain, chronic sprained ankles, chronic traumatic myositis due to postural strain, stiff joints, and as one of three methods in reduction of fractures, the other two being traction and surgery.[1] Wiles used manipulation to treat tennis elbow, chronic arthritis of the feet, painful hip joints in early cases of osteo-arthritis, shoulder bursitis after the early stages, and chronic mid-tarsal pain in the foot.[1] Kuhns and Potter, in the treatment of arthritis, used manipulation when there were adhesions within and about the joints or where there were contractures in muscles or fascia.[12]

Wesson, commenting on corrective manipulation, pointed out that it could: (1) stretch or rupture adhesions—intra- or extra-articular (joints); (2) reduce subluxations (partially slipped joints) and regain normality; and (3) stretch shortened muscles and fascia.[6] He also used it in treating chronic postural fault cases of cervical lordosis and lumbar lordosis, stating: "...in long-standing cases, so much contracture has taken place in the non-expansile elements of the muscles and in the capsules and ligaments of the underlying joints, that forcible manipulation is the essential foundation on which we can rebuild—architecturally and mechanically—a well-balanced, efficient, and erect animal." Cyriax used forced movements to: (1) break adhesions; (2) reduce intra-articular cartilage displacement; (3) stretch capsules of joints; (4) stretch tendons or muscles; (5) reduce subluxations; and (6) correct a deformity to maintain joint range of movement in the presence of paralyzed muscles.[3]

Watson Jones, who was highly critical of the use of manipulation in treating actual stiffness of elbow and finger joints caused by adhesions, commented that very localized adhesions of certain joints which caused discomfort and weakness and only a slight limitation of movement could be successfully treated by manipulation.[10] These included tennis elbow, sprained back, twisted knee and ankle, and painful flat foot.

In the treatment of foot disorders, Dickson and Diveley used manipulation in treatment of rigid flat foot;[4] Lake, in treatment of dropped metatarsal arch and flexed toes;[13] Hauser, in treatment of club foot, the spastic type of foot vagoplanus and flat foot, and painful and subluxated sub-astragaloid and mid-tarsal joints (see Chapter 17, Figures 21 and 22).[8]

This writer has been able to uncover only one statistical study on results of manipulative therapy applied to musculo-skeletal disorders. Wiles, in 1933, used this technique in the treatment of painful feet due to adhesions resulting from micro-trauma imposed on the foot muscles, fascia, and ligaments over a number of years due to foot faults and chronic foot strain.[16] A great percentage of the persons treated suffered from postural pes valgus or pseudo flat foot, which caused chronic foot strain under the stress of weight bearing. Wiles treated 100 patients, 87 with chronic foot strain and 13 with chronic arthritis of the feet. Of the arthritis patients, three were "cured," six were "much improved," and four "improved." Of the 87 cases of chronic foot strain, 72 (83%) were "cured," 13 (15%) were "much improved," one was "improved," and one was "unchanged." The mobility of the feet was the most important single prognostic factor. The more mobile the feet to start with, the better were the results. Wiles stated that the mid-tarsal foot joints were the most commonly affected joints and reported that results of manipulation on these joints are almost uniformly good, if only the patients can be persuaded to throw away their supports and maintain the suppleness and improve the strength of their feet by exercises.

The authorities cited above have emphasized the value of manipulation as a therapeutic tool in treatment of chronic after-effects of syndromes that occur from two causes: (1) improperly treated or untreated acute traumatic injuries; and (2) repetitive micro-trauma resulting from faulty alignment of the skeletal structure. They have ruled out, however, the use of joint manipulation to restore loss of movement in body joints that is due to gout, acute infectious arthritis, ankylosis (joint fusion), osteomyolitis, tuberculosis, infection, toxic poisoning, or actual fractures of joints or bones.

## MANIPULATION IN TREATMENT OF ACUTE INJURIES

The body reacts to traumatic injuries exactly as it does to infection and with the same inflammatory response. In injuries, this response takes the form of traumatic effusion (escape) of fluids into tissue spaces. These fluids consist of blood oozing from sound capillaries, bleedings from torn blood vessels, and—if a synovial membrane is injured—an excess of synovial fluid. Effusion may cause the development of fibrous tissues (adhesions). It is these adhesions that can lead to restriction of joint motion and that cause pain when stretched. The combination of fluid accumulations results in swelling at the site of the injury, with added congestion that impedes their absorption.

This stage of the injury is the acute or negative phase. Immediately the swelling and the products of tissue disintegration are absorbed or removed, the positive healing phase commences. Too vigorous active treatment in the early negative phase can often cause aggravation and further effusion.

The immediate non-surgical treatment to hasten reabsorption and reduction of the swelling generally consists of elevation of the limb w`ere possible, cryotherapy (ice treatment), gentle massage of the injured part directed toward the heart, and pressure bandaging. In the more serious injury accompanied by a large amount of swelling, however, the medical specialist may remove the products of swelling by aspiration or expression.

When this has been accomplished, the positive and active therapeutic approach can be put into effect. It is in this phase that manipulative therapy, as one tool of physical therapy, plays an important part in increasing circulation and preventing the formation of adhesions.

Wesson, in discussing the use of therapeutic manipulation, called attention to the fact that in internal medicine it is usually impossible to put the affected organ absolutely to rest.[6] He maintained that recovery occurs not because the treatment has stopped the normal function of the organ, but because it has reduced the organ's work to a *minimum*—which happens when the patient is kept flat in bed. Wesson contended that in the treatment of acute joint conditions there should not be an attempt to completely stop the joint and its muscles from moving, but only to reduce its work to a minimum. In treatment of joint injuries, this means: (1) relief from weight bearing; (2) support of the limb from the effects of gravity or imbalance of antagonist muscles; and (3) manipulation or daily assisted active movements of the joint.

Sir Robert Jones maintained that if an inflamed joint is kept at rest too long after inflammation has abated, then the process of healing may lead to the formation of unnecessary bands of fibrous tissue with associated restriction of movement in the joint.[11]

Tucker pointed out that reactionary muscular spasm and swelling limit the range of full movements—both active voluntary and accessory involuntary.[15] Unless gentle manipulations, which restore both types of movement, are performed frequently throughout the course of treatment, full function of the joint for vigorous use will not be restored quickly.

Tucker also outlined the rules that must be strictly followed when recommending the use of therapeutic manipulation:[15]

1. X-rays must be carefully examined before manipulation is used.

2. No force is employed and gentleness is stressed.

3. The amount of reaction by the patient must be anticipated and controlled.

4. The use of short lever movements is employed.

5. There must be no excessive swelling or edema of the tissues if controlled manipulation under anesthesia is being used.

Watson Jones cautioned that manipulation is a two-edged sword.[10]

Manipulation breaks down adhesions; but the same process, if forcible and vigorous during after-treatment, can produce further adhesions. Jones maintained that it is the recurrence and persistence of sero-fibrinous effusions from the damaged tissues which provides the key to the problems of adhesion formation. His advice should be taken to heart by athletes, joggers, and coaches who believe that a minor ankle sprain or knee twisting that tears one or two tissue fibers will disappear in continued activity. On the contrary, the repetitive weight-bearing activities tear more fibers, and the effusion process begins. The following morning, there is a slight swelling and a little stiffness, which tend to disappear during the day. This may go on for one or two days. Then the athlete begins to limp a little. By the time he seeks medical attention, some adhesions have formed. He is then compelled to rest. Application of ice therapy and rest from activity for a day at the start would have eliminated the acute or negative phase of the injury and allowed the positive healing phase to begin promptly.

## MANIPULATION IN PREVENTION AND WARM-UP

Dr. Wayne Dooley, a currently practicing osteopathic physician, contends there would be far fewer athletic injuries if during the off season the athlete would engage in self-manipulation, stretching programs, and some form of constant activity.[5] Dooley also maintains that assistive joint manipulation to increase the circulation of blood in the joint capsules and surrounding tissues would substantially reduce the amount of time spent in warming up. He points to the amount of throwing done by the baseball pitcher to warm up prior to a game, as a result of which the pitcher begins to suffer from arm and shoulder fatigue in the sixth or seventh inning. In Dooley's view, five to seven minutes of shoulder, elbow, and wrist joint manipulation followed by eight to ten warm-up pitches would save the pitcher's energy and time spent in warming up and would prevent the occurrence of elbow or shoulder strains.

## REFERENCES

1. Armstrong, J. R., and Tucker, W. E., *Injury in Sport* (London: Staples Press, 1964).
2. Bick, Edgar M., *Source Book of Orthopedics* (New York: Haffner Publishing co., 1968).
3. Cyriax, James, *Textbook of Orthopedic Medicine, Treatment by Manipulation, Massage and Injection*, Vol. 2, 8th edition (Baltimore: William and Wilkins Co., 1971).
4. Dickson, Frank D., and Diveley, Rex L., *Functional Disorders of the Foot* (Philadelphia: J. B. Lippincott Co., 1953).

5. Dooley, Wayne, in a personal communication of March, 23, 1975.

6. Douthwaite, A. H., and Wesson, a. S., "Discussion on Manipulation in Rheumatic Disorders," *Proceedings of Royal Society of Medicine,* Vol. 32.

7. Ferguson, A. B., and Bender,Jay, *The ABC's of Athletic Injuries and Conditioning* (Baltimore: William and Wilkins Co., 1964).

8. Hauser, Emil D., *Diseases of the Foot* (Philadelphia: W. B. Saunders Co., 1941).

9. Hood, Wharton, "So-Called Bone Setting, Its Nature and Results," *The Lancet,* March 11, 18 and April 1, 15, 1871.

10. Jones, R. Watson, "Adhesions of Joints and Injury," *British Medical Journal,* May 9, 1936.

11. Jones, Sir Robert, "The Problem of the Stiff Joint," *British Medical Journal,* December 5, 1931.

12. Kuhns, J. G., and Potter, T. A., "Painful Feet," *Comroe's Arthritis and Allied Conditions* (Philadelphia: Lea and Febiger, 1953).

13. Lake, Norman C., *The Foot* (London: Balliere, Tindall and Cox, 1952).

14. Lewin, Philip, *The Knee* (Philadelphia: Lea and Febiger, 1952).

15. Tucker, W. E., "Athletic Industrial Muscle and Joint Injuries," reprint from *Traumatic Medicine and Surgery for the Attorney* (New York: Matthew Bender and Co., Inc., 1969).

16. Wiles, Philip, "The Manipulative Treatment of Painful Feet," *British Medical Journal,* September 23, 1933.

17. _____ , *Essentials of Orthopedics* (Boston: Little, Brown and Co., 1959).

## RECOMMENDED READING

*Textbook of Orthopedic Medicine, Treatment by Manipulation, Massage and Injection,* by James Cyriax, Vol. 2, 8th edition (Baltimore: William and Wilkins Co., 1971).

*The Science and Art of Joint Manipulation,* by J. B. Mennel (London: Churchill, Livingstone, 1949).

*Home Treatment and Posture in Injury, Rheumatism and Osteoarthritis,* by W. E. Tucker (London: Churchill, Livingstone, 1973).

# 23

## Screening and Pre-Participation Physical Examination

Preventive and corrective exercise programs must be based on two basic principles: individuality and specificity. This requires that the individual athlete be subjected to a complete medical and physical examination.

### ROLE OF COACH, TRAINER, AND TEAM PHYSICIAN

As soon as the prospective athlete enters the athletic world, it is the responsibility of coach, trainer, and team physician to correct the muscle imbalance and the postural and foot faults the athlete brings with him and to prevent their further development. They can only accomplish this by:

1. Recognizing that the problems discussed in this book do exist.

2. Possessing or acquiring a knowledge of muscular anatomy and joint structure.

3. Adhering to the premise that the earlier in the athlete's career the program of correction or prevention is stated, the better will be the results obtained.

4. Remembering that any postural or foot fault that cannot be corrected by the voluntary effort of the prospective candidate himself is a structural fault and that no type of exercise or conditioning program should be recommended until the candidate is first examined by an orthopedic physician, preferably one who is posture conscious. A great many orthopedic specialists pay little attention to the feet unless a deformity is visually apparent. As Cerney commented (see Chapter 16), a podiatrist, preferably one who has had experience with athletes, is an invaluable aid to a coach in detecting foot faults and defects.

5. Bearing in mind that many hidden cogenital anomalies or defects

in the spine, pelvis, and feet cannot be detected by visual observation, only by X-ray. Ideally, every prospective athlete or candidate for a physical fitness jogging program should undergo an X-ray analysis for his spine, pelvis, and feet.

## ROLE OF COACH OR JOGGER IN SCREENING

Very few junior high schools, if any, have a trainer assigned to the coaching staff. Medical assistance for team sports is generally provided on the day of a contest, while in individual sports like Track and Field, injured athletes are simply referred to a doctor. The same situation exists as to high schools. Some large municipal high schools do have a corrective physical education teacher on the staff who can be of assistance to the coach; but in the majority of cases, the coach alone must carry out the physical screening.

Organized industrial physical fitness programs are usually headed by a director of recreation who provides facilities, but in most instances does not hire a specifically trained person to lead the program. In the non-industrial jogging clubs, the jogger is entirely on his own. Their advocates stress only testing for heart deficiencies or reduced oxygen provision due to disease or other factors.

It is the responsibility of physical fitness participants and joggers themselves to carry out a screening process to protect themselves from the troublesome injuries and overuse syndromes that interfere with their progress or enjoyment. Several hundred books and pamphlets have been written on the subject of physical fitness, conditioning, and jogging. Some stress examination by the reader's personal physician for signs of cardiovascular disorders. In addition, some recommend tests of strength and flexibility of the low back and stomach muscles.

The following discussion is intended to be of benefit to the coach who must work alone in screening athletes or to the physical fitness jogger who must rely on his own initiative and arrange to undergo a screening process administered by a physician or physical therapist.

## PRE-PARTICIPATION PHYSICAL EXAMINATION

A pre-participation physical examination is the basis of a preventive or corrective program. In a 1959 lecture, Slocum maintained that the physical examination is most important in the pre-adolescent period, and becomes progressively less important throughout high school and college years, since the repeated examinations to which persons at these levels are subjected eliminate the majority of the unfit.[10] Slocum recommended—as very few others have—that examination of posture and flexibility is essential to the athletic physical. Like others, however, he failed to mention testing for muscular imbalance, one of the basic causes of muscular strains (muscle pulls).

Most of the medical and athletic writers discussing pre-participation physical examinations stress testing of the cardiovascular-pulmonary systems and questioning of the prospective athlete about any previous disturbances in the digestive, genito-urinary, and neurological body systems; previous childhood diseases; loss of consciousness; and serious injuries (sprains, fractures). Some emphasize testing for acute infectious diseases not symptomatically apparent at the time of the examination.

Others endorse identification of body build (endomorph—fat ectomorph—slim, mesomorph—muscular) and general muscular development in relation to calendar age for the purpose of eliminating the prospective athlete from participation in sporting activities for which he is unqualified and instead directing him to those activities for which he is best qualified. With respect to postural faults and injuries, Slocum pointed out that the questions which the physician must ask himself are: Can an athlete with a malaligned, deformed, weakened, or previously injured skeletal condition withstand the trauma inherent in a given spot? Can he be rehabilitated to a point where he can safely return to that sport?[10]

In physical fitness jogging programs, the emphasis has been on questioning about and testing of the cardiovascular-pulmonary systems, with relatively little attention to other internal body systems or the musculo-skeletal system. In the past few years, however, *Runner's World* magazine has emphasized the importance of foot faults and defects in fitness joggers and recreational runners, and Allman, Blazina, Corrigan, Liljedahl, and Lowman have all written articles about orthopedic factors and problems encountered in calisthenic fitness programs, as well as in jogging.

## MUSCULAR IMBALANCE

Tests for muscular imbalance in running athletes and physical fitness joggers should include testing of the following muscle groups: (1) neck flexors and extensors; (2) upper back adductors and chest flexors; (3) lower back extensors and abdominal flexors; (4) hip extensors (buttocks) and hip flexors; (5) hip abductors and hip adductors; (6) upper leg extensors and hamstring flexors—with each leg tested separately and the strength of one leg compared with the opposite leg; (7) lower leg calf flexors and the shin dorsiflexors; (8) ankle and foot invertor-adductors and evertor-abductors.

In the majority of cases, it will be found that the neck flexors, chest flexors, lower back extensors, hip flexors, hip adductors, upper leg extensors, calf flexors, and foot-ankle invertor-adductor muscles will be stronger than their antagonist muscle groups. The greatest imbalance found in runners and joggers generally involves the neck flexors, lower back extensors, hip flexors, leg extensor and calf flexor muscles, which are stronger than their antagonists.

The objective is to determine the degree of imbalance between the muscle groups and to reduce the ratio to a degree that falls within the normal range of some of the figures quoted in Chapter 6. Testing is by three methods: (1) manual (dual resistance); (2) mechanical; and (3) functional. The manual method is generally used by physical therapists, physical medicine specialists, and corrective physical education teachers; the mechanical means, by physical education research technicians; and functional testing, by coaches and physical education teachers.

Methods of manual testing are illustrated in *Muscle Testing— Techniques of Manual Examination*, by L. Daniel and C. Worthington,[2] and *Muscle Testing and Function*, by Henry and Florence Kendall.[6] Physical education researchers testing for static (isometric) strength use dynamometers, strain gauges, and hydraulic systems. For testing dynamic strength, they use cable tensiometers. This equipment is generally found in universities and colleges with well-staffed physical education departments. Its use is illustrated in H. Harrison Clarke's *Muscular Strength and Endurance in Man*.[1]

Coaches and physical education teachers employ functional testing, using weights and calisthenics for testing strength; the vertical jump, for height; and the 60-yard dash and standing broad jump, for testing power.

The use of weights includes barbells, dumbbells, iron boots, and head strap. Usually, three attempts are made to determine the RM (maximum load lifted or pushed on one attempt). Weights can be used to test all the muscle groups listed above except the hip adductor muscles, the foot and ankle invertor and evertor muscles, and the upper leg internal and external rotator muscles.

The important points to remember in testing with weights or dual resistance methods are to warm up throughly first and to perform the movements at a slow pace (a count of three to four for the entire movement).

It should be noted that the new mini-gym isokinetic exerciser now on the market provides an excellent functional method of testing strength in muscle groups.

Functional testing for muscular imbalance using weight-training movements of the muscles groups listed above is described later in this chapter and illustrated in Chapter 27. The same movements can be used for prevention and correction of muscular imbalance.

The best way to prevent muscular imbalance is to design training programs for strength development so that both prime mover muscles and their antagonists are equally developed. The way to correct imbalance is to strengthen the weak muscles on one side of the joint and stretch the strong muscles on the opposite side.

## FLEXIBILITY OR MOBILITY

Flexibility has been defined as mobility, mobilization, freedom to move, or the measure of range of motion in the joints. Davis *et al.* maintained that there is an optimum range of flexibility for prevention of injury.[3] Extreme flexibility can be a predisposing cause of injury to joints and a less than normal range of motion can result in tearing of connective tissues. Several studies have shown that flexibility is highly specific in nature and not a general factor. Athletes display a greater or lesser flexibility in specific body joints depending on the sports involved.

### Measuring Joint Range of Motion

Several different types of instruments have been devised to make precise clinical measurements of the range of joint motion. These include goniometers (protractor and pendulum), flexo-extensio-meters, and spinal fleximeters. One of the latest developments is the fleximeter. This instrument, the technique of using it, and an example of a homemade device are dealt with in articles by Leonard[7] and Sigerseth.[9] Lately, electro-goniometers, known as elgons, have been developed for clinical measurement of joint range of motion. An elgon is a goniometer in which a potentiometer has replaced the protractor. The manual goniometer measures angles of joints in a stationary position only. The elgon can record continuously in degrees in changes in the angles of joints during movement. The cheapest commercial instrument on the market is an orthodial protractor sold by Reedco, Inc., of Auburn, New York.

In an extensive review of the literature on flexibility, Holland pointed out that norms of average range of joint movement have not been standardized, maintaining that some clinicians use 0° for measurement in the neutral position.[5] The standard, however, is usually 180° in the neutral position. This is confusing to the reader, but is really only a matter of semantics. What Holland meant is that some use 0° for the starting position and proceed to the end result of 180°, while others reverse the procedure. The end results are the same.

Many orthopedic physicians, physical medicine specialists, physical therapists, and most corrective physical education teachers, coaches, trainers, and physical fitness authorities use a functional method of testing flexibility, in place of the more highly specialized mechanical equipment. This method is more practical and such tests are far easier to administer. It involves movement into a static held position. The same movements are used in prevention and correction of restricted range of movement. Examples of functional testing methods using body movements are illustrated in Figures 51 to 54.

Sigerseth, however, cautioned that the measurements of joint movement thus derived are influenced by variations in the lengths of body segments, and can only be applied to movement in a few joints.[9] In contrast to this, Harper, an English physical education authority and a national track coach, maintained that clinical instruments record only measurements of joint motion in static positions, and that athletes pass through positions too quickly and involve many joints at a time.[4] He pointed out that A. D. Munrow was clearly cognizant of this when he wrote of the shoulder not as a specific joint, but of the "shoulder joint complex."

### Joints to Be Tested

In determining range of motion in body joints as specifically related to the flexibility required of runners and joggers and the elimination of postural and foot faults, the following should be tested: (1) pectoral muscles of the chest; (2) hip flexors; (3) lower back extensors; (4) hamstrings—for antereo-posterior upper body and pelvis faults; (5) gastrocnemius-soleus calf flexors and inability to dorsiflex the foot with the leg straight beyond the 10° mark for ankle flexibility; (6) foot adductors and abductors for foot flexibility; and (7) the tensor fascia latae muscle (see Chapter 14, Figure 17)—if there is visual evidence of a lateral pelvic tilt not caused by a short leg.

### Ranges of Joint Movement

For those who have access to the clinical mechanical methods of measuring ranges of joint motion, the following figures compiled from numerous references using different base lines of measurement reflect average norms. However, the reader should keep in mind that—whether the neutral 0° starting position starts at the foot, head, or midline of the body in either the supine, prone, side lying, sitting, or standing erect position—or at the opposite 90° or 180° neutral position—the figures are an average of the different base line methods of measurement.

*Shoulder—to test pectoral flexibility:*
    Shoulder flexion to overhead position—0° to 170-180°
    Shoulder extension, hand moving behind body—0° to 50°
    Shoulder abduction outward—0° to 90°
    Shoulder adduction inward—0° to 90° (to midline of body)

*Hip—to test lower back, hip flexor, and extensor and hamstring flexibility:*
    Hip flexion supine, bring knee to chest—0° to 115-130°
    Hip flexion supine with straight leg—0° to 90°
    Hip extension prone lying—0° to 10-15°
    Hip abduction side lying—0° to 45°
    Hip adduction side lying—0° to 45°
    Hip lateral rotation standing—0° to 45°

Hip medial rotation standing—0° to 45°
*Ankle—to test calf flexor and extensor flexibility*:
    Plantar flexion lying—0° to 40°
    Dorsiflexion lying 0° to 10°
    Dorsiflexion standing—0° to 15°
*Foot—to test front and rear foot flexibility*:
    Foot abduction outwards—0° to 10°
    Foot adduction inwards—0° to 40°
    Foot eversion and plantar flexion—0° to 35°
    Foot eversion and dorsiflexion—0° to 25°
    Flexion of toes—0° to 25-30°
    Extension of toes—0° to 80°
    Rearfoot varus or inversion—0° to 20°
    Rearfoot valgus or eversion—0° to 10°

## POSTURAL FAULTS AND THEIR EVALUATION

Postural evaluation by visual observation can reveal faults existing in the pelvis and upper body and whether any visible faults can be corrected by the voluntary effort of the athlete himself. If deviations from normal alignment are due to structural defects or anomalies, however, they must nearly always be detected by X-ray. A good example of a non-structural fault that can be corrected voluntarily is a lateral asymmetry of the spine that resembles a structural scoliosis. If the curve disappears when the athlete is hanging from a bar, the curve is due either to muscular imbalance or a short leg, which can be corrected by exercise or a heel lift.

The most difficult problem in postural evaluation is to determine the degree of pelvic tilt. However, if there is an exaggerated inward curve of the lower back (lordosis), it is almost a foregone conclusion there is an associated forward tilt of the pelvis. If the lower back is flat, without a normal curve, there is a strong possibility of an associated posterior tilt of the pelvis.

## EVALUATION

The following points should be checked in postural evaluation of upper body and pelvis: (1) body type; (2) body balance or total body lean in the antereo-posterior and lateral planes; and (3) alignment of body segments, including (A) forwards and sidewards head position, (B) shoulder level, (C) scapula level, (D) hip level laterally and antereo-posterior pelvic tilt, and (E) spine (antereo-posterior lateral).

A postural evaluation chart displaying examples of normal posture and deviations from the norm can be of great assistance to the coach and trainer. Figure 50 illustrates a commercial posture evaluation chart that can be purchased at a very low cost from

259

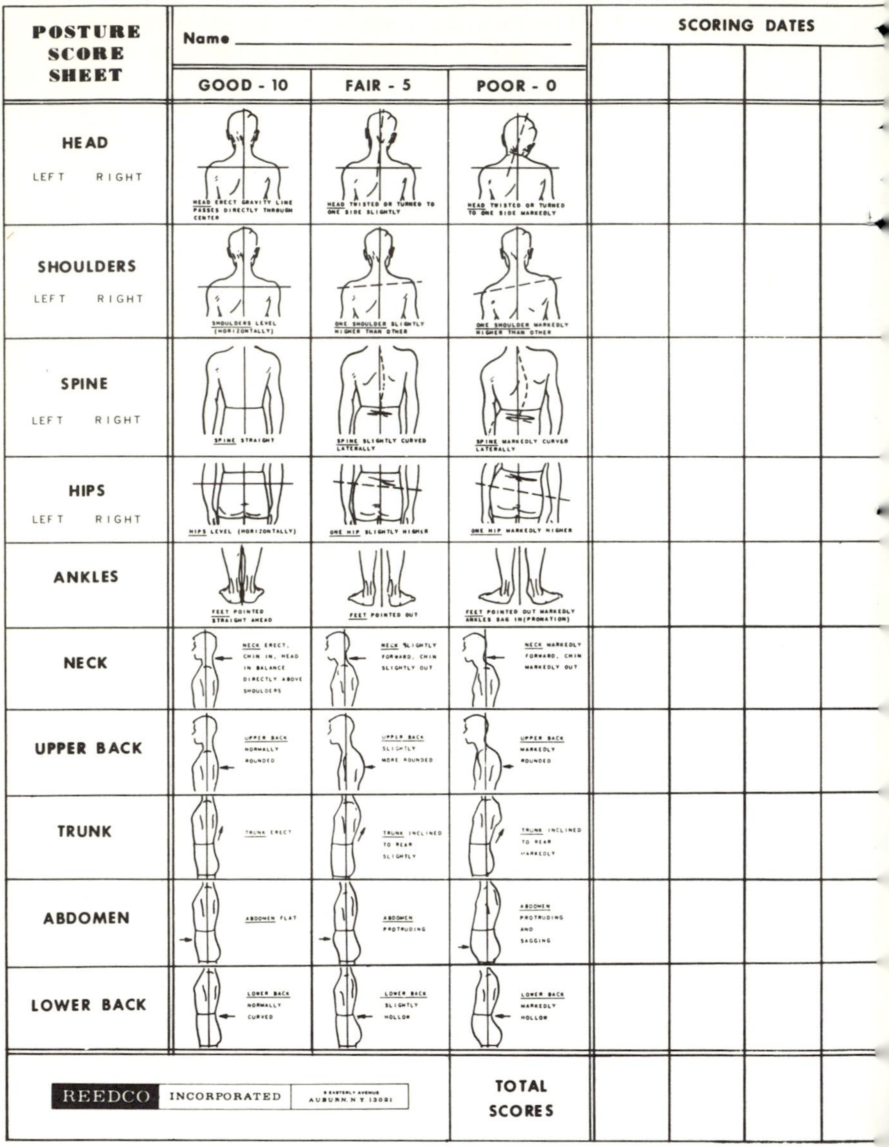

**Figure 50**
REEDCO POSTURE EVALUATION CHART

260

**Figure 50**
REEDCO POSTURE EVALUATION CHART

Reedco, Inc., 5 Easterly Avenue, Auburn, New York 13021. One dozen pads, each containing 50 individual postural evaluation sheets (600 total), 8 × 11½ inches, currently cost approximately $20. With such a chart and referral to postural faults illustrated in this volume (Chapter 10, Figure 7, antereo-posterior and Chapter 12, Figure 9, lateral shoulder, spine, and pelvis), the coach and trainer should encounter no problem in determing postural deviations in young adolescent athletes when they first enter the athletic world. Exercises for prevention and correction of upper body postural faults are illustrated in Chapter 27.

## FAULTY LEG ALIGNMENT AND FOOT FAULTS

In the screening and testing pre-participation examination, leg alignment and deviations in foot alignment must be considered as an entity. In most cases, a deviation in one is associated with a deviation in the other. This excludes certain congenital anomalies, such as an accessory scaphoid bone, that can be detected only by X-ray.

### Leg Alignment

Internal rotation of the thigh associated with pronation of the feet or excessive outward rotation of the thigh associated with toeing out, along with knock-knees or bowlegs, indicates deviations in abnormal leg alignment. In Chapter 14, Figures 13, 14, 15, and 16B show normal leg alignment and deviations from the normal weight-bearing line, including internal thigh rotation, functional knock-knees and foot pronation, outward thigh rotation and abducted toed-out foot position, and hyperextended knee joints. Tibial varum (Chapter 18, Figure 48) may be associated with a rear-foot varus (Chapter 18, Figure 47).

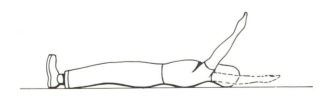

*Figure 51*

Lie on floor face up. Keep small of back on floor. Try to lay arms straight on floor behind head (dotted line). If arms do not lie flat on floor or if back rises from floor so as to rotate shoulders down, the pectoral (chest) muscles will be tight and shortened.

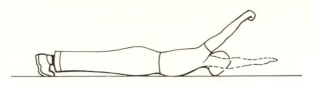

*Figure 51A*

Lie on floor face down, chin in contact with floor. Arms straight overhead grasping a pole or yard stick at shoulder width. Keeping the chin on the floor, raise arms as high as possible. Objective: a 45-degree angle.

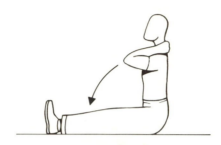

*Figure 52*

Sit on floors, legs straight, hands clasped behind neck. Attempt to touch elbows to knees, keeping legs straight. If elbows do not touch knees, and the lower back displays a flat rather than a rounded appearance, it indicates a tight low back. If the lower back is rounded but elbows do not touch knees, it indicates tight hamstrings.

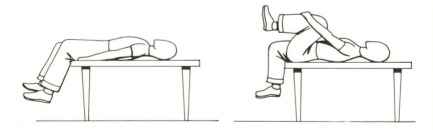

*Figure 53*

Lay flat on a table with legs over the end as shown. Bend left knee toward chest. When leg is pulled as tight as possible, then attempt to press back of right thigh on top of table, keeping lower leg at right angles to upper body. Repeat with other leg. Not being able to touch entire thigh to table indicates tight hip flexors.

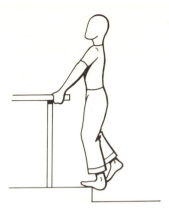

*Figure 54*

Place toes on edge of box or step, legs straight, knees locked. Lower heel as far as possible. If pull is felt in calf muscles, heel tendon is normal in length. If felt behind knee or ankle, it indicates a tight heel tendon.

## Tests for Foot Faults and Function

The simplest test to determine if the foot is being used normally is the weight-bearing line (Chapter 14, Figure 13), which displays the relation of the foot to the leg. Standing with the kneecap pointing straight ahead while maintaining the normal position of the foot, drop a line from the center of the kneecap, projecting it forward over the foot. If the line falls directly over the big toe or the inner side of the foot (Chapter 18, Figure 42), the body weight is being improperly borne and this reflects a foot fault (pronation or abduction) or poor leg alignment (internal thigh rotation). A second test is to view the Achilles tendon line from the rear (Chapter 18, Figure 42). If tilted outwards, it reflects rear foot valgus (Chapter 18, Figure 46) and/or pronation (Chapter 18, Figure 42). If tilted inwards, it reflects a rearfoot varus (Chapter 18, Figure 47), associated with tibial varum, internal tibial torsion, or muscle imbalance. If there is evidence of pronation, see how far inwards the mid-portion of the foot is misplaced. There may be bulging or tenderness on the inner side of the foot below the internal malleoli (Chapter 17, Figure 24) and a rearfoot valgus (Chapter 18, Figure 46) position.

Inability to dorsiflex (Chapter 17, Figure 32) the foot 10° beyond a right angle with the leg extended and the knee locked indicates a short Achilles tendon or calf muscle.

A wide spread of the forefoot (splay foot), sometimes with callouses under the metatarsal heads, indicates strain of the metatarsal (anterior arch). It also suggests the possibility of a hypermobile first metatarsal (Chapter 18, Figure 40) or a spread of the metatarsal bones due to laxity of the ligaments. The latter can be positively determined only by X-ray. There may be a burning sensation under the sole of the foot and a slight swelling about the internal and external malleoli (Chapter 17, Figure 24). Splay foot in a prospective female athlete or physical fitness jogger means there is a strong possibility of an associated hallux valgus, due to the wearing of narrow shoes. The big toe will be bent inward towards the second metatarsal. The broad forefoot and hallux valgus and the short metatarsal (Chapter 18, Figure 39), called Morton's toe, places the stress of weight bearing in walking and running on the second, third, and fourth metatarsals. The added stress on these more fragile bones leads to metatarsal stress fractures and Morton's neuralgia, an inflammation of the plantar nerves between the metatarsal bones. The forefoot should also be examined for evidence of valgus or varus faults (Chapter 18, Figures 44 and 45).

Testing should include observation of the medial longitudinal arch for height or lowness (Chapter 17, Figure 19). It should be noted that a completely flat arch may be a strong arch with no symptoms of pain even when subjected to extreme or strenuous use. If, however, a flat arch is associated with any degree of foot pronation (Chapter 18, Figure 42), it is a sign of a strained foot that can lead to a weak foot. A high arch (pes cavus)—Chapter 17, Figure 19—indicates a weak foot and an unstable heel that can lead to forefoot pains and stress fractures.

Foot position in standing and walking should also be observed. An excessively toed-out position in standing or toeing out more than five degrees from a median line (Chapter 18, Figure 38) is a sign of abduction in the foot or rotation of the foot at the ankle with associated outward tibial torsion, or total leg outward rotation at the hip joint. Running and walking with a toed-out foot position places tremendous strain on the medial aspects of the foot.

### Structural Defects

The one structural defect that can be easily observed on visual examination is the short first metatarsal (Chapter 18, Figure 39), called Morton's toe. As in the case of the spine or pelvis, other structural defects or anomalies of the foot or ankle can be detected only by X-ray.

### Weak Feet

Most corrective physical education authorities classify an abducted (pronated) foot as a weak foot. Some indicate that the presence of pain is the main indicator of weak feet. Morrison and Chenoweth developed a functional test of four exercises to determine if the feet are weak.[8] These include: (1) Rise on toes, foot pointing outward. (2) Walk on toes with the soles of the feet nearly vertical to the floor. (3) Hop on the toes. (4) Jump into air and land on toes with knees relaxed and feet pointing outward. If any pain is felt in the feet after completing any or all of these exercises, it is a sign of weak feet.

Exercises for the prevention and correction of foot faults are illustrated in Chapter 27.

## NEUROMUSCULAR TENSION

It has always been recognized that the highly successful athlete possesses the ability to muscularly relax prior to competition or between active movements during competition. Many prospective athletes, because of basic emotional tension, enter the athletic world with various levels of neuromuscular tension which denotes an inability to relax the muscular structure of the body. This inability to relax subjects muscles to constant tension and strain, creating a predisposition to muscular strains. Residual neuromuscular tension is defined as muscular tension that persists in spite of an athlete's conscious effort to relax.

Functional testing for residual muscular tension can be done in the following manner. The athlete or jogger lies on a hard level surface on his back. He is advised to make himself as "limp as a rag." Then he is cautioned not to do a thing; when he feels the tester lift an arm or leg, he is not to assist, but is to let the arm hang heavy in the tester's hand. The muscles to be tested are those of the neck, wrist, elbow, shoulder, ankle, and hip joint.

The tester should detect whether the subject is assisting in the movement by observing whether the body part postures itself by maintaining an attitude resisting gravity, and whether—when the tester removes the support—the athlete resists the former's attempts to move various other body parts or keeps the motion going after the tester starts the movement.

## TESTING FOR MUSCULAR IMBALANCE

As mentioned earlier in this chapter, resistance type exercises with weights provide the most practical method of testing for muscular imbalance. Certain muscle group testing, however, requires the use of special equipment or dual resistance.

1. *Neck flexor versus extensor muscles:* Use a head strap with attached weights. Lie prone or seated on bench to test neck extensors (Chapter 27, Figure 61). Lie on back or be seated to test neck flexors.
2. *Chest flexor muscles:* Use straight arm supine lateral raise (Chapter 27, Figure 154) versus *Upper back shoulder adductor muscles:* Bent over lateral raise (Chapter 27, Figure 67).

3. *Abdominal flexor muscles:* Use bent knee sit-up (Chapter 27 Figure 87) versus
   *Lower back extensor muscles:* Good morning exercise (Chapter 27, figure 79).
4. *Hip flexor muscles:* Supine bent knee leg raise (Chapter 27, Figure 127) versus
   *Hip extensor muscles:* Prone double straight leg raise (Chapter 27, Figure 84.
5. *Knee extensor muscles:* Knee extension (Chapter 27, Figure 119) versus
   *Knee flexor muscles:* Leg curl (Chapter 27, Figure 121). Test legs separately.
   N.B.: Both extensor and flexor muscles can be tested separately with use of an iron boot on one leg.
6. *Calf flexor muscles*: Heel raise (Chapter 27, Figure 130A) versus *Calf dorsiflexor muscles:* Shin raise (Chapter 27, Figure 115).
7. *Ankle and foot abductor muscles:* Abductor movement (Chapter 27, Figure 142, and adductor movement, figure 143).
8. *Internal hip rotator muscles:* Dual resistance, internal movement exercise (Chapter 27, Figure 129) versus
   *External hip rotator muscles:* Dual resistance, external movement exercise (Chapter 27, Figure 129).

If pulley weights with ankle attachments are available, they can be used for testing hip adductor versus hip abductor muscles. If pulley weights are not available, these muscles must be tested by dual resistance methods, with the subject lying on his side or back.

## REFERENCES

1. Clarke, H. Harrison, *Muscular Strength and Endurance in Man* (Englewood Cliffs, N.J.: Prentice Hall, Inc., 1966).
2. Daniel, Lucille, and Worthington, Catherine, *Muscle Testing— Techniques of Manual Examination* (Philadelphia: W. B. Saunders Co., 1972).
3. David, E. C., Logan, G. A., and McKinney, W. C., *Biophysical Values of Muscular Implications for Research* (Dubuque, Iowa: William C. Brown Co., 1961).
4. Harper, Peter R., *Mobility Exercises* (London: British Amateur Athletic Board, 1971).
5. Holland, George J., "The Physiology of Flexibility," *Kinesiology Review* (American Association of Health, Physical Education and Recreation), 1968.
6. Kendall, Henry O., and Kendall, Florence P., *Muscle Testing and Function* (Baltimore: William and Wilkins, 1949).

7. Leonard, J. R., "A Simple Objective and Reliable Measure of Flexibility," *Research Quarterly,* 13:205-216, 1942.

8. Morrison, William R., and Chenoweth, Laurence B., *Normal and Elementary Physical Diagnosis* (Philadelphia: Lea and Febiger, 1955).

9. Siegerseth, Peter O., "Flexibility," *An Introduction to Measurement in Physical Education* (Indianapolis: Phi Epsilon Kappa Fraternity, 1970).

10. Slocum, Donald B., "Prevention of Athletic Injuries," *American Academy of Orthopedic Surgeons: Instruction Lectures,* Vol. 16, 1959.

# 24

## Prevention and Corrective Exercise Principles

Certain objectives are common to the prevention and correction of both muscular imbalance and postural and foot faults. They are: (1) a balanced strength development around body joints; (2) normal mobility (flexibility of body joints); (3) postural reflex and foot gait development; and (4) prevention or reduction of residual neuromuscular tension.

### MUSCULAR IMBALANCE

The goal involved in the prevention or correction of muscular imbalance is a relative balance of muscle and connective tissue on both sides of a body joint, i.e., a relative balance between the strength of the prime mover muscles and that of their antagonist muscles. Muscle fibers and connective tissue on one side of a joint that are contracted and shortened must be stretched and muscles and connective tissue on the opposite side of the joint that are stretched beyond their normal length must be strengthened and shortened.

If postural faults are associated with muscular imbalance, however, postural reflex training will also be required to correct both conditions. If there is any evidence of residual neuromuscular tension, reduction of this factor through training will also be necessary.

### POSTURAL FAULTS

Several orthopedic and physical education authorities have commented on the principles of postural fault prevention and correction. Flint wrote: "Within a postural program there are five essential and interdependent factors to be used as guides in developing an exercise program."[8] These factors are:

1. Accurate diagnosis of the deviation and the determination of all contributing factors, such as muscle tension or weakness, congenital anomalies, and mental attitude.

2. Full awareness by the athlete of his own special problems and stimulation of him in every way to carry out the prescribed program.

3. Assistance to the athlete in kinesthetic perception by him of the feeling of the corrected body position so his new neuromuscular patterns will become automatic and habitual.

4. Minimum muscular tension in maintaining the corrected position. This may require a lesson in tension awareness, or it may necessitate prolonged training in controlled relaxation.

5. Flexibility and muscle strength, of which both are highly individualized and must be carefully controlled to assure that the joint mobility remains within the normal range for the individual and that a proper ratio of strength is developed between the muscles and their antagonists.

Burt commented that features constantly found in association with faulty posture are; (1) inability to relax muscles; (2) loss of agility; and (3) loss of mobility of the spine.[4] He pointed out that five factors which vary from patient to patient must be considered in treatment: (1) improvement of agility; (2) improvement of mobility; (3) re-education of muscular relaxation; (4) strengthening of weak muscles; and (5) re-education of the postural reflexes.

In 1937, Wiles warned against over-reliance on strength and flexibility exercises alone to correct postural faults.[19] He maintained that the establishment of new postural reflexes is the final aim of all remedial treatment, and stated that remedial work requires "postural fixation" not "postural change," so when it is possible to make a voluntary correction, exercises that move the parts of the body principally concerned can be no good. Exercises must be directed toward keeping *those* parts as still as possible, while the rest of the body is moved. Thus the patient is taught to maintain a good posture during every type of movement.

Caillet mentioned this factor in his comments on posture training 30 years later.[5] He maintained that the greatest failures occur in patients who carry out exercises faithfully, but fail to "carry over" correct posture to everyday activities. Exercise for one hour a day coupled with a faulty stance during the other 15 waking hours will not bring about correction of posture faults.

Stressing relaxation in the correction of postural faults, Brunnstrom in 1940 cited the principles proposed by Elin Falk in 1911.[3] She advocated an easy erect carriage, with relaxation of all those muscles not directly involved in maintaining the upright position. Brunnstrom insisted that training in proper relaxation is of fundamental importance. Alignment of various body sections has to be brought about by the easy balancing of body parts, requiring control and coordination, but not forceful muscle action.

McClurg Anderson, one of the first to relate postural faults to athletic injuries, based his concept of *lock actions* on the principles of postural reflexes.[1] He defined a *lock action* as the placing of a body part into a position which automatically stabilizes other parts of the body and leads to more efficient action with a minimum of effort. He maintained that the foot *lock action* of pointing the foot straight ahead stimulates a chain of muscular actions on the entire body, and claimed it is probably the most actively developed postural reflex in bipeds, and therefore dominates most muscular actions performed in the erect position. The second important *lock action* is the tucking in of the chin to elevate the head and straighten the cervical spine. The development of these two basic *lock actions,* along with the correction of muscular imbalance, forms the basis of Anderson's successful approach to the correction of postural faults among athletes.

## FOOT FAULTS

Lowman who first demonstrated the relationship between upper body faults and foot faults in 1908, spent a greater part of his career attempting to convince physical education authorities of the necessity of paying attention to the posture of young children.[14] In an article written in 1940 on the feet and body mechanics, he stated:

> From your standpoint, you should base your corrective practice on a few fundamentals recognized as sound. They are chiefly:
>
> 1. A pelvic segment balanced in both anterior posterior and lateral planes.
>
> 2. Leg rotation balanced to maintain the kneecap in the sagittal plane (straight ahead).
>
> 3. Weight should be carried on the foot from the heel around the outer border to the forefoot; the thrust of propulsion forward in walking should be mainly off the first and second metatarsals in a reasonably straight foot position.
>
> 4. Recognize the postural needs of feet and legs as simply a part of the whole problem of body mechanics, and not as an isolated matter to be handled by any set method of muscular exercise, mechanical aids, or corrective shoes.
>
> 5. Learn to recognize hereditary, congenitally faulty feet; do not waste your time and that of the student doing useless exercises in an effort to correct a structural fault that only surgery can accomplish, i.e., any extreme flat, contracted, or club foot.

In discussing physical therapy and foot disabilities and their treatment, Kuhns noted three factors that must be considered: (1) the way the foot is used in standing and walking; (2) the posture of the whole body; (3) the shoe that is worn habitually.[12]

Lewin pointed out that the objectives in the treatment of postural defects of the feet should include a balance of muscle pull between evertor and invertor muscles controlling the balanced posture of the foot.[13] In some, the intrinsic muscles of the foot must be strengthened.

According to Rex Diveley, in an article in the *Journal of the American Medical Association* entitled "Foot Imbalance," correct walking with a heel-toe gait and the foot pointed straight ahead is important to the development of good foot posture and prevents the development of foot faults.[7] Correcting a poor walking gait, particularly toeing out of more than five degrees for each foot, requires training in the correct walking gait. This is accomplished by having the person walk with feet pointed straight ahead, or it may be necessary to overcompensate by walking with the feet turned slightly inward. This habit pattern must be continued during the entire day for a couple of months. Its constant repetition can result in the person's subconsciously adopting it as a correct walking gait.

In conclusion, the basic value of exercises for foot faults and weak feet lies in: (1) improved circulation; (2) increased mobility (flexibility); (3) strengthened muscles; (4) promotion of better gait. Depending on the diagnosis, various types of exercises will be appropriate: passive exercises, active exercises, non-weight-bearing exercises, and/or weight-bearing exercises. It is usually considered a good policy to employ non-weight-bearing exercise movements in the early stages of treatment for foot faults.

## BALANCED STRENGTH DEVELOPMENT

Strength is the capacity, demonstrated or potential, or a muscle to exert or resist force without any reference to motion, time (speed), or distance (endurance). The potential of a muscle to produce maximum force is dependent upon three characteristics of the organism:

*Anatomical*—In general, the greater the size (cross-section) of the muscle and the greater its number of muscle fibers, the greater its potential strength. Muscles having the same circumference may not possess the same strength potential. One may contain a large percentage of fat tissue, which lacks contractile power, while another may consist of pure muscle tissue.

*Neurological*—The greatest strength a muscle can produce is determined by the total number of muscle fibers that contract when the frequency and timing of impulses directed to the motor units is great enough to cause a sustained and simultaneous contraction in all fibers of the muscle.

*Psychological*—The upper limit of a person's strength is largely determined by the degree to which psychologically induced inhibitions (fear, lack of confidence, unwillingness to face pain, etc.) consciously or subconsciously limit maximum expression of strength.

When motion is introduced into its definition, we find there are two basic kinds of strength: *Isotonic* (dynamic or kinetic) and *Isometric* (static).

*Isotonic strength* involves two types of muscular contraction: (1) *Concentric*—A muscle develops tension sufficient to overcome a resistance or load and produce work, so that the muscle visibility shortens and moves a body part despite the resistance (raising a weight from the ground). (2) *Eccentric*—A specific resistance or load overcomes the muscle tension and the muscle actually lengthens. In this case, the muscle does negative work (lowering a weight to the ground).

*Isometric strength* contractions occur when the muscle develops tension within itself insufficient to move a body part against a given resistance or load and the length of the muscle remains unchanged (pushing against an immovable object).

Whatever type of resistance movement is used by athletes to develop strength, they must adhere to the following precepts if they expect to gain maximum results for the time, energy, and effort expended:

1. Tension in the muscle created by resistance is the basic stimulus for strength development. Maximum tension must be exerted throughout the entire range of motion if the strength of the entire muscle is to be developed. All strength development exercises should be carried out at a slow pace to eliminate as far as possible the factor of velocity, which converts the exercise to a power movement. The maximum tension in a power movement comes at the beginning of the movement. Velocity compensates for tension as the movement continues to its conclusion.

2. The dominating principle in strength development is *overload*. Muscles must be compelled to carry out work beyond that which can be performed comfortably, easily, and without strain.

3. The second outstanding principle of strength development is *progression*. The amount of resistance (load) used in an exercise must be reset whenever the athlete becomes able to complete a required number of repetitions with less than all-out effort. To fulfill the principle of *progression,* resistance of loads must be increased at regular intervals as the strength of the muscle increases. In exercise, for improvements in strength to continue, the overload level must keep pace with the body's adaptive changes. To achieve

the best results, the training program must be individualized and progressive.

4. Closely allied to the principle of *progression* is the *rate of progression*. The body adapts slowly. Steinhaus stated, " ... rapid training induces only a loosely anchored adjustment of the muscle to the measured demands made on it. If, however, the increased strength is maintained for a time it becomes fixated or anchored in the muscles."[18] When the exerciser completes a certain number of repetitions with a given load without strain, he should continue using that load for two weeks before increasing the resistance. This is the reason why strength gains that are made rapidly tend not to be retained for any length of time.

5. Since tension is the basic stimulus for strength increase, the athlete must remember to maintain maximum tension throughout the entire exercise movement if he expects to increase the strength of the entire muscle. The greatest tension a muscle can produce occurs at a slow rate of contraction. This requires that dynamic (isotonic) resistance movements used for pure strength development be performed in a smooth and even manner, at a slow rate of speed.

6. The muscle produces its greatest tension when it is on stretch. In this respect, flexibility or mobility contributes to the strength potential in that it permits a stretch on the prime mover muscles; thus, it allows a stronger contraction and permits the force of contraction to be applied over a greater distance. Each dynamic resistance movement should begin from a position in which the joint is fully extended and should end with full contraction. Utilization of a full range of motion with complete flexion and extension of the muscle develops strength in all areas of the muscle.

7. The will to exert a physiologically maximum (all-out) effort must never be overlooked in a strength development exercise. Gains in strength will occur only if the athlete is willing constantly to put forth greater efforts at regular intervals, with the intention of exceeding his previous level of strength growth and accomplishment. Deep concentration on the muscles being used in the resistance exercise improves the neurological processes (number and frequency of stimuli sent to muscles) that are an important factor in the development of maximum tension contractions.

8. The principle of *specificity of training* applies in strength training. Gains in strength are specific to the exercise and the method of training. Strength does not carry over from one exercise to another. Specific training programs develop or improve specific strengths. Training for strength is an entirely different matter than training for power, endurance, speed, balance, reaction time, or coordination.

9. The *specificity* principle in resistance training for the prevention or correction of muscular imbalance, postural faults, and

foot faults is based on the pre-participation physical examination, screening for postural and foot faults, and testing for a high ratio of muscular imbalance.

## FLEXIBILITY DEVELOPMENT

Flexibility or mobility has been defined as the full range of movement around a joint (shoulder, ankle, etc.) or the normal range of movement of an anatomical segment (arm or leg) about the joint. Physiologists maintain that there are two major kinds of flexibility: (1) *Static*—involving the maximum range of motion in a joint during a slow controlled stretching movement and (2) *Dynamic*—involving the amount of resistance offered by a joint in maximum range movements at various speeds.

### Limiting Factors

Anatomically, the limiting factors in the range of movement of body parts are connective tissue, tendons, and ligaments. Tendons are not meant to be stretched. Ligaments adapt to stretching, but once stretched will not return to their normal length. The connective tissue surrounding the muscle fibers, interspersed among the fibers, and surrounding the entire muscle is know as fascia. It has the ability to contract or stretch, and it can become permanently contracted due to inactivity, enforced bed rest, injury, muscular imbalance, and postural faults. However, it is the one connective tissue that can be stretched and maintain its stretch permanently through activity or planned flexibility programs.

The neurological limiting factor in range of movement is the myostatic (stretch) reflex. Nerve receptors in the muscles, tendons, and ligaments are sensitive to stretch and tension. When the muscle is stretched beyond its limit, these receptors send impulses to the central nervous system, which reacts immediately by sending back impulses to the muscle to resist further stretching by contraction, thereby protecting it from tearing loose from the bone. In fast stretch movements, the myostatic reflex protects the joint from injury.

Other limiting factors include muscular imbalance, lack of physical activity, age, sex, muscle and body temperature, and muscle bulk.

### Principles

Adherence to the following premises is essential to the development of flexibility.

1. There is no such thing as general flexibility. Flexibility is highly specified to each joint. Participation in various sports results in development of rather specific patterns of joint flexibility that parallel the skills and body movements peculiar to the sport.

2. The athlete and jogger should be aware that there is an optimum range of flexibility in muscles and joints. Extreme flexibility of a joint, if not corrected by surgical intervention, requires great strength in the surrounding muscles for protection from injury. A lack of strength in muscles surrounding an extremely flexible joint is a predisposing cause of strains, sprains, and ruptures because it causes the primary responsibility for support and stabilization of the joint to fall to the ligaments and tendons, which have very limited ability to stretch when the habitual range of movement in the joint is exceeded. Nicholas tested the mobility of the lower extremities of 139 professional football players.[15] They were classified as having either loose or tight body joints. He found that independent of many other factors responsible for injury in football, there existed an increased likelihood of ligamentous rupture of the knee in loose-jointed football players and of muscle tears in tight-jointed football players. He recommended that specific exercises be designed to increase the strength of "loose" players and the mobility of "tight" players.

3. It has been well established that the range of motion in body joints and the extent of muscle mobility are adjustable through a planned flexibility training program.

4. In flexibility training programs, the athlete must make sure that the muscles he is exercising are consistently being used beyond their present habitual limits or the exercise will be of no value in increasing flexibility.

5. Muscle fibers and muscle fascia (sheaths) are the anatomical limiting factors that can be most easily modified through a planned training program. Tendons cannot be stretched. Ligaments can be stretched to some degree, particularly in the young, but such stretching will weaken joint stability.

6. When a muscle contracts (protagonist or prime mover), there is always an equal and opposite reaction in the antagonist muscle. In physiology, this is known as the "reciprocal innervation process" which is the key to neuromuscular coordination. In flexibility development exercises, emphasis must be placed on relaxing the muscles that are being stretched, particularly the antagonist muscles.

## POSTURAL REFLEX TRAINING

Sherrington, a great English neurosurgeon, was the first to demonstrate that the upright posture of the body is maintained by continuous tonic reflex muscular activity. The muscles which perform this important function are capable of acting continuously for long periods of time without showing any of the usual signs of fatigue. The postural muscles are plastic. They adapt themselves to a greater or shorter length, as required, without any change of tension, and they maintain that length, apparently without effort, until some other length is imposed upon them. Postural reflexes are acquired in early life, and are developed by practice, that is, by voluntary effort constantly repeated, until an action becomes involuntary or automatic. The ordinary standing tonic reflex of the upright position is essentially a continuous act of extension—extension of the head and neck, the spine, the hips and knees—with adduction and inversion of the feet.

Postural reflexes stem from impulses received from proprioceptor sensory nerve terminals which provide information concerning movements and positions of the body. They are located chiefly in the muscles, tendons, and labyrinth (inner ear). It is the constant pull of gravity on the extensor muscles that acts as a stretching force, and the proprioceptors of the extensor muscles stimulate the muscles' reflex tonic contraction to maintain upright posture. The extensor muscles concerned with the upright posture are the posterior muscles of the neck, the muscles of the upper and lower back, the buttocks, the quadriceps or knee extensors, and the plantar flexor muscles of the foot.

Bankart maintained that the first point to be emphasized is that postural activity is not a question of muscle.[2] The real purpose of exercises or gymnastics in the treatment of postural faults is the re-education of postural reflexes, not the strengthening of weak muscles.

"We are also convinced that exercises alone have little effect on posture," stated Carnett and Bates.[6] However, they pointed out that special exercises do constitute an essential first step in the correction of faulty posture or body mechanics in three main directions: (1) They improve the tone and power of flaccid feeble muscles, particularly those of the abdominal wall and buttocks; and they help to elongate contractured muscles, particularly the spinal and pectoral (chest) muscles; and for these reasons they should be continued daily for months or years. (2) They educate the person in voluntary muscle control by training his brain and nervous mechanisms. (3) They make the person posture conscious.

Haynes pointed out that in the correction of postural faults the person must obtain all or several of the following: (1) inversion of the feet; (2) extension of the knee and hip; (3) reduction of the lumbar lordosis; (4) extension of the dorsal spine; (5) elevation and widening of the thoracic cage; (6) straightening of the cervical spine; and (7) leveling of the head.[9] He emphasized full extension of the hip and knee joints as the basis for correction of faulty antereoposterior posture, and he stressed the development through exercises of consciousness of the anti-gravity muscles. Haynes contended that when a child learns to make a bilateral gluteal muscle contraction in the erect position, his thighs become abducted his knees extend and turn outward, and weight is borne on the outer side of the foot and on the outer four toes, leaving the big toe hardly touching the ground, and the feet held in the inverted or strong position.

The basic principle of postural reflex re-education is *continuity*. Improvement is directly dependent upon and proportionate to the amount of time in which the individual holds his body in the corrected position between exercise periods, which may occur for only fifteen or twenty minutes once or twice daily. Development of a posture-conscious attitude between exercise periods greatly facilitates maintenance of good mechanics. To hold the body in the corrected position may at first require such extreme mental and physical strain that it should be attempted on a part-time basis only; but the longer it is persisted in, the easier it becomes, until the better posture is maintained without conscious effort. It has been repeatedly observed that if a posture is maintained long enough by conscious effort, the increase of reflex muscle tones obtained by such practice will eventually serve to maintain the same attitude without need of thought or attention.

### RELAXATION TRAINING

Successful athletes are generally assumed to relax under the stress of competition. Nevertheless, studies cited in Chapter 20 of this volume showed that even the most successful athletes in top flight competition may suffer from anxiety and apprehension. This is particularly true of those who are using sports participation in fulfillment of neurotic needs.

Sainsbury and Gibson, summarizing numerous studies in addition to their own, demonstrated that symptoms of anxiety and tension resulted in muscle overactivity (residual neuromuscular tension), particularly in the arms, shoulders, neck, chest, and lower back.[17] Ogilvie and Tutko devoted an entire chapter of their book *How to Handle Problem Athletes* to the hyper-anxious or "psyched out" problem athlete who displays elevated levels of tension and literally "burns himself out" prior to competition.[16]

Jacobson, the pioneer in relaxation training, tested ten college-level athletes untrained in relaxation against control groups of ten non-athletic college students untrained in relaxation and ten trained in relaxation.[10] Of the ten athletes tested, four could relax the flexor muscles of the forearm completely (sometimes, at least), but six consistently failed to reach this stage. Marked failure to relax was noted in two or three of them, and over-all their success was less marked than that of the students who had been trained to relax.

Jacobson later outlined his method of progressive relaxation, based on his theory that relaxation should be cultivated according to physiological methods:[11]

277

1. The subject lies face up on a comfortable couch or bed with a pillow, or at least a thin cushion, under his head.

2. Under direction, the patient increases the tensions in specific muscle groups noted by the doctor during the testing period. For example, if his teeth are clenched tightly, or he is frowning excessively, he increases the jaw clenching or frowning to a degree where he becomes aware of it.

3. As a rule, most of the first hour of instruction is devoted to repeated contraction and relaxation of the muscles that flex and extend the left arm, to recognize the tensions.

4. After becoming aware of his tension in a specific group of muscles, the patient is then instructed to discontinue what he was doing both (A) abruptly and (B) slowly and progressively.

5. The patient learns that whenever he contracts a muscle group it is he who is doing it, i.e., there is always effort involved; but discontinuing that doing negates the effort.

6. Repeated practice takes place until the overactive muscle groups have become manifestly more relaxed.

7. The subject learns to relax principal muscle groups individually and in succession. With each new group, he simultaneously relaxes such body parts as have received practice in previous sessions. As the subject practices, he progresses toward a habit of repose and a state in which quiet is automatically maintained.

8. In conditions of chronic neuromuscular tension, the relaxation procedure follows an anatomical order—including the chief muscle groups of the limbs, trunk, neck, and head—often as follows: Total left arm muscle groups; right arm similarly; total left leg and foot muscle groups; right leg similarly; anterior and posterior trunk muscles; respiratory muscles; neck groups, frontalis (wrinkling); corrugator (frowning); lid and eye muscles; facial muscles; and speech muscles. Relaxation of those muscles involved in seeing and speaking requires more detailed instructions, as these characteristically participate in mental activities.

Jacobson proved the validity of his concept of "progressive relaxation" in numerous experiments. In one, he electrically recorded residual neuromuscular tension of subjects in a sitting position. Relaxation methods were applied to the chief muscle groups, and the subjects reported that they practiced 30 to 50 minutes daily. When retested in the same position, ten to twelve weeks later, all of them displayed greater degrees of relaxation and reduced residual neuromuscular tension.

Jacobson noted with regard to relaxation during activity, known in the physiological literature as "differential relaxation" in contrast to the general notion of relaxation in a lying posture, that " . . . evidently, training procedures administered in the lying posture can recondition the neuromuscular state in other postures. Training in general relaxation can contribute towards differential relaxation." .

The relaxation techniques practiced in *Hatha Yoga* are similar to those of Jacobson's "progressive relaxation." Each of two active *asanas* assumes a pose of complete relaxation—called *savasana,* or the "dead pose." The technique of *savasana* is simple to understand, but somewhat difficult to practice. The student is to lie on his back and fully relax his muscles, group by group. This requires concentration and an effort of will.

Numerous writers in the field of competitive running have emphasized the importance of relaxation during running to conserve energy or increase speed, advocating the use of "differential relaxation" training while the athlete is running. However, they make use of the principles of generalized progressive relaxation postulated by Jacobson, although they concentrate on the relaxation of the upper body only.

Physical fitness runners, too, are faced with the problem of learning to relax while they run if they desire to increase their running times. Nor should the jogger, despite his concern for distance rather than speed, fail to note that exercise *per se* is an excellent method of reducing residual neuromuscular tension.

## REFERENCES

1. Anderson, McClurg, *Human Kinetics and Analyzing Body Movement* (London: William Heinemann Medical Books, Ltd., 1951).
2. Bankart, Blundell, "On Postural Deformities," *Journal of Scientific Physical Training,* Vol. 14, 1921-22.
3. Brunnstrom, Signe, "The Changing Conception of Posture," *Physiotherapy Review,* Vol 2, 1940.
4. Burt, H. A., "Effects of Faulty Posture," *Proceedings of the Royal Society of Medicine,* Vol. XLIII.
5. Caillet, Rene, *Low Back Pain Syndrome* (Philadelphia: F. A. Davis Co., 1972).
6. Carnett, John Berton, and Bates, William, "Some Phases of Body Mechanics," *The Journal of Health and Physical Education,* April 1933.
7. Diveley, Rex, "Foot Imbalance," *Journal of the American Medical Association,* November 17, 1934.
8. Flint, Marilyn, "Selecting Exercises," *Journal of Health, Physical Education and Recreation,* February 1964.

9. Haynes, Royal, "Postural Reflexes," *American Journal of Diseases of Children,* December 1928.

10. Jacobson, Edmund, "The Course of Relaxation in Muscles of Athletes," *American Journal of Psychology,* Vol. 48, 1936.

11. _____, "The Cultivation of Physiology Relaxation," *Annals of Internal Medicine,* Vol. 19, 1943.

12. Kuhns, John G., "Physical Therapy in Disabilities of the Foot," *The Physiotherapy Review,* Vol. 21, No. 3, 1941.

13. Lewin, Philip, "Flat-foot in Infants and in Children," *American Journal of Diseases of Children,* May 1926.

14. Lowman, Charles L., "Feet and Body Mechanics," *Journal of the American Medical Association,* June 24, 1970.

16. Ogilvie, Bruce, and Tutko, Thomas A., *Problems Athletes and How to Handle Them* (London: Pelham Books, Ltd., 1966).

17. Sainsbury, Peter, and Gibson, J. G., "Symptoms of Anxiety and Tension and the Accompanying Physiological Changes in the Muscular System," *Journal of Neurosurgery and Psychiatry,* Vol. 17, 1954.

18. Steinhaus, Arthur H., "Strength from Morpugo to Muller—A Half Century of Research," *Journal of Physical and Mental Rehabilitation,* Vol. 9, No. 5, September-October 1955.

19. Wiles, Philip, "Postural Deformities of the Anterior-Posterior Curves of the Spine," *The Lancet,* April 17, 1937.

# 25

## Strength and Flexibility Training Procedures

Strength and flexibility development through exercise is the basis for prevention or correction of muscular imbalance and postural or foot faults. From research and empirical findings, certain procedures have evolved that if followed will guarantee to the athlete or jogger maximum benefit from time and effort expended in preventive or corrective exercise.

### STRENGTH DEVELOPMENT

Whatever the method used to increase strength, e.g., self-resistance, dual resistance, weight training, gymnastics, etc., the athlete or jogger should be guided by the principles cited in the previous chapter, as well as the following procedures.

### Number of Work-Outs

Work-outs three times a week are accepted practice. This allows a day of rest between each two work-outs, which provides the body with an opportunity to recuperate. This procedure, however, does not apply to postural or foot correction exercises that do not employ external resistance of any degree. Such exercises should be performed six days a week.

### Time of Training Session

Strength development exercises for prevention purposes should be performed following any running or other athletic activity. Exercises performed for corrective purposes should be performed when the muscles are rested. If such exercises—particularly foot ones—do not employ heavy external resistance, they should be done before retiring or after a night's rest.

## Selection of Exercises

In meeting the objectives of a strength development program, two points should be kept in mind: (1) Strength development should be balanced on both sides of a body joint. In a preventive program, an exercise for muscles on one side of a joint should be followed by an exercise for muscles on the opposite side of the joint in order to insure this balance. (2) Exercises should be periodically changed every two months to avoid boredom.

## Exercise Cadence

Strength development exercises should be carried out at a slow controlled pace and in a strict manner, with complete flexion and extension of the muscle groups involved. There should be no "swinging" or "rebound" movements. The use of such movements is too common among athletes, both in strength development and injury rehabilitation programs. Perhaps the most frequent example of this improper practice is in the use of the leg extension movement for the prevention of knee injuries or rehabilitation of an injured knee, when the athlete or jogger swings the weight with velocity and does not complete a full movement of extension. This writer has observed such misuse of strength development exercises with weights in numerous gymnasiums throughout the world. A classic example of it was published recently.[2] Ernie DiGregorio, a former all-American and a prominent professional basketball player, suffered a knee injury that required an operation. His progress in rehabilitation and return to playing was considerably slowed down due to his failure to perform strength development rehabilitation exercises correctly. Following the surgery, he was supposed to lift 30 pounds of weights with his legs. "But," said he, "I lifted them the wrong way for four or five weeks. It was my fault." The mistake made was in not locking (extending to its fullest) his knee while lifting. At the time the story was published, he was working with 10-pound weights and confessed: "Some days, I can't even lift that much."

## Rest Pause

In performing strength development exercises, rest periods between exercises or sets are based on the muscle groups involved. In the normal athletic or physical conditioning program, standardized rest pauses have been developed. However, in this book, we deal in particular with weakened stretched muscles on one side of a joint. Above all, fatigue in the weakened stretched muscles should be avoided. Because of their weakened condition, they are highly susceptible to strain when subjected to overload resistance training. Rest periods of up to two minutes or longer between exercises may be required.

## Maximum Load

The amount of resistance that can be moved for one repetition of a specific movement equals maximum load. Near maximum load would be 85 to 90 percent of maximum. In any case, the maximum load should relate not to one some other person is using or to some hypothetically established one, but to the exerciser's own level of strength at the beginning of a program.

## Starting Weight

Trial and error is still the best method of determing the initial starting resistance for an exercise. Development of strength demands an all-out effort against resistance. If he is using near maximum resistance, the person performing the exercise will find himself straining to complete it. A word of caution, however: Again, we are dealing with weakened muscles. The exercises may have to start with a resistance that is far less than a near maximum load.

## Increasing Resistance

Resistance should be added when the exerciser can complete the required number of repetitions of the last set, without strain for four successive exercise sessions.

## Repetitions

Exercises used in prevention, correction, or rehabilitation should be *isotonic* in nature, because circulation to the muscles is as important as strength and *isometric* exercises impede circulation. *Isotonic* (concentric-shortening) strength development requires use of low repetitions (three to eight) at a slow controlled pace (three to four seconds) and a number of sets based on the number of repetitions—three sets times six repetitions; five or six sets times three repetitions; etc. Generally, three sets times six to eight repetitions is favored.

## Weight Increases

If barbells, dumbbells, or iron boot(s) are used, weight is added when the exerciser can complete the required number of repetitions on the *final* set for the specific exercise without strain for three successive work-outs. It is the final set that provides the greatest gain in strength and muscular endurance. In general, two and one-half to five pounds are added for arm and shoulder exercises; five pounds for lower back, side, and abdomen exercises; ten pounds for leg exercises; and two and one half pounds for ankle exercises.

> *N.B.:* Foot exercises employ the use of calisthenics, self-resistance, dual resistance, body weight, and mechanical equipment. Persons with foot faults or weak feet should employ non-weight-bearing exercises

until the feet are strong enough to handle weight-bearing ones. If the only fault is widely abducted (toed-out) feet, gait training and stretching of the peroneal muscles on the outer side of the ankle only are required.

### Dual Resistance Exercise

Dual resistance exercises will develop strength. Their main drawbacks, however, should be considered:

1. There is no objective way to determine or gauge the amount of resistance used during the exercise.

2. There is no way to accurately gauge the amount of increased resistance that is required to exceed the previous resistance used, so as to insure a development of increased strength.

3. Motivation is many times lacking, due to lack of visual evidence that the level of strength is increasing.

In performance of an exercise, the resister should slowly yield to the force exerted by the exerciser through a full range of movement. To fulfill the overload principle, the person providing the resistance should at regular intervals increase the resistance to the force exerted by the exerciser.

## FLEXIBILITY DEVELOPMENT

In the previous chapter, both *static* and *dynamic* flexibility were mentioned. As yet, however, little is known about the development of *dynamic* flexibility. In general, the formalized methods used by doctors, physical therapists, trainers, and coaches have been designed to increase *static* flexibility, i.e., the maximum range of motion in a body joint. These methods have been classified as ballistic (fast), static (controlled or slow), and spring (bobbing) in nature.

### Ballistic Method

Limbs or body parts are put into movement by the contraction of a protagonist (mover) muscle, and momentum is stopped at the end of the movement by contraction of the antagonist muscle. During the movement, the antagonist muscle is being stretched by the action of the protagonist muscle.

Those who do not favor this method maintain that this movement is actually a controlled movement instead of a free swinging movement. If it is carried out without control and using maximum velocity, as in high kicking or arm swinging, the athlete or jogger risks damage to the muscles and joints involved.

Further, the use of great momentum invokes a strong "myostatic reflex" reaction. The stretch receptor nerves in the contracting (mover) muscle and tendons send messages to the brain telling the antagonist muscle to begin to slow down and halt the movement so as to protect the muscle and joint from going too far past their habitual range of motion and causing injury to the muscle or joint. A muscle being stretched with a ballistic (fast) movement develops a tension (resistance to stretch) increase more than double that of a slow static stretch.

The increased tension in the antagonist muscle being stretched prevents development of relaxation in the muscle and increases its resistance to stretch. Also, because the stretched muscle is not at the end of the movement held for any time in a static controlled position beyond its habitual length, the movement fails to condition the stretch receptor nerves to tolerate the increased muscle length without invoking the myostatic reflex action.

### Static Method

The key point in static stretch exercises is the end or "held" position at the completion of the movement where the muscle is stretched beyond its habitual length. This method involves a slow controlled stretching of the muscle. The athlete holds a static position while for a stated period of time he locks the joint into a position beyond the habitual length of the muscle. Those who favor static stretching methods contend they are superior in that they (1) permit greater relaxation in the antagonist muscle being stretched; (2) do not provoke the "stretch receptor" nerves to the same degree as do fast ballistic movements; and (3) cause the static position, with steadily applied tension at the completion of the movement, to be held for a period of time—which conditions the "stretch receptor" nervers to tolerate the new position.

Two methods of reaching the end position in static stretching exercises have been advocated: (1) *Active*—where the stretch position is achieved by active contraction of the protagonist (mover) muscle throughout the movement; and (2) *Passive*—where the limb or segment of the body in the final range of movement is not being moved by active contraction of the protagonist muscle.

An *active* stretching movement takes place when an athlete or jogger, seated on the floor, legs locked at the knee, reaches slowly forward and grabs his feet, applying steady tension for 30 seconds in that position, and concentrating on relaxation of the hamstring and lower back muscles in order to stretch them beyond their habitual length.

A *passive* stretching movement includes the use of an external force (partner or weights) or gravitational pull (position of body or weights). In the exercise described in the immediately preceding paragraph, external force would take the form of a partner slowly and gradually pushing the seated athlete's or jogger's shoulders forward to a position a little beyond the existing habitual length of the muscles involved. Hanging from a bar to stretch the shoulder joint and muscles is an example of a gravitational pull stretching exercise.

*Active* static stretching exercises are generally employed by athletes or joggers working out alone or during warm-up activities. *Passive* static stretching exercises with use of a partner are more common to team participation sports, both in formalized flexibility programs and warm-up activities.

### Spring Method

This method of stretching also includes both *active* and *passive* forms. The *passive* method is employed by a partner who is assisting the person stretching. The partner would move a joint through its entire range of motion, as far as the muscles would permit. Then a slight swinging or bobbing motion exerting pressure to extend the joint further would be applied by the partner.

*Active* spring stretching is performed by the individual himself. For example, a person standing erect bends downward with knees straight to touch the floor with his fingertips. When he has bent over as far as possible, he bobs up and down with a spring-like motion, exerting power in the downward direction, repetitively decreasing the distance from fingertips to floor.

### Comparison of Methods

What little evidence has been obtained from comparisons of ballistic and static stretch methods reveals that both are equally effective in increasing a joint's range of motion.[1] Most doctors, therapists, trainers, and coaches, however, favor the static stretch method because violent ballistic-type movements are more liable to damage the joint and strain muscles, especially if practiced by an over-zealous athlete. In addition, less muscle soreness is experienced after a static stretch session than after a ballistic one.

Weber and Kraus found the spring stretch method superior to static stretching in low back cases resulting from muscular imbalance.[3] Their comment follows:

> The spring stretch may be dangerous in conditions with pain and muscle spasm as there is greater possibility of provoking increased pain with subsequent limitation of motion and increased muscle spasm. On the other hand, the large group of patients with imbalance of muscle power and elasticity but no pathologies can be treated with the spring stretch method.

Weber and Kraus tested 50 patients with foreshortened hamstring and back-hamstring-gastro-soleus muscle groups. In 25 of them, the spring stretch method was used, and in the control group of patients the static stretch method was employed. The results revealed that the spring stretch method was 200 percent more efficient than the static stretch method in the hamstring muscle cases and 100 percent more efficient in the back-hamstring-gastro-soleus muscle cases.

## Warm-Up

A flexibility training program should be preceded by a warm-up period to raise muscle temperature—a very important factor in increase of muscle flexibility and reduction of residual neuro-muscular tension. Studies have shown that a rise in deep muscle temperature affects relaxation of the muscles three times as much as does muscle contraction. A warm-up also helps to prevent injuries and helps to relax the antagonist muscles.

## REFERENCES

1. DeVries, H., "Evaluation of Static Stretching Procedures for Improvement of Flexibility," *Research Quarterly,* 33, 1962.
2. "DiGregorio Sore," Associated Press Release, New York, February 24, 1975.
3. Weber, Sonya, and Kraus, Hans, "Passive and Active Stretching of Muscles," *Physiotherapy Review,* Vol. 29, 1949.

# 26

## The Holistic Approach to
## Preventive or Corrective Exercise

T he holistic approach to the prevention or correction of muscular imbalance and postural and foot faults was emphasized in the Introduction to this book. Nevertheless, its importance warrants bringing it again to the reader's attention. The athlete or jogger who uses exercise to prevent or correct these hidden factors must do so in an integrated "total body" manner.

To rely on orthotic appliances or exercise for prevention or correction of foot faults alone, while neglecting leg or upper postural faults, or attempt prevention or correction of upper body postural faults without considering faults in leg alignment or the foot constitutes a serious mistake. Sports literature has thoroughly established that upper or lower body postural faults rarely if ever exist alone without some concommitant effect on a body segment above or below the original fault—whether the latter is a congenital or acquired defect.

In a discussion on faulty weight bearing with special reference to the position of the thigh and foot, Brunnstrom summarized the holistic approach to the treatment of faulty body mechanics: [1]

> Anybody attempting to correct faulty body mechanics must take the whole individual into consideration, studying the relationships between the different parts of the body and determing for each case the particular malalignment present. Correction of thighs and feet must be emphasized for all cases, regardless of the original trouble which caused the child to be sent to the clinic. The position of feet and legs greatly influences the position of the pelvis, and through the pelvis, acts on the spine, shoulders and head. Vice versa, a faulty position of the pelvis may produce incorrect position of the feet. The whole weight-bearing problem must be followed up through all parts of the body, if any results are to be expected.

In preventing muscular imbalance, all conditioning or strength development programs should be organized on the principle of balance, instead of concentrating on the development of strength in the muscles that are the prime movers in the sport for which the athlete is conditioning himself.

In correcting muscular imbalance, to rely on the use of flexibility exercises to stretch shortened contracted muscles on one side of a body joint, without strengthening the stretched weakened muscles on the opposite side of the joint is a serious mistake. From the standpoint of injury prevention, flexibility around a body joint without accompanying strength on both sides of the joint is just as hazardous as extreme flexibility on one side of a joint with little or no flexibility on the opposite side.

## REFERENCES

1. Brunnstrom, Signe, "Faulty Weight Bearing," *Physiotherapy Review,* May-June 1935.

# 27

## Preventive and Corrective Exercise

P revention and correction of postural and foot faults involve the use of postural reflex training movements and strength and flexibilty development exercises. Various methods of exercise are presented in this chapter, including those of dual resistance and weight training for development of strength and solo and partner type activity for development of flexibility. Of equal importance is the avoidance of exercises that are specifically contra-indicated in postural and foot fault programs, and the last section of the chapter includes a cautionary discussion of these faults.

### UPPER BODY POSTURAL FAULTS

Andry maintained that upper body postural faults were the result of muscular imbalance. However, most of the orthopedic and corrective physical education authorities of the past century have argued that poor upper body posture was due to failure to develop adequate postural reflexes, a failure which resulted from malnutrition, laziness, disease, or psychological factors in early childhood.

### PRINCIPLES OF POSTURAL REFLEX TRAINING

Temporary modification of poor posture can be obtained by conscious control, but any permanent change must be associated with an alternation in the postural reflexes. Postures are not achieved through body movements, but through static positions held frequently. Strength and flexibility exercises are a supplement to postural reflex training, but they will not aid in training the nervous system. The only way to permanently acquire a desired postural attitude is to repeat it until it becomes reflex in nature.

Posture training must be continuous throughout the day. In addition, adherence to the following principles is of utmost importance.

1. The person engaging in postural reflex training is taught to train his reflexes in the horizontal position (crook lying, Figure 56). He then progresses to a sitting position (Figure 59A-B) and finally to a standing position (Figure 59C).

2. Progression to another position should not be carried out until the person can maintain a correct posture in the previous position without excess effort and while performing simple arm and leg movements.

3. The success of reflex training depends on whether the person has the determination to practice the training techniques on his own and to try and hold himself correctly in the ordinary movements of everyday life.

4. In corrective upper body postural reflex training, supplementary flexibility exercises should be used wherever necessary to stretch shortened muscles and fascia. Correction of antereo-posterior faults generally involves one or more of the following muscle groups: hip flexors, lower back extensors, chest muscles, or front neck flexors.

5. The strength development exercises used in postural reflex training include isometric exercises at the start, as the objective is to train the nervous system in static posture positions.

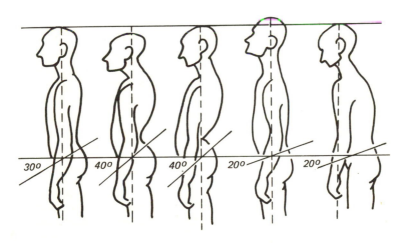

*Figure 55*
NORMAL POSTURE AND FOUR POSTURAL FAULTS

## POSTURAL REFLEX TRAINING FOR
## ANTEREO-POSTERIOR FAULTS
### Mobility in Spinal Exercise

Sway back (Figure 55C) and round back (Figure 55E) are the most difficult types of antereo-posterior postural fault to correct, according to Wiles, who stated: "From this point of view of treatment, sway back differs from simple lordosis in that the correction of the pelvic angle does not enable the spinal curves to be restored to normal. Treatment has therefore to be directed at first to increasing the mobility of the spine—one of the most difficult problems of postural correction."[10]

Wiles maintained that the weakest part of the extensor mechanism of the spine is in the upper lumbar and lower dorsal regions (Chapter 9, Figure 3A). Loss of tone in the spinal extensors will allow the whole of the upper part of the body to come on to the spine and produce one of the commonest faults, a dorso-lumbar kyphosis (sway back, Figure 55C). In its early stages, the fault can be straightened by strengthening of the spinal extensor muscles and retraining of postural reflexes. Later on, however, the ligaments on the inner (anterior) side of the spinal column become contracted and the spine loses its mobility in this region, which is the least mobile part of the normal spine.

### Postural Reflex Training Techniques

Postural reflex training techniques are started from the crook lying position (Figure 56). This position discourages the person who is training from hollowing the lumbar (lower) back. He must learn to contract the extensor muscles of the hip joints (gluteals or buttocks) in an isometric contraction maintained for at least three minutes. These muscles decrease the forward pelvic inclination associated with lordosis. Next, forward and backward tilting of the pelvis is practiced and subsequently carried out in the sitting and standing positions.

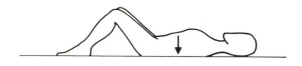

**Figure 56**
CROOK LYING POSITION

The exercises illustrated below are excellent for teaching a person to master the reflex training movement of the lumbar spine. Each exercise should be performed for 10 repetitions.

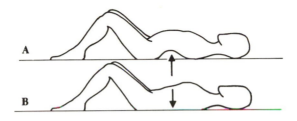

*Figure 57*
REFLEX TRAINING MOVEMENT OF LUMBAR SPINE

(A) Arch back, keeping buttocks on floor. (B) Press spine downwards and flatten lower back against mat or floor.

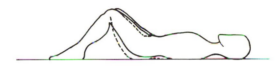

*Figure 58*
Tense buttocks and raise off floor about three inches. Then lower back to floor.

The thoracic (dorsal) spine, along with the scapulae (shoulder blades), will be straightened to some degree by lateral rotation of the shoulder joints in the crook lying position. Figure 59A illustrates lateral rotation of the shoulders with upward extension of the arms in the seated position.

Postural reflex training of the cervical spine is accomplished by a person's drawing his head up toward a wall and attempting to press the back of the neck gently against a pad or mat. He maintains this position for three minutes, and then allows his neck to relax. Throughout the period, the chin should be level and no effort made to pull it in.

After the person has mastered each individual movement in the crook lying position, he should combine them and hold all the separate movements for at least three minutes.

Once he has mastered the techniques of the reflex training positions presented, he should then carry out simple arm and leg movements in the crook lying position while maintaining the reflex training postures. Listed below is a series of exercises that should be used:

1. Raise the left arm to the position illustrated in Figure 59A. Then raise it directly overhead with arm pressed against mat on floor. Return arm to sides in an extended position.

2. Stretch left leg downwards to an extended position, with the heel skimming the surface. Then return leg to the original crook lying position in the same manner. Repeat with right leg.

3. After both the above movements have been mastered with the individual arm and leg raise both arms overhead simultaneously, and then extend both legs at the same time.

4. Once the double arm or leg movements have been mastered separately while maintaining the postural reflex positions, perform them together.

When the person can control his posture in the crook lying position while moving his arms and legs, he progresses to a sitting position, preferably on a stool. The stool should be placed against a wall so the lower (lumbar) back can be pressed against the wall.

Performed in the sitting and standing positions, postural reflex training positions for the thoracic (dorsal) spine, shoulders, and head can be much more productive than when performed in the crook lying position. Figure 59A and B illustrates two exercises—A and B—to accomplish this objective.

A. Place hands up beside head, with arms in elbow bent position. Flatten lower back against wall by pulling up and in with the lower abdominal muscles and tightening gluteal muscles. Straighten the upper back, press the head back with chin down and in, and pull the elbows back against the wall.

B. Repeat same exercise, but from elbow bent position move arms upward to a diagonal overhead position, keeping arms flat against wall. Sometimes, straighten arms to a straight overhead position.

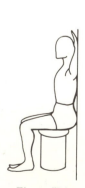

*Figure 59A*

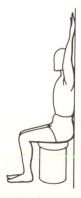

*Figure 59B*

After mastering exercises A and B in the seated position, perform them in the standing position with heels, lower back, upper back, and head held against a wall. In both exercises, the final position should be held for three minutes.

After mastering exercises A and B in the standing position, hold the standing static posture of the pelvis and upper body while walking around a room or gymnasium. Figure 59C shows an excellent starting position for walking posture reflex training.

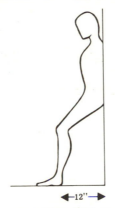

*Figure 59 C*

Stand one foot away from wall. Sit against wall with slightly bending knees. Tighten abdominal and buttock muscles and flatten lower spine against wall. Inch up the wall with upper back and head against wall, with the eyes level and chin pulled inwards, until legs are straight. Then walk around room maintaining the correct posture. After doing this for three minutes, place entire back against wall to see if the correct posture was held for the three minutes.

After practice in maintaining a correct antereo-posterior upper body posture, both in a stationary position and during walking, balance exercises are of considerable value in postural reflex training. They provide practice in maintaining and controlling posture while the body is moving under varying conditions of balance.

Lowman maintained that all remedial exercises in the standing position should be carried out on a tilted balance board.[4] His contention was that with a very high proportion of faulty foot and leg positions exercises could not be carried out in a total correct position. Traditionally, a flat balance board has been used in Swedish gymnastic drills for the teaching of balance. He devised the Lowman tilted balance board (Figure 60) in which the treads are slanted downward about 15 degrees. In Lowman's opinion, standing on this type board forces the leg to rotate outwards while the feet go into a mild varus or inversion position (Chapter 18, Figures 45, 47),

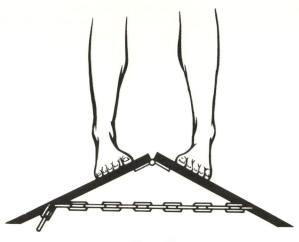

**Figure 60**
TILTED BALANCE BOARD

which assists in correction of the pronated or valgus foot (Chapter 18, Figures 44, 46) found so commonly among the general population. He has used the board to correct pronated ankles, knock-knees, inward rotation of the thigh, and lordosis. Trickett adopted this type board for use in strengthening the ankles of football players at Tulane University.[8]

Details for construction of the balance board are set forth in Chapter 28, Figure 166.

Exercises on the balance board include walking with arms swinging and knees raised high from one end to the other. Eventually, one end of the board can be elevated on a chair, thus increasing the difficulty of the exercise. Other board exercises include tossing a basketball from one hand to the other while walking or walking with a book or sandbag on the head. The correct upright posture should be maintained, with the eyes level, chin in, lower back flattened, and stomach and gluteal muscles slightly contracted. Balance activities are strenuous and should be engaged in for only a short period of time before general strength and flexibility exercises.

## STRENGTH AND FLEXIBILITY EXERCISE FOR ANTEREO-POSTERIOR FAULTS

Every postural or foot fault is accompanied by various degrees of muscular imbalance. Shortened muscles and fascia on one side of a joint must be stretched, while stretched and weakened muscles and fascia on the opposite side of the joint must be strengthened.

296

In Chapter 25, amounts of resistance, weight increases, and number of repetitions used in weight training exercises were discussed. The repetitions used in dual resistance are similar to those used in weight training. With respect to flexibility exercises, each should be repeated five times and the final holding position maintained for 30 seconds.

The following exercises are grouped according to the faults they relate to, with strength development exercises preceding flexibility exercises in each case.

## TO PREVENT OR CORRECT

### FORWARD HEAD POSITION
### Neck Extensor Strength Exercises

The muscles in the back of the neck should be strengthened, just the same as the muscles in the front of the neck.

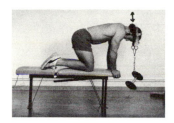

**Figure 61**
REAR NECK RAISE

With a headstrap on the head, kneel on a bench. Head should be lower than the shoulders as shown. Then raise the head slowly upward as far as possible without leaving bench.

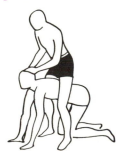

**Figure 62**
POSTERIOR NECK PUSH

With white down on his hands and knees, black sits on his back as shown. Black then pushes whites head down against his resistance.

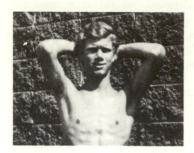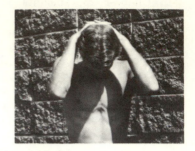

**Figure 63**
HEAD-NECK EXERCISE

Stand with head erect and hands clasped behind neck. Slowly pull head forward until chin touches chest while resisting the pull with back of neck. As head is raised, the hands maintain their pull until head comes to erect position. The resistance is regulated by the athlete himself. It is best to go very easy at first with light resistance being applied so the neck is not strained. Begin with 5 repetitions and gradually work up to 15 repetitions before applying greater resistance.

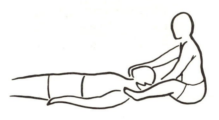

**Figure 64**
NECK FLEXIBILITY EXERCISE

Partner pulls neck backwards; also pulls to the right and to the left.

### Forward Shoulders, Round Upper Back, or Winged Scapulae

1. In treating a round upper back or forward shoulders where no structural defects are present, the key is to stretch the pectoral muscles, strengthen the adductor muscles of the upper back, and strengthen the spinal extensor muscles.

2. *If a lumbar lordosis is also present, avoid all upper back exercises that will aggravate the lordosis condition, particularly hyperextension exercises in the prone (face down) position.*

3. If winged scapulae (protruding shoulder blades) are present, it is necessary to strengthen the serratus anterior muscles (Chater 9,

Figure 5). These muscles originate from the first eight or nine ribs and are inserted into the medial border of the scapula. Their function is to pull the scapula forward in throwing, pushing, or forward elevation of arm. Normally, floor push-ups, bench presses, and similar exercises are given for strengthening these muscles. These exercises, however, also strengthen the chest (pectoral) muscles and should not be used because *all pectoral exercises are contra-indicated in preventing or correcting round shoulders or upper back*. The shoulder push exercise presented in this section will strengthen the serratus anterior muscles without further strengthening the pectoral muscles.

## UPPER BACK AND SHOULDER EXERCISE

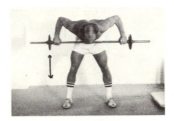

*Figure 65*
WIDE GRIP ROWING

With legs slightly bent, with upper body near horizontal to floor, grasp bar in a wide grip position and pull up weight until bar touches body at chest as shown.

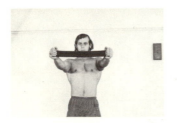 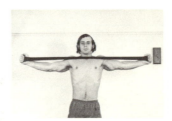

*Figure 66*
CHEST EXPANDER FRONT PULL

Hold expander out directly in front at arms length as shown. Begin by moving the arms out sideways, pulling on the rubber belt. Force the arms well back, which works the deltoids and the upper back adductor muscles. Hold and slowly return to the starting position and repeat.

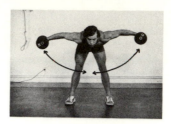

*Figure 67*
BENT OVER LATERAL RAISE

Bend over from the hips with flat back and legs locked at knees. Pick up dumbbells and, without swinging the body, raise dumbbells sideways as high as possible. Hold a second, then lower to starting position.

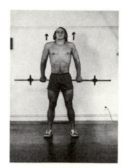

*Figure 68*
SHOULDER SHRUG BEHIND BACK

Pick by barbell with a grip position so hands will be at sides as shown. Raise the weight of the barbell as high as possible, using only the muscles of the shoulder and make a rotation movement of the shoulder in a shrug. Lower to starting position.

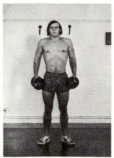

*Figure 69*
DUMBBELL SHOULDER SHRUG

Grasp dumbbells and hold at the sides as shown. Pull up and make a shoulder shrug as if trying to touch your ears with the shoulders. Lower to the starting position.

300

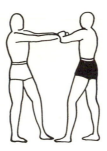

**Figure 70**

FRONT PULL SIDEWAYS

White moves arms sideways against blacks resistance.

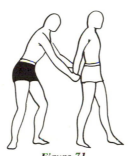

**Figure 71**

POSTERIOR SHOULDER PUSH

White pushes arms backwards against resistance of black.

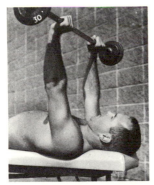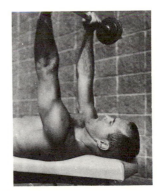

**Figure 72**

SHOULDER PUSH

Lie on bench, weight overhead, hands shoulder width apart. Raise weight upward with shoulder movement only (about 3 to 4 inches) maintaining straight arms, locked at the elbows. Develops serratus anterior muscles.

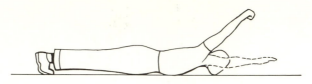

**Figure 73**
SHOULDER JOINT AND CHEST EXERCISE

Lie on floor face down, chin in contact with floor. Keep arms straight overhead grasping a pole or yardstick at shoulder width. Keep chin on floor. Raise the arms as high as possible. The objective is a 45-degree angle.

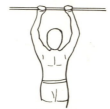

**Figure 74**
CHEST EXERCISE

Stretch the body by hanging from an overhead bar. Straighten body and relax arms. Weights can be attached to body for greater stretch.

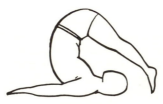

**Figure 75**
UPPER BACK STRETCHING EXERCISE

Lay flat on the floor with hands at the sides. Raise legs up and over head. Leave hands and arms flat on the floor.

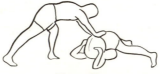

**Figure 76**
UPPER BACK EXERCISE

Assume position as shown. Partner applies pressure by pushing downward on lower back area.

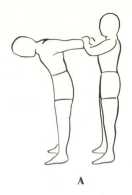
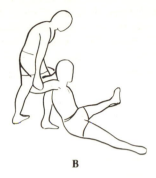

A                                                    B

**Figure 77**
SHOULDER CHEST EXERCISE

(A) Partner applies pressure to bring hands together behind back. (B)
Sit with legs spread, fingers locked behind neck. Partner grasps elbows
and pulls arms back.

## To Prevent or Correct Sway Back and Total Round Back

Wiles pointed out that mobility exercises for the dorsal spine
make up the most important factor in correcting sway back and
total round back. Two of the three flexibility exercises presented in
this section have proved to be highly effective in stretching the
contracted anterior spinal ligaments associated with these types of
faulty posture. They are also effective in stretching the intercostal
muscles that lie between the ribs. These muscles are shortened as a
result of the flat-chested condition associated with sway back and
total round back. The rotational flexibility exercise is excellent for
preventing loss of mobility in the dorsal spine.

The best exercises for the prevention and correction of these
postural faults are round back dead lifts and round back good
morning exercises. Orthopedic physicians and corrective physican
education specialists, however, will not agree with that statement.
They have recommended the use of straight back lifting from the
floor and hyperextension exercises for development of the spinal
muscles, maintaining that round back lifting exercises place
abnormal stress on the inter-vertebral disks that lie between the
vertebrae.

It is well-evidenced by today's literature, however, that the
hyperextended lifting position of the Olympic weightlifter and
hyperextended forward charge of the interior lineman in American
football have proven to be major predisposing causes of low back
pains and development of acquired defects in the vertebrae of the
spine.

303

By contrast, old time strong men, who lifted bulky and heavy weights from the floor to the shoulders with rounded backs and performed full deep knee bends in the same manner developed massive spinal extensor muscles in the lumbar and dorsal areas of the spine. This, when combined with the use of the chest expander front pull popular in those days, resulted in an erect upright posture. Further, the medical and strong man literature never mentioned a case of a strong man suffering from low back pain or being treated for an injury of the back due to lifting.

The round back exercises they performed developed the spinal extensor muscles in the dorsal area of the back, whereas straight back and hyperextension exercises primarily strengthen the lumbar extensor muscles.

## DORSAL SPINE EXERCISE

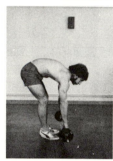 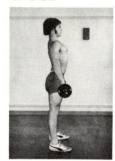

*Figure 78*
ROUND BACK DEAD LIFT

Stand erect holding barbell at arms length in front of body with palms facing body, and hands shoulder width apart. Bend forward and lower weight to a point half way between ankles and knees. Never bend knees more than shown.

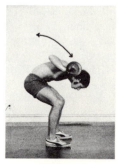

*Figure 79*
ROUND BACK FORWARD BEND

With barbells on shoulders and hands shoulder width apart, bend forward as far as possible. Never bend knees more than shown.

## DORSAL SPINE STRENGTH EXERCISES
## TO PREVENT OR CORRECT

### Lordosis and Forward Pelvic Tilt

1. Correction of the forward pelvic tilt is of primary·importance in the correction or lordosis.

2. The hip extensors (buttocks) and abdominal muscles must be strengthened.

3. The hip flexor and lower back extensor muscles must be stretched in the correction of lordosis and forward pelvic tilt. If the hamstring muscles are also shortened, which is manifested by flexion of the knees, they should be stretched.

4. Strength development exercises should be carried out at first without added resistance or with very little resistance, with gradual increase in resistance as strength increases.

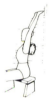

*Figure 80*
DORSAL SPINE STRETCHING EXERCISE

Hang passively from stall bars high enough to raise the body a few inches above the stall. The sand bag or pillow should extend approximately 3½ to 4 inches from rungs, and should be in contact with the mid-dorsal spine. This thrusts the trunk forward as the body hangs passively, with head erect.

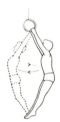

*Figure 81*
DORSAL SPINE STRETCHING EXERCISE

Stand under rings at tiptoe height. There should be circumduction (rotation) around the toes and rings, with shoulders facing directly forward. The position of toes should not change. The direction of body movement should be changed frequently.

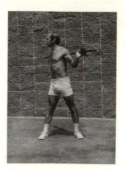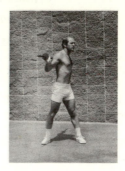

**Figure 82**
TRUNK ROTATION

Place light barbell about 12 inches below the shoulder blades. Twist from side to side as far as possible without moving the buttocks.

## HIP EXTENSOR STRENGTH EXERCISES

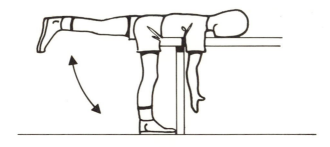

**Figure 83**
SINGLE LEG EXTENSION

Place a pillow under the pelvis. Raise one leg and then raise the other as high as possible. Do not raise above the horizontal position.

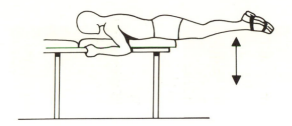

**Figure 84**
DOUBLE LEG EXTENSION

Place a pillow under the pelvis. With iron boots or some weight on the feet, lower the legs. Do not raise legs above the horizontal.

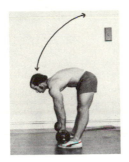

**Figure 85**
STRAIGHT LEG DEAD LIFT

Hold barbell, palms turned inward, arms hanging straight. Without bending knees, bend forward and lower barbell as far as possible. Perform exercise slowly.

## ABDOMINAL STRENGTH EXERCISES

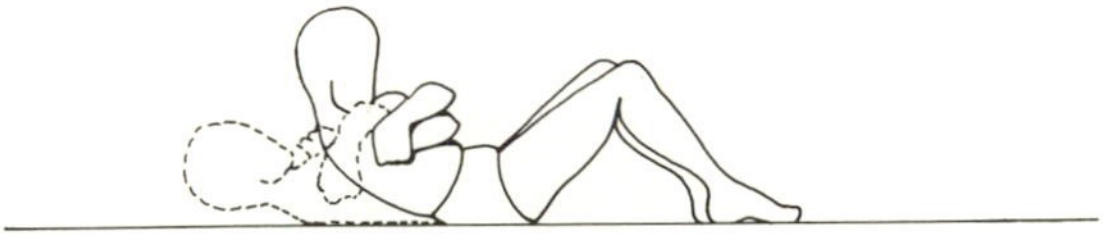

**Figure 86**
TRUNK CURL

Lay flat on floor, bring up knees and fold hands across the chest. With hands still folded, raise the head only as high as possible to chest as shown.

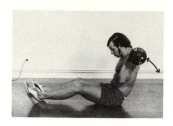

**Figure 87**
BENT KNEE SIT-UP

Lay flat on floor with barbell behind the neck. With knees bent. Bend head forward. Hold and return to floor.

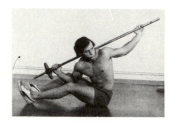

**Figure 88**
TWISTING SIT-UP

With a weight on one end only, raise body to a twisting sit-up. Repeat on the other side.

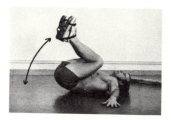

**Figure 89**
REVERSE ABDOMINAL SIT-UP

Lay flat on the floor with iron boots on the feet. Bring up legs with knees to chest and also raise the hips about six inches off the floor as shown. Spread hands for balance. Lower and repeat.

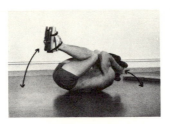

**Figure 90**
DOUBLE CURL

Lay flat on the floor with iron boots on the feet. Place hands behind neck. Bring legs up to chest and raise head at the same time so knees and elbows touch.

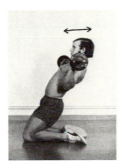

**Figure 91**
BACKWARD LEAN

Get down on knees with barbell on the chest. With the body straight, bend as far back as possible from the knees.

## GROIN STRETCHING EXERCISES

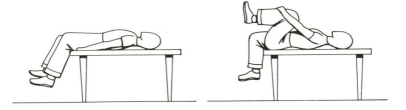

**Figure 92**
GROIN STRETCHING EXERCISE

Lie flat on back on a bench with buttocks on the edge. Bring the right leg to chest and grasp it just below the knee. Hold until stretch pain is felt and continue for 10 seconds. The opposite leg should hang relaxed over edge of bench. Repeat 3 times with each leg.

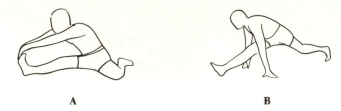

A                                        B

**Figure 93**
GROIN STRETCH

(A) Reach forward and touch toes of extended front foot. Reverse position of legs and repeat. (B) Bring chest directly over thigh. Try to widen leg spread as far as possible.

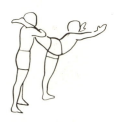

**Figure 94**
GROIN STRETCH

Partner lifts the lower leg of partner and places leg on shoulder as shown. He then places his left hand on partners lower back and applies pressure.

## LOWER BACK STRETCHING EXERCISES

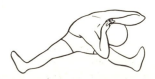

**Figure 95**

Sit on floor with legs spread apart and hands behind the neck. With knees straight, lower head to one leg and then the other as shown.

*Figure 96*

Sit on floor as shown, then grasp the feet and pull head downwards.

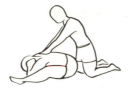

*Figure 97*

Sit on floor with legs spread as shown. Partner on knees applies pressure forward and downwards.

## HAMSTRING STRETCHING EXERCISES

### To Prevent or Correct a Flat Back Posture

In treatment of a flat back posture, hyperextension exercises for the lower back should be used. In addition, strengthening of the hip flexors is required to assist in tilting the pelvis forward. Generally, there is tightness in the hamstring muscles also, and they must be stretched (see Figures 98 and 99).

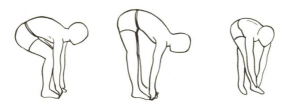

*Figure 98*

(Left-Right) Bend knees and grasp toes. Straighten legs, keeping feet flat on the floor while maintaining grasp of toes. Cross the legs while keeping rear leg locked at the knee. Repeat with other leg crossed over.

311

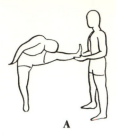
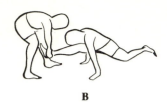

A                                    B

*Figure 99*

(A) Place heel in partners hands. Keep legs straight as possible. Attempt to touch nose to knee. (B) Legs split, front knee locked with toe up. Rear leg knee is locked with toe to side. Partner lifts front leg off floor.

## HYPEREXTENSION STRENGTH EXERCISES

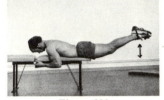

*Figure 100*
HIP EXTENSION

With iron boots on the feet, lay on a heavy bench as shown. While keeping legs straight and together, raise and lower the legs.

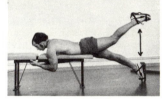

*Figure 101*
ALTERNATIVE HIP EXTENSION

Perform like the exercise above, however, alternate leg raises while keeping the legs straight.

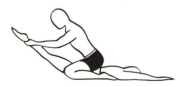

*Figure 102*
HIP EXTENSION

Perform exercise with partner. White lays face down on a mat and raises legs upward as black resists.

312

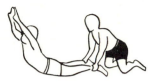

**Figure 103**
BACK HYPEREXTENSION

White lays face down on a mat or floor. Black holds white's legs as he attempts to raise body upwards.

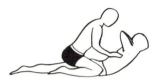

**Figure 104**
UPPER BACK RAISE

White lays face down on a mat with hands behind the neck. White attempts to raise upwards against black's resistance.

## HIP FLEXOR STRENGTH EXERCISES

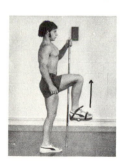

**Figure 105**
BENT KNEE LEG RAISE

Stand erect with iron boot on one foot. Keeping in balance, raise leg as high as possible. Aim to touch chest.

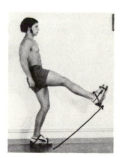

**Figure 106**
STANDING LEG RAISE

Stand erect with iron boot on one foot. Keeping in balance, swing leg as high as possible. Bend legs slightly as shown. Repeat with other leg.

313

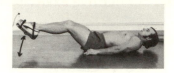

**Figure 107**
SUPINE BENT KNEE LEG RAISE

Lay on mat with iron boots on legs. With arms at the side for balance, raise legs with knees slightly bent.

## A TOTAL BACK EXERCISE

In 1782, Tissot first recommended the practice of walking with a light object on the head as an excellent method of creating good upper body posture. This was, of course, a custom among African natives and the peasant populations of Asia. In a study of 77 mill workers who habitually carried heavy weights (about 200 pounds) on their heads, South African researchers found that they displayed amazing stability of the lower spine, erect carriages, and extremely strong backs.[2] From this, the researchers postulated the theory that this practice contributed to a thickening of the rupture-prone lumbar intervertebral disks which allowed greater space for the nerves leaving the spinal cord.

Walking with a progressively heavier sandbag on the head will correct forward head and round upper back, and if the abdomen is pulled inward while walking it will assist as well in preventing or correcting a lordosis condition of the lower back. If the athlete toes straight ahead at the same time, the action becomes a "total body posture" exercise. Details relating to the construction of sandbags can be found in Chapter 28.

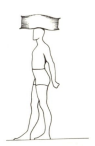

**Figure 108**
WEIGHT ON HEAD

With a sandbag on the head, walk slowly keeping the sandbag in balance.

314

## PREVENTIVE AND CORRECTIVE EXERCISES FOR LATERAL ASYMMETRY

Lateral asymmetry may be reflected in uneven shoulder height, a spinal curvature (scoliosis), or a lateral pelvic tilt (Chapter 12, Figure 9). As pointed out in Chapter 12, there are three types of lateral asymmetry of the spine: (1) *functional scoliosis,* which has not affected the skeletal structure of the spine; (2) *transitional scoliosis,* which is beginning to affect the spinal column; and (3) *structural scoliosis,* which has affected the spinal column and resulted in a permanent structural deviation. Chapter 12 also explained how a lateral pelvic tilt could result from a scoliosis, a muscular imbalance, or a short leg.

The reader should bear in mind that in *transitional* and *structural scoliosis* there is a rotation of the vertebrae in addition to the lateral flexion. For this reason alone, any symptoms of a lateral curvature imply a complicated orthopedic problem. Therfore, *no type of exercise should be prescribed for any athlete displaying any symptoms of lateral asymmetry until he has been examined by an orthopedic physician.*

The fact that muscle imbalance resulting in functional lateral asymmetry can be corrected by exercise is well-established. This type of imbalance is commonly found in athletes participating in sports wherein one side of the body only is used, such as tennis and javelin throwing. It is manifested in an uneven shoulder height and/or a simple C curve of the spine. A lateral pelvic tilt due not to a short leg but to a one-legged standing posture can also be corrected by exercise.

Authorities maintain that a simple functional curve of the spine should be corrected by symmetrical exercises. Asymmetrical exercises (one-sided ones) should only be undertaken at the direction of an orthopedic physician. For this reason, exercises for correction of lateral curvature of the spine will not be presented here. A list of texts by orthopedic physicians, physical therapists, and corrective physical education specialists describing symmetrical and asymmetrical exercises for correction of lateral curvature of the spine is, however, presented at the end of this chapter.

1. A lateral pelvic tilt due to a short leg can be easily corrected by a heel lift in the shoe of the foot associated with the short leg.

2 Uneven shoulder height or lateral pelvic tilt due to muscular imbalance can be corrected by use of asymmetrical (one-sided) strength and flexibility exercises.

3. A lower shoulder can be corrected by a one-handed shoulder shrug (Figures 68 and 69), a one-handed rowing motion with dumbbell (Figure 65), or a one-handed bent over lateral raise (Figure 67).

4. A lateral pelvic tilt can be corrected by strengthening the stretched abductor muscles of the hip on the high side of the pelvic tilt, and stretching the shortened muscles (tensor fascia latae and gluteus medius) of the hip on the lower side of the pelvic tilt.

315

## LEG ABDUCTOR STRENGTH EXERCISES

In 1935, Ober pointed out that a tight tensor fascia latae muscle (Chapter 14, Figure 17) that blends into the ilio-tibial band on the lateral side of the thigh could create sciatica pains and was also a factor in creating a knock-knee alignment of the legs and a lateral tilt of the pelvis.[5]

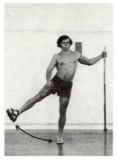

**Figure 109**
STANDING SIDE LEG RAISE

Standing erect with an iron boot on one leg, raise weighted foot to the side while keeping balanced. Repeat with other leg.

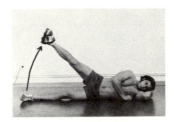

**Figure 110**
PRONE SIDE LEG RAISE

Lay on mat with iron boot on one leg. Raise weighted leg while keeping legs straight. Repeat with other leg.

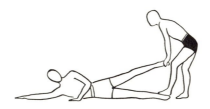

**Figure 111**
HIP ABDUCTION

White lays on the floor on one side, then raises legs upward as black resists.

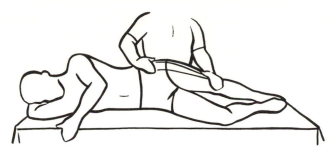

*Figure 112*
TENSOR FASCIA LATAE STRETCH

To stretch the left tensor fascia latae muscle, lie on the right side with the right hip and knee bent. Have a partner hold the pelvis firmly with one hand. Then draw the thigh slightly backwards and have the partner press it downward towards the table. The knee should not be allowed to rotate inward. If the right tensor fascia latae is short and contracted on the low side of a lateral pelvic tilt, reverse the position by lying on the left side during the exercise.

Ober suggested a standing stretch exercise for a contracted tensor fascia latae muscle (Chapter 14, Figure 17) and ilio-tibial band. The athlete or jogger stands with the affected side about two and one-half feet away from a wall, with his arm extended horizontally toward the wall and the palm of his hand placed flat on the wall. The athlete or jogger then bends the affected hip toward the wall as far as he can, with his entire figure forming an arc. This position is held for five seconds and then repeated five times the first day, with an increase of one repetition per day until the exercise is being performed 25 times daily.

## PREVENTIVE AND CORRECTIVE EXERCISE IN HIP AND LEG ALIGNMENT

### To Prevent or Correct Inward Thigh Rotation, Functional Knock-Knees, Foot Pronation, Hyperextended Knees, and Total Outward Leg Rotation and Foot Abduction

1. To prevent or correct inward thigh rotation, strengthen the hip abductors and the six outward hip rotators. Exercises for this purpose will also correct functional knock-knees due to inward thigh rotation, and will assist in correction or prevention of pronation of the foot (Chapter 18, Figure 42). Stretch the thigh adductor muscles (inner ones), as well.

317

2. To prevent hyperextended knees (Chapter 14, Figure 16B), the athlete must strive for a balanced development of the quadriceps muscles on the front of the thigh and the hamstring muscles on the back of the thigh. The method used to correct hyperextended knees depends upon whether the quadriceps are weak and stretched and the hamstrings strong and shortened, or vice versa. The athlete should strengthen the stretched muscles and stretch the strong ones.

3. To prevent total outward rotation of the leg and the outward abduction of the feet, the athlete should develop the correct walking habit of toeing straight ahead at all times. To correct the rotation and abduction, he should strengthen the inward rotators of the hip and the adductors of the thighs and stretch the outward rotator hip muscles.

## LEG ADDUCTOR STRENGTH EXERCISES

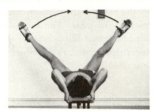

*Figure 113*
SUPINE LEG SPREAD

Lay flat on bench with an iron boot on both feet. Raise feet and spread to each side as shown.

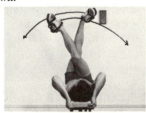

*Figure 114*
SUPINE LEG SCISSORS

Lay flat on a bench with iron boot on each foot. Raise feet the same as above exercise, then perform scissor action as shown.

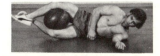

*Figure 115*
MEDICINE BALL SQUEEZE

Lay on mat with medicine ball between the legs as shown. Squeeze the legs around the medicine ball as hard as possible.

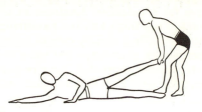

*Figure 116*
Hɪᴘ Aᴅᴅᴜᴄᴛɪᴏɴ

White lays on mat with one arm outstretched the other at waist to balance. White attempts to lower raised leg while black resists.

## LEG ADDUCTOR STRETCHING EXERCISES

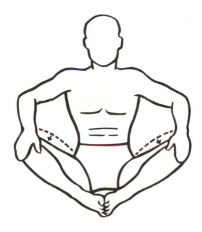

*Figure 117*
Place hands on knees and push slowly downwards. Hold for 30 seconds and repeat.

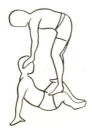

*Figure 118*
While sitting on a mat, spread legs, bend at the knees and place feet together. Partner stands on the inside of legs, gradually applying pressure.

# UPPER LEG STRENGTH EXERCISES

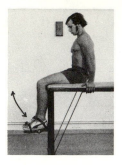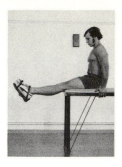

**Figure 119**
LEG EXTENSION

Sit on edge of bench with iron boots on the feet. Lock knees for count of one as legs are extended.

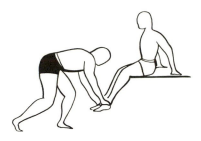

**Figure 120**

KNEE EXTENSION

White sits on end of bench. White raises his legs upward as black resists.

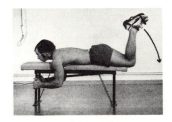

**Figure 121**
LEG CURL

Lay flat on bench with iron boots on feet. Raise legs to buttocks as shown, and repeat.

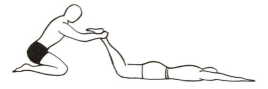

**Figure 122**
KNEE FLEXION

White lays face down on mat with arms stretched out in front. White curls legs toward hips as black resists.

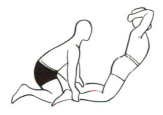

**Figure 123**
LEG CURL

White lays face down on mat with hands behind the head. White raises and lowers body as shown, while black keeps body steady.

## UPPER LEG STRETCHING EXERCISES

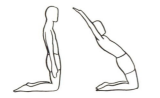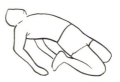

**Figure 124**
FRONT THIGH EXERCISE

Come erect on knees as shown. Raise hands above head and lean backwards. Tuck arms towards feet so trunk is in line with thighs.

# HAMSTRING EXERCISES

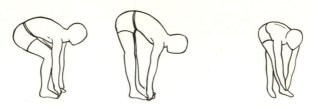

**Figure 125**

(Left-Right) Crouch down and grab toes. Straighten legs, keeping feet flat on the floor while maintaining grasp on toes. Keep rear leg locked at knees. Repeat with other leg crossed over.

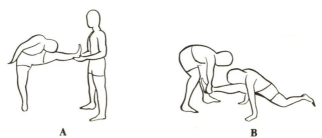

A                                                                B

**Figure 126**

(A) Place heel in partners hands. Keep legs as straight as possible. Attempt to touch nose on knees. (B) With legs split, partner picks up the right leg and slowly lifts leg up off the floor. Hands should be on the floor for support as shown.

## LEG ROTATION STRENGTH EXERCISES

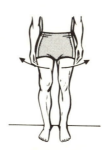

**Figure 127**
OUTWARD HIP ROTATION

While standing, hold onto a chair or stall bars for support. Place feet straight ahead, three to five inches apart. While keeping toes pressed down hard and legs straight, rotate hips outward, contracting buttocks at the same time. Under no circumstances move the feet.

322

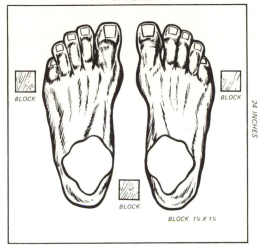

*Figure 128*
LEG ROTATION BASE

This is the baseboard of the leg rotation base. Details of construction of the baseboard used to keep the feet stationary during the hip rotator exercise are found page 342, figure 161.

## INTERNAL—EXTERNAL LEG ROTATION

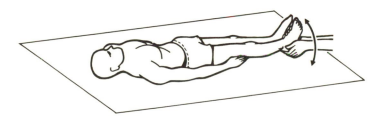

*Figure 129*
The legs should be straight with the knee locked and the partner applying the resistance while grasping the heel of the foot with one hand and the forefoot with the other hand. This dual resistance exercise can be used to strengthen or to stretch the inward or outward rotator muscles of the hip. To stretch the muscles, the athlete relaxes his leg muscles and allows the partner to rotate the entire leg inward and outward. The end position of the stretching should be held for 15

seconds and repeated five times. To strengthen either group of rotator muscles, two methods are available: (1) The athlete may turn his entire leg inward or outward while resistance is being applied by the partner holding the foot. (2) The partner applying the resistance may rotate the entire leg inward or outward while the athlete resists his efforts to do so.

## EXERCISE IN LOWER LEG, ANKLE, AND FOOT DEVELOPMENT

Any exercise designed for the development of the feet or ankles involves most of the muscles of the foot, ankle, and lower leg because of the complex manner in which the tendons of the extrinsic (calf) muscles cross each muscle within the foot—extrinsic or intrinsic—acts upon several joints at once.

Most of the abduction and adduction of the foot takes place in the sub-astragaloid joint (Chapter 17, Figure 22), which is freely movable in all directions and in a position to be affected by nearly all the muscles, particularly the extrinsic lower leg muscles. The intrinsic muscles of the foot tend to contract simultaneously with the extrinsic muscles, supplementing the action of the latter. Thus it is almost impossible to devise exercises which will provide isolated action of any one muscle or even one group of muscles in the foot. As a result, the foot, ankle, and lower leg are treated as a whole in preventive or corrective exercise programs.

1. Exercises for the feet serve three major purposes: (A) ankle flexibility; (B) strengthening of the muscles (and their tendons) that support the medial longitudinal arch; and (C) strengthening of the metatarsal (forefoot) region. Depending on the individual case, these objectives are best obtained by passive exercise, active exercise, non-weight-bearing exercises, weight-bearing exercises, and/or resistance exercises.

2. While foot exercises are important in attaining the afore-mentioned flexibility and strength, they cannot by themselves prevent or correct foot faults. Just as postural reflex training is highly important in the prevention or correction of upper body postural faults, so a person's manner of walking, standing, and/or sitting is crucial to foot fault prevention and correction.

In walking, the foot should be pointed straight ahead and the greater part of the motion carried out by the forefoot. The athlete or jogger should swing his leg forward on the ball of the foot and, as the weight is carried by his toes, press down upon the sole of the foot, gripping the ground with his toes.

In standing, a person should avoid a foot attitude of abduction (toeing outward) or pronation (inward sagging of ankle).

In the sitting position, the feet should be crossed and resting upon their outer borders. This assists in prevention or correction of shortened peroneal (outisde of ankle) muscles, which accompany abducted and pronated foot postures.

3. Foot exercises should not be prescribed before a careful diagnosis of the problem within the foot itself and the relationship of the foot to the total leg alignment has been made. In one case, the thigh may be internally rotated due to a forward pelvic tilt—with the foot pointed straight ahead, but in a pronated foot posture. In another, the entire complex of thigh, lower leg, and foot may be rotated outward, with the foot in an abducted (toed-out) pronated posture. If we accept Cerney's statement that 80 percent of American athletes have weak feet, Morton's statement that 50 percent of the population suffers from first degree pronation, and Lowman's statement that 80 percent of children display postural faults, particularly in the lower legs and feet, the importance of leg alignment in relationship to foot posture comes into focus.

4. A shortened Achilles tendon or shortened posterior calf muscles restrict ankle flexibility, and each has been identified as a major cause of the abducted toed-out foot position and pronated feet. In addition, running athletes tend to overdevelop the posterior calf muscles, which are normally five times stronger than their antagonists, the shin muscles. When the foot is turned outward due to a congenital or acquired short Achilles tendon or calf muscle, the lateral side of the Achilles tendon or of the calf muscles is shortened more than the inner side. Stretching exercises for shortened calf muscles should be carried out with the feet pointed inward, and repeated five times with the end position held for 30 seconds each time. The same repetition and maintenance of position applies to stretching exercises for the lateral muscles of the calf, ankle, and foot. Strengthening exercises for the extrinsic (calf) muscles should be repeated in three sets of six to eight repetitions each.

5. With the foot in contact with the floor, any exercise used to develop the medial longitudinal arch should be executed in terms of "press toes to floor," rather than "curl the toes." Curled toe exercise causes the big toe to be forced upward and the shin muscle (anterior tibialis) to be overactivated. Overactivation of the shin muscle in the correction of pronated feet tends to produce oversupination of the forefoot, which is referred to as forefoot varus in today's podiatric literature (Chapter 17, Figure 37B). To correct forefoot varus, activation of the peroneus longus (Chapter 17, Figure 30) is required, wherein the muscle holds the big toe down against the floor while its antagonist muscle, the anterior tibialis (shin), whose action would raise the big toe off the ground, remains relaxed.

6. In preventing or correcting valgus heel (Chapter 18, Figure 46), pronated foot with lowered medial longitudinal arch (Chapter 18, Figure 42), and varus forefoot posture, emphasis should be placed on strengthening the plantar flexors (posterior tibialis, flexor hallucis

longus, flexor digitorum longus) whose tendons support the medial longitudinal arch (Chapter 17, Figure 27), along with the peroneus longus muscle whose tendon holds the big toe flat on the ground.

Exercises should first be executed in the non-weight-bearing position. When the muscles have been strengthened sufficiently, weight-bearing exercises can be substituted. Note, however, that in the correction of weak feet, heel raises in the weight-bearing position should not be used. The powerful (gastrocnemius) (calf) muscle depresses the medial longitudinal arch, unless the plantar flexors are strong enough to counteract its pull.

7. In the abducted toed-out foot position, the muscles on the lateral side of the ankle and foot are shortened and contracted, and correction involves stretching them. In addition, the adductor-invertor muscles on the inner side of the ankle should be strengthened and a straight ahead foot position should be emphasized during walking and running.

8. Foot exercises should be executed barefoot, to allow freedom of movement for the flexors of the toes. Indeed, the most effective preventive exercise for the development of the plantar flexor muscles is walking barefoot in sand or soft dirt—with the feet pointed straight ahead—and concentrating on curling the toes downward on each step.

9. In the prevention or correction of a lowered forefoot metatarsal arch, the emphasis should be placed on strengthening the intrinsic foot muscles that flex the toes. Exercises for intrinsic foot muscles to strengthen the metatarsal arch (forefoot) should be performed slowly and deliberately and repeated six to ten times.

10. Correct performance of many localized foot exercises requires patience and practice in learning the proper technique. An athlete or jogger should therefore thoroughly master one foot exercise before proceeding on to a second one. Osgood, who as an orthopedic physician experienced great success in the correction of weak pronated feet, insisted that his patients learn one exercise at a time, and learn it well![6]

### To Prevent or Correct a Valgus Heel Posture, Pronated Foot with Lowered Medial Longitudinal Arch, and Varus Forefoot

1. Figure 130A and 130B illustrate the seated heel raise with the feet toed inward. This exercise strengthens the extrinsic plantar flexor muscles.

2. Figure 131 illustrates an exercise that strengthens the adductor muscles of the foot and ankle, assisting in correction of toed-out foot position.

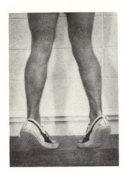

**Figure 130A**
INVERTED FEET

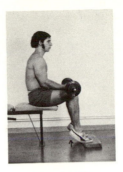

**Figure 130B**
SEATED HEEL RAISE

Use two and one-half inch block of wood under the toes. With barbell on knees, raise heels as shown. Those with weak or pronated feet perform without weights.

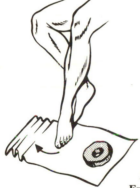

**Figure 131**
FOOT ADDUCTION

While seated in a chair, place the right foot behind the left foot for balance. Lift the forefoot and move to the left. Press the ball of the foot on the towel as shown. Pull the towel to the right until weight reaches foot. Repeat with other foot.

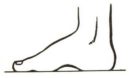

**Figure 132**
BOWING THE ARCH

Spread the foot and toes flat on the floor. Press down with the pads of the toes and contract front part of foot. This raises the arch as shown. Do not curl the big toe. Press with the big toe.

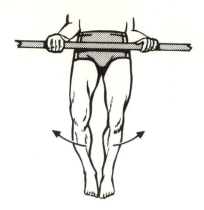

*Figure 133*
OUTWARD KNEE ROTATION

Hold back of a chair or stall bars, etc. With the heels about three inches apart, big toes together, flexed knees, then slightly rotate knees outward as if to bring heels together against the floor. Do not let heels move and press big toe on floor.

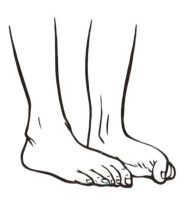

*Figure 134*
INVERSION CURL

Stand with feet parallel, with toes pointing straight ahead. Roll feet outward on lateral border, but keep all toes touching the ground as shown. As feet become stronger, take steps forward while holding the position.

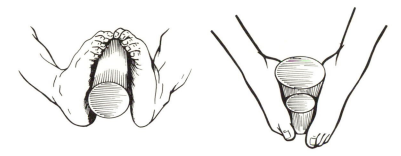

| Figure 135A | Figure 135B |
|:---:|:---:|
| SINGLE RESISTANCE | DOUBLE RESISTANCE |

Lie flat on the floor. Heels should be touching the floor while the forefoot grasps a cylinder held between the feet. Now raise the feet 6 to 12 inches from the floor, then bend the knees bringing the feet towards the abdomen. Then extend the legs outward and lower heels to the floor. Do not use the lying position if lordosis of back is present. Instead perform exercise in a seated position. Once you master the single resistance exercise, try with two cylinders.

3. Figure 132 illustrates an exercise to strengthen both the extrinsic plantar flexor muscles and the intrinsic foot muscles that flex the toes.

4. Figure 133 illustrates an exercise to strengthen the peroneus longus muscle that holds the big toe on the ground and corrects forefoot varus.

5. Figure 134 illustrates an exercise that strengthens the plantar flexor muscles, assists in stretching the lateral ankle muscles, and—like the tilted balance board (Figure 60)—helps to train postural foot reflexes.

6. Figures 135A and 135B illustrate a progressive resistance method of exercising foot muscles devised by Chepesuik to rehabilitate plantar flexors and toe flexors after injuries in which the lower leg, ankle, and foot were placed in a cast for healing purposes.[1] He deplored the fact that little effort had been made to apply the heavy resistance principle to mobilizing the forefoot and foot before and during early ambulation and devised for the purpose cement-filled metal cylinders of varying heights and diameters which he made from ordinary household grocery tins. The cylinders weighed one-half, one, two, three, five, and eight pounds respectively—their diameters and heights generally increasing with their weight. Wire hooks for handling were imbedded in the cement. Heavier weight combinations could be made by strapping the cylinders together with adhesive tape, and additional resistance could be added by attaching small barbell plates to the smaller cylinder.

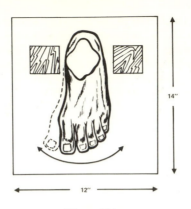

*Figure 136*
FOOT ADDUCTION

This exercise is fully described in the text below.

Chepesuik instructed his patients to lift the weight 20 to 30 times during a 10-minute period six times daily. Under this regime, heavy resistance to the forefoot begins after the first week. While the exerciser is gripping a large cylinder at mid-foot level, a smaller diameter cylinder is placed anterior to the large one, where it is gripped by the toes and forefeet, as illustrated in Figures 135A and 135B. No strapping together of the forefoot and mid-foot weights is permitted. The larger diameter of the mid-foot cylinder provides a purposeful obstacle to the forefeet as the toes are being forced to curl around it in order to grasp the smaller cylinder. Progressively, on a weekly basis, weights are added to the lower forward part of the smaller cylinder. This can be accomplished by means of the hooks imbedded in the ends of the cylinders or by use of adhesive tape, leaving the upper part of the cylinder clear for forefoot and toe grasping.

7. Figure 136 illustrates an exercise devised by Wiles to train the foot in attaining a correct foot posture by moving the forefoot inward without twisting the rearfoot.[9] A mark is made about one and one-half inches internal to the big toe, and the patient is told to move the front of the foot inward to the mark. The big toe is depressed—with or without the assistance of the hand. Usually, there is little pressure under the big toe because its antagonist, the tibialis anterior (shin muscle), is in action. The patient must learn to contract the peroneus longus, which holds the big toe down, while relaxing the tibialis anterior. This writer has devised a piece of equipment to assist in this difficult exercise, construction details for which appear in Chapter 28.

8. Figure 137 illustrates a non-weight-bearing exercise for strengthening the plantar flexor muscles and toe flexors and

increasing the circulation of the foot. The seated patient extends his foot as far as possible, then inverts it (turns it inward) and flexes the toes downward. With the foot in the inverted position, toes flexed and in plantar flexion, he then dorsiflexes the foot strongly (raises it toward shin). The foot should not be moved outward (abducted) in the course of this dorsiflexion.

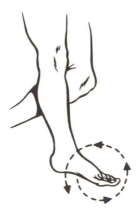

**Figure 137**
FOOT CURLING

Extend and plantar flex the foot, then invert foot, then dorsiflex the foot, and finally move straight down to the original starting position. Do not move the foot outward.

9. An excellent exercise for strengthening the medial longitudinal arch which is not illustrated herein goes as follows: With the feet side by side in slight adduction, rise on toes while ten is being counted. Hold the tip-toe position for approximately the same time. Then lower gradually upon the outer borders of the feet to a count of ten while the feet are inverted (Figure 130A). If the feet are weak (pronated), or there is a depressed metatarsal arch, the exercise should at first be carried out in the seated position and not executed in the standing position until the muscles are greatly strengthened.

## FOOT AND ANKLE STRENGTH EXERCISES

### To Prevent or Correct
### Metatarsal (Transverse) Arch Depression

Strengthen the intrinsic foot muscles that support the metatarsal arch and flex the toes, and tighten the forefoot ligaments that bind the metatarsal bones together.

Additional exercises for the metatarsal arch area and the toe flexors are as follows:

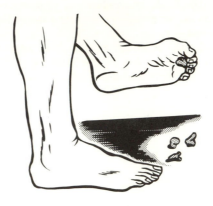

*Figure 138*
MARBLE PICK-UP

While standing or seated in a chair, pick up marbles or wads of paper by curling the toes. As the foot is raised up and across the mid-line of the body, curl foot inward to the final position with soles facing upward.

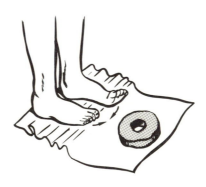

*Figure 139*
BUILDING MOUNDS

Place a towel on floor with a weight on it. Sit down on a chair and grip towel with toes. Pull towel backward toward the heels. Keep heels on floor. Alternate with each foot until weight is reached.

1. Stand barefooted on a thick wide book, so that the toes overlap the edge of the book. With slow but regular motion, bend the toes down as far as possible over the edge of the book. Repeat about 50 times.
2. Place a golf ball or small rubber ball on a rug. Place the metatarsal area of the foot on the ball with the toes flexed. Roll the ball back and forth and sidewards for one minute. Repeat five to ten times.

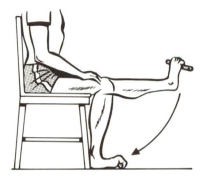

**Figure 140**
PENCIL PICK-UP

While seated in a chair, grasp a pencil or some other long object with the toes. Then raise legs as shown.

## To Prevent or Correct Pronated Ankles and Feet

Strengthen the lateral sides of the ankles, the invertor-adductor and evertor-abductor muscles of the ankle and foot, and the anterior tibialis (shin) muscles.

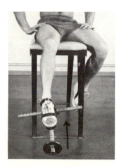

**Figure 141**
ANKLE DORSIFLEXION

Using an "Ankle-Shin Exerciser" sit down on a high table with the exerciser hanging down as shown. Raise exerciser toward shin until level or higher.

Details for construction of exerciser may be found on page 343, figure 163.

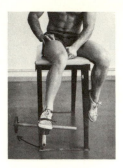

**Figure 142**
ANKLE INVERSION

Place weight on right side and raise weight to the exerciser's right.

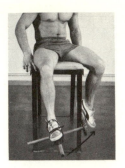

**Figure 143**
ANKLE EVERSION

Place weight on left side and raise weight to the exercisers as shown.

## ANKLE EXERCISES WITH ANKLE EXERCISE BASE

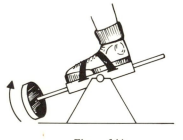

**Figure 144**
ANKLE DORSIFLEXION

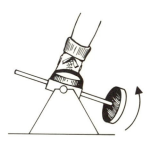

**Figure 145**
ANKLE INVERSION

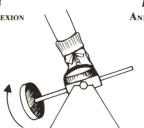

**Figure 146**
ANKLE EVERSION

Details for construction of Ankle-Shin Exercise Base may be found on page 344, figure 164.

334

## DUAL RESISTANCE EXERCISES

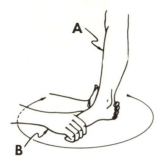

# Ankle Inversion

(A) pulls foot in and up while (B) resists.

# Ankle Eversion

(A) raises foot out and up while (B) resists.

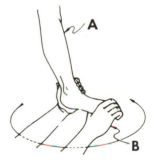

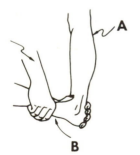

# Ankle
# Dorsi Flexion

(A) raises foot towards shin while (B) resists.

NOTE: (B) places free hand behind heel of (A) to stabilize ankle.

*Figure 147*

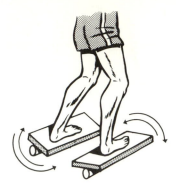

**Figure 148**
ANKLE BALANCE BOARD EXERCISE

Tilt balance boards from side to side, inverting and everting the ankles. Keep feet flat on the board at all times and press down with the toes.

Details for the construction of an ankle balance board may be found on page 346, figure 167.

## ANKLE-SHIN FLEXIBILITY EXERCISES
## CALF AND ACHILLES TENDON

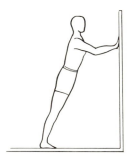

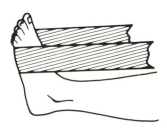

**Figure 149**

Place the feet about three feet from a wall as shown. Bend the elbows and move toward wall until stretch is felt in the calves and tendons. Be sure to keep feet flat on floor.

**Figure 150**

While in a seated position on the floor, place a towel around the metatarsal area of the foot. Relax the calf muscles and pull backwards on towel.

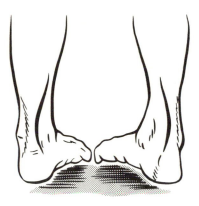

**Figure 151**
INVERTED CALF MUSCLE STRETCH

Use this exercise with an outward curve of the achilles tendon indicates valgus heels and pronation of the feet.

## SHIN AND ANTERIOR ANKLE

Lateral and medial flexibility of the ankle can be attained by use of the ankle exercises illustrated in Figures 142 and 143. Let the weight hang without any resistance of the muscles for 30 seconds, in either the eversion or inversion starting position. Lateral flexibility can also be developed through use of the tilted balance board (Figure 60) or by walking on the lateral borders of the feet (Figure 134).

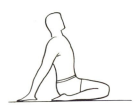

**Figure 152**
Sit on the legs as shown. Raise knees slightly as body bends backwards. Note the position of the toes.

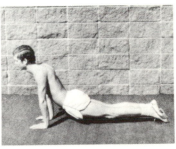

**Figure 153**
Lay face down on hands and toes as shown. Bounce feet alternately from instep to tip of toes and back to instep with swaying motion of the body.

There are several weight training and calisthenic exercises used effectively for testing muscular imbalance that should not be employed in postural and foot correction programs.

Lowman has campaigned for several years in physical education journals on the dangers of consistently using such exercises in physical education classes for young children and adolescents, maintaining that they further the development of existing faults and in many cases do permanent damage to the skeletal structure of the body.[3]

His contention, as an orthopedic physician, is that 80 percent of all school children suffer from postural deviations. The most common are increased lumbar lordosis and increased forward tilt of the pelvis. From 40 to 50 percent manifest a lateral pelvic tilt, and a very high percentage have drooping shoulders—with or without round back—together with a forward head position. Practically 60 to 75 percent will also have some foot and leg deviations: pronated ankles, knock-knees, bowlegs, back knees, or tibial torsion with toeing out of the feet and inward rotation of the thighs.

It has been well established that the average human being possesses greater strength in the chest muscles that pull the shoulders forward than in the shoulder adductor muscles that pull the shoulders back, and this imbalance is common among athletes.

Lowman, and Allman and Rasch after him, have emphasized that floor dips, parallel bar dips, bench presses, and supine lateral raises (Figure 154), all of which develop the chest muscles (pectorals), should be used guardedly in conditioning programs and should be prohibited absolutely in postural correction programs.[7]

Another postural fault frequently found among average human beings, and particularly among runners, is overdevelopment of the hip flexor muscles that tends to tilt the pelvis forward and increase the tendency toward lordosis. The above authorities also condemn the use of supine straight leg exercises (Figure 159), sit-ups with straight legs, or sit-ups with legs held down by a partner if there is any evidence of shortened hip flexors and lordosis of the lumbar spine.

With respect to foot exercise, the use of the toes pointed straight ahead heel raise (Figure 160) in a standing weight-bearing position is contra-indicated in cases of relaxed medial longitudinal arches, valgus ankles, inward rotation of the thighs, and pronated feet. This exercise depresses the medial longitudinal arch, unless the plantar flexor muscle and intrinsic muscles of the foot are sufficiently developed to resist the powerful pull of the calf muscles. It is a fact that the natural muscle imbalance of five to one between the posterior calf muscles and the shin muscles is increased by running, jogging, and walking.

Other exercises rejected by nearly every authority in the

orthopedic and athletic injury fields are deep knee bends (going below a parallel position), the duck waddles and the Russian bounce. These exercises place abnormal strains on knee ligaments and will eventually stretch the medial collateral ligaments.

Rasch and Allman have also commented on the use of back hyperextension exercises in corrective exercise programs. They maintain that these exercises increase the inward curve of the lower back when there is an overdevelopment of the hip flexors and evidence of a forward pelvic tilt and lordosis.

Thus the exercises illustrated below *should not be used* in corrective postural or foot programs. They are presented only for use in testing muscular imbalance.

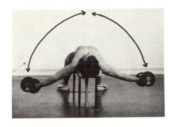

**Figure 154**
STRAIGHT ARM LATERAL RAISE

Lay on back on a lifting bench. With a dumbbell in each hand, raise to the center above body. Now lower dumbbells to sides keeping arms straight.

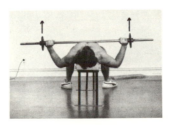

**Figure 155**
WIDE GRIP BENCH PRESS

Lay on back on a lifting bench. In a wide grip grasp barbell and place on chest as shown, then raise in a regular bench like lift and return to chest.

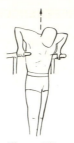

**Figure 156**
ELBOW WIDE DIP

In a regular grip position, grasp bar with hands pointing inwards towards each other, elbows wide, as shown. Then perform dips.

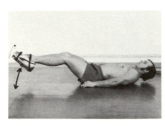

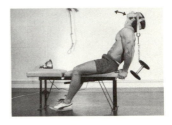

**Figure 158**
SUPINE BENT KNEE LEG RAISE

Lay on mat with arms at the sides and iron boots on the feet. Raise legs together as shown.

**Figure 157**
FRONT NECK RAISE

Sit on a bench with dumbbell attached to a head strap. While holding on to end of bench, pull head forward as shown.

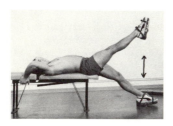

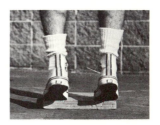

**Figure 159**
SUPINE ALTERNATE LEG RAISE

Lay on bench with iron boots on the feet. Perform alternate leg raises as shown.

**Figure 160**
HEEL RAISE

Stand erect with barbell on shoulders, with feet spaced about 10 inches apart. Place the toes on a 2x4 inch wood block as shown. Raise body by elevating heels. Raise, hold, then lower.

# REFERENCES

1. Chepesuik, Maurice W., "Progressive Heavy Resistance Exercises for the Forefoot and Lower Limb," *Canadian Medical Association Journal,* January 15, 1955.
2. "Comments," *Strength and Health,* September 1967.
3. Lowman, C. L., "Analysis of Exercises Commonly Misused," *Physical Educator,* October 1967.
4. Lowman, C. L., "Colestock, Claire; and Cooper, Hazel; *Corrective Physical Education for Groups* (New York: A.S. Barnes and Co., 1932).
5. Ober, Frank R., "Back Strain and Sciatica," *Journal of the American Medical Association,* May 4, 1935.
6. Osgood, Robert B., "An Important Etiologic Factor in So-Called Foot Strain," *The New England Journal of Medicine,* April 2, 1942.
7. Rasch, Philip J. and Allman, Fred L., "Controversial Exercises," *Corrective Therapy Journal,* July-August 1972.
8. Trickett, Paul C., *Prevention and Treatment of Athletic Injuries* (New York: Appleton-Century-Crofts, 1965).
9. Wiles, Philip, "Flat-feet," *The Lancet,* November 17, 1934.
10. _____, "Postural Deformities of the Antereo-posterior Curves of the Spine," *The Lancet,* April 17, 1937.

## RECOMMENDED READING

The following texts illustrate asymmetrical exercises used by corrective physical education, physical medicine, and physical therapist authorities for the correction of functional and transitional scoliosis of the spine.

*The Kinesiology of Corrective Exercise,* by Gertrude Hawley (Philadelphia: Lea and Febiger, 1949).

*A Manual of Corrective Gymnastics,* by Louisa C. Lippit (New York: The Macmillan Company, 1923).

*Scoliosis,* by Beatrice Woodcock (London: Stanford University and Oxford University Press, 1946).

# 28

## Exercise Equipment
## for Lower Extremity Exercises

$S$pecial equipment is required to properly strengthen the muscle on both sides of the ankle, the shin, and the feet, as well as the outward hip rotator muscles. Homemade equipment that can be constructed at little cost is illustrated in this chapter. One piece of commercial equipment for foot exercises which in this writer's opinion is the best on the market is also presented. Many of the homemade pieces are adapted from those of, or reproduced with permission of, others who conceived the original idea.

Set out in Figure 161 is a piece of equipment to assist in strengthening the outward hip rotators adapted from an idea first presented by Dr. Charles Lowman in 1912.[3] Figure 162 illustrates equipment designed by this writer. The exercise itself was first suggested in 1933 by Dr. Phillip Wiles.

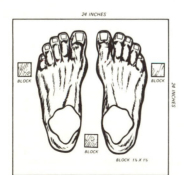

*Figure 161*
HIP ROTATOR EXERCISE BASE

Base should be one-inch in thickness. Attach blocks to base with two-inch wood screws. Set the rear blocks first. Then with the heels tight against the blocks and pointing straight ahead, fix forward blocks next to outside borders of feet.

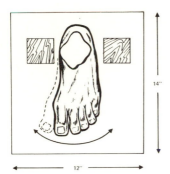

*Figure 162*
FOREFOOT ADDUCTOR
EXERCISE BASE

Baseboard should be one-inch in thickness. Attach blocks to base with two-inch wood screws. The stationary blocks should set close to the heels at a point covering the front portion of heel and posterior area of metatarsal area. After the exercise is mastered, perform without equipment.

Specifications for construction of equipment for development of strength in the medial and lateral muscles, tendons, and ligaments of the ankle joint and the shin muscle (anterior tibialis) similar to that designed by Drs. James G. Dunkleberg and Gene A. Logan are set out in Figure 163.[2] It is used for the exercises illustrated in Figures 141, 142, and 143 of Chapter 27.

The base that goes with this equipment is illustrated in Figure 164. It permits a more localized application of the exercises, as it eliminates any movement of the total lower leg, and it is used in the exercises illustrated in Chapter 27, Figures 144, 145, and 146.

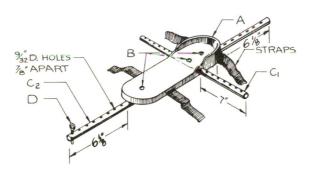

*Figure 163*
ANKLE-SHIN EXERCISER

Obtain a pair of iron boots (A) with straps from a sporting goods store. Only one, however, is needed. Obtain three bolts (B) ¼"x3½" in length, two pieces of water pipe ($C_1$, $C_2$) with a one-inch outside diameter and 3/4" inside diameter and each piece 20 inches in length. Obtain and cut at a hardware store. Obtain a pin or stovebolt (D) 2½" in length to hold barbell weight plates. Drill holes in pipe as prescribed on the drawing. Pipe steel is hard so you may have to have these drilled at a machine shop. Attach pipe to boot with the ¼" bolts.

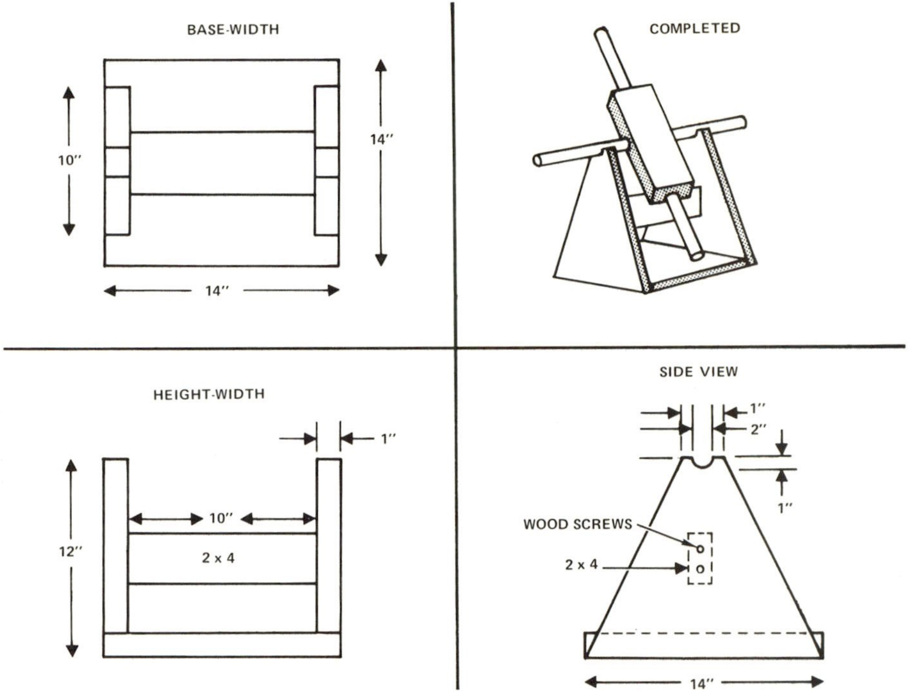

COMPLETED

BASE-WIDTH

14"

14"

10"

SIDE VIEW

WOOD SCREWS

2 x 4

1"

2"

1"

14"

HEIGHT-WIDTH

1"

10"

2 x 4

12"

*Figure 164*
ANKLE-SHIN EXERCISER BASE

Figure 165 illustrates an ingenious method of exercising the ankle and shin muscles, tendons, and ligaments in rehabilitation designed by Dr. John H. Arnett.[1] The equipment can be used for ankle rotation exercises.

Figure 166 illustrates a tilted balance board designed by Dr. Paul C. Trickett which is similar to that originally designed by Dr. Charles Lowman in the early 1920's.[4] It permits adjustment of the angle of the tilt. Lowman pointed out the advantage of its use in postural reflex training and correction of pronated feet.

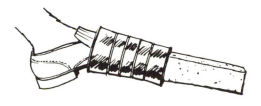

*Figure 165*
ANKLE-SHIN EXERCISER

To make the exerciser obtain a 46-ounce food can open at both ends. Force a standard brick in one end for a distance of two inches by pushing down can to form a more oval shape. When pressure is released, the metal can will hold the brick firmly. A shoe the right size for the exerciser to use the base should be slipped into the other end of the can. A brick weighs approximately five pounds. If more weight is required, as strength progresses, additional bricks may be tied to or strapped to the original brick. For small or large feet, obtain a can to fit or fasten to the can with adhesive plaster.

## TILTED BALANCE BOARD

Figure 167 illustrates details of construction of an ankle balance board to be used with the exercise shown in Chapter 27, Figure 148.

Figure 168 illustrates an easier method of performing knee extension and leg curl exercises at home with barbell equipment. A barbell handle tends to be unwieldy. A 24-inch to 30-inch water pipe one inch in diameter can be used with any type of barbell plates, collars, or iron boots.

Figure 169 describes a method of constructing various sizes of sandbags for use in postural reflex training and strengthening of all the muscles supporting the spinal column. The sandbags are used in the exercise shown in Chapter 27, Figure 108.

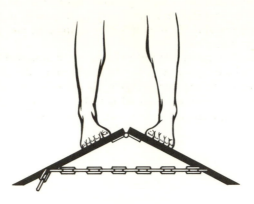

**Figure 166**
**TILTED BALANCE BOARD**

Obtain two good boards without knots or splits one-inch thick and ten inches long and hinge together securely in the center as shown. Place a screw at both ends of the boards, as shown, and chain the boards together to form a pyramid. Apply additional screws along sides to permit adjustment of tilt to various angles.

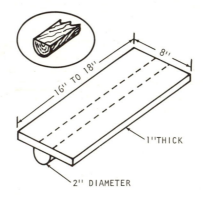

**Figure 167**
**ANKLE BALANCE BOARD**

Make two ankle balance boards to the dimensions in the above drawing. Be sure the wood has no knots or splits which might break under pressure. Obtain a 2-inch dowel or pole from a lumber yard and cut off a portion as shown, to form the balance roller. Glue with extra strong bonding cement.

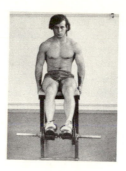

**Figure 168**
IRON BOOTS LEG RAISE

Obtain a 30-inch length of water pipe from the hardware store and run it through the holes of two iron boots as shown. Run a barbell adjustment clamp on each end to hold boots in place. Now perform leg raises. If weight is required, place a barbell weight plate on each end next to the boot and tighten with the plate clamps.

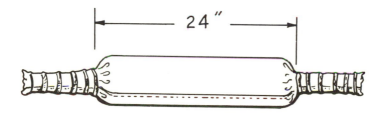

**Figure 169**
SAND BAG

Use canvas type material 34 inches long and 16½ inches wide. Sew one end together, leaving other end open to fill in sand. A strong seam is essential so don't spare the needlework. A shoe repair or luggage repair shop can do the job easily. Use twine to tie unsewn end and form handles for both ends. Fill finished bag with dry sand to a weight of 25 pounds. Fine sand tightly packed will increase weight. A heavier sandbag may be obtained by increasing the width and length of canvas material. A 3-inch increase in length and 19½ inches in width will increase the weight capacity by five pounds.

## COMMERCIAL FOOT EXERCISE EQUIPMENT

Illustrated here is the "Vimulator Conditioner." The writer first observed this equipment in a book about the feet written by Dr. John C. Mennel, a physical medicine specialist. The writer personally recommends this equipment for athletes and joggers who suffer from weak feet and for people whose occupations demand standing in a relatively stationary position during the working day or walking on hard surfaces or pavement all day.

Not only podiatrists treating the foot problems of athletes, but the general population and particularly senior citizens should experiment with this equipment. It eliminates foot fatigue, improves circulation, and strengthens the muscles and tendons of the foot.

Inquiries concerning the "Vimulator Conditioner" can be directed to Foot King, Inc., 19415 Pacific Highway South, Seattle, Washington 98188.

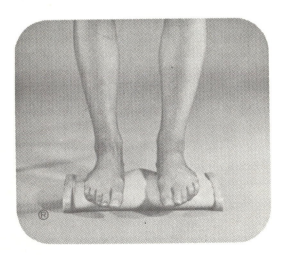

*Figure 170*
VIMULATOR - FRONT VIEW

The six exercises used with the "Vimulator Conditioner" strengthen the muscles supporting the arches of the foot and improve circulation. The equipment is also used to stretch shortened foot muscles. It can be used in a standing position as shown or seated in a non-weight-bearing position.

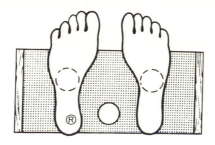

**Figure 171**
Vimulator - Top View

## REFERENCES

1. Arnett, John H., "Device for Strengthening Ankle Joints," *Journal of the American Medical Association,* Vol. 213, No. 7. Reprinted by permission of the publisher.
2. Logan, Gene A. and Dunkleberg, James G., "Ankle Strenghening," *Athletic Training News,* Vol. 1, No. 5. Reprinted by permission of the authors.
3. Lowman, Charles L., "Relation of Thigh and Leg Muscles to Malpostures of the Feet," *Boston Medical Journal,* January 18, 1912. Reprinted by permission of the publisher.
4. Trickett, Paul C., *Prevention and Treatment of Athletic Injuries* (New York: Appleton-Century-Crofts, 1965). Reprinted by permission of the publisher.

# 29

## Conclusion

The hidden factors discussed in this book represent only a small part of the total picture of prevention and reduction of athletic or jogging injuries. Little progress will be made toward solving the problem of athletic injuries, however, until the tunnel vision specialist approach is abandoned and a multi-disciplinary or holistic approach adopted. The holistic concept emphasizes all factors in the athlete's environment or within himself that contribute to and affect his development as a successful performer, and it applies equally to the prevention and reduction of injuries.

A national committee should be established that will act as a policy-making, planning, and coordinating group in directing a holistic approach toward the problem of athletic injuries. It should be headed by a full-time paid chairman, thoroughly supportive of holistic methods and trained as an administrator.

Representatives of every discipline, specialty, or interest in which athletic injury and the health of athletes are factors should be appointed to such a committee. These representatives should include: (1) members of all the medical specialities, including internal medicine, cardiovascular medicine, neurology, surgery, orthopedics, osteopathics, physical medicine, dermatology, and podiatry; (2) members from allied professions, including exercise physiology, kinesiology, biochemistry, psychology, nutrition, and physical therapy; (3) coaches from contact and non-contact sports for both males and females, and from professional, college, high school, and little league levels; (4) trainers, corrective physical education specialists, and industrial physical fitness directors; (5) rule makers, equipment, shoe, and running surface manufacturers.

This committee should convene at least once a year to formulate policy in relation to areas of future research, studies, and statistics gathering. Representatives from each discipline should be assigned responsibilities in the collection of the latest and most advanced research information developed during the year in their respective fields of interest. These compilations should be submitted to the chairman every three months.

Findings should be published semi-annually and made available to every person in the country involved in the handling of young persons engaged in athletic competition in the schools, professional athletic organizations, and directors of industrial physical fitness programs.

A major problem in the dissemination of such information is the highly technical language peculiar to all the professions and scientific specialties. Such terminology should be abandoned, and material distributed to the practitioners who deal with the athletes should be presented in simple easy-to-understand language.

With respect to financing a project of this type, the federal government could sponsor the program as it presently finances the President's Council on Physical Fitness. The project could also be financed by contributions from professional athletic organizations and equipment manufacturers, and small portions of the monies received by college teams from television appearances.

# APPENDIX

# Ligament
# Strengthening Program

These are the fundamentals of the Ligament Strengthening Exercises. (A) Exercises for the knee joints should not be performed until the athlete can perform a leg extension (both legs) with 120 pounds for 10 repetitions, and leg curls (both legs) with 75 pounds for 10 repetitions; (B) Added resistance can be applied by a workout partner pressing on the joint involved.

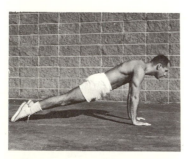 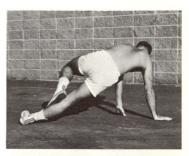

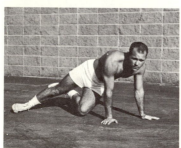 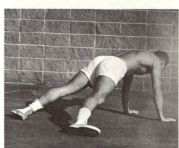

*Figure 172*
ANKLE LIGAMENTS EXERCISE

The starting position is a front leaning rest, with feet extended, resting on the toes. The action is (A) Bounce up and down on toes three times; (B) Turn the trunk to the left, supporting feet on the lower side of ankle. Bounce three times; (C) Do the same to the right side; (D) Turn back to front, leaning rest and supporting feet on the inner borders, and bounce up and down three times.

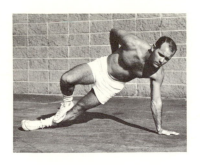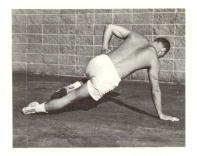

**Figure 173**

OUTER KNEE LIGAMENTS EXERCISE

The starting position is a side leaning rest on the left hand and left foot, while the right foot rests on the inner side of the left knee. The action is (A) Raise the outer side of the left ankle from the floor and bounce up and down three times; (B) Counterlike same action.

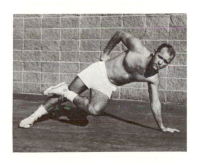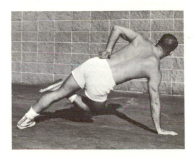

**Figure 174**

INNER KNEE LIGAMENTS EXERCISE

The starting position is a side leaning rest on the left hand and the right foot, the left foot (outer side of ankle) resting atop the right knee. The action is (A) Raise the outer side of the right ankle, bounce up and down three times. (B) Counterlike same action.

*With the kind permission of Dr. Michael Yessis, the following article is being added to the manuscript, as it was received from him after completion of the book. Yessis translates articles from various Soviet athletic publications and publishes them in his Yessis Review of Soviet Physical Education and Sports. Subscriptions can be obtained by contacting Dr. Yessis, Dept. of Physical Education, California State University, Fullerton, California.*

# Postural Disorders

*Track and Field*, 5:24-5, 1972
G. Vorobiev
National Track & Field Team Physician
(Yessis Translation Review, Vol. 9. Dec., 1974)

Among athletes, and even among "all-rounders," who are considered to be paragons of physical perfection, one sometimes encounters individuals with certain postural disorders. In spite of this, and because of their determination and persistent training, sportsmen still attain high athletic accomplishments. Such facts more than indicate the great compensatory capacity of the human organism.

Physical loads have a pronounced formative effect on the support-motor system, including the vertebral column. Rational use of physical loads produces positive changes. Irrational use of physical loads, however, brings about adverse effects on the spinal column, which are manifested by various pathologies (scoliosis, lordosis, kyphosis, and other forms of posture disorder).

The problem has been given considerable attention in the literature. The efforts of a large group of scientists (Turner, 1927-1929; Handelsman, Boikova, Zenkevich, 1951; Kuslik, 1956; Golovinskaya, 1960; Kaptelin, 1956; Grokh, 1967-1971; Franke, 1966; Akkerman, 1964, and others) have developed the diagnosis, treatment, and prophylaxis of postural disorders. However, most of this research deals with serious disorders. In this article we are concerned with deviations which usually are of no consequence, but which—for athletes subject to modern training loads—result in changes in habitual biomechanics of movement and various microtraumas.

The causes of postural disorders are very wide-ranging. We will note here only the exogenous causes related to shortcomings in physical education and irrational application of physical loads. For example, incorrect posture of students or asymmetric exercises for the torso (discus, javelin, shotput, triple jump) can lead to scoliosis;

attraction to exercises for the spinal and ilio-pectinal muscles encourages development of increased lordosis, etc. Hence, athletes may acquire one or another form of spinal curvature. Since the compensatory capacity of the young organism is so great, complete functional compensation takes place for these deficiencies. The athlete may not be aware of the deviations in his body until they bother him.

As training loads increase and athletic participation lengthens, decompensation may take place, showing various signs of pathology, with corresponding complaints from the athlete. Urgent treatment begins, which usually is of a symptomatic nature. The true cause of the trauma (deformation of the spine) is substituted for by attendant conditions (cold weather, poor warm-up, breakdown in discipline, poor equipment, etc.). But if only symptomatic treatment takes place, with no removal of the causes of the trauma, pathological changes can materially alter the athlete's sports career.

We will examine the most commonly seen posture disorders among track and field athletes and their influence on the sportsman's health and athletic results.

*Scoliosis*—a form of posture disorder characterized by spinal curvature in the frontal plane (Drawing 1). Athletes with scoliosis typically have more heavily developed muscles on the concave side of the spine, and frequently there is asymmetric development of the muscles of the trunk. The normal position of the spine is disturbed and as a consequence, the position of the axis of the shoulder and pelvis is changed. The axis of the pelvis is tilted in the frontal plane and dramatically changes the biomechanics of athletic skill.

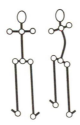

**Drawing 1**
**Scoliosis. Left is the normal position.**

As a result of the tilted axis of the pelvis, one leg becomes seemingly shorter than the other, and this is seen in a different stride length for the right and left foot. Running becomes asymmetric and less effective. Rotation of the pelvis axis by 5 degrees leads to a difference in "leg length" up to 3 cm.; rotation of 2 degrees, to a difference of 1.5 cm. Correspondingly, stride length from the "long" leg to the "short" leg will be 4-5 cm. less in the first case and 2 cm. less in the second case. The axis of the pelvis can be kept in the physiological position by additional effort of the muscles of the corresponding side of the torso, but this is not economically warranted, causes tightness and lowers the effectiveness of motor skill.

The medical aspects of scoliosis are even more perilous. Scoliosis causes redistributed effort in sections of the spine: on the one side there is stretching of tissues, and on the other side—compression. The load increases on the non-mobile sacroiliac articulation. As a result, various sorts of pains arise in the lumbar and pelvic regions, which can be spread by the sciatic nerve.

Scoliosis easily leads to microtraumatization of intervertebral nerve ganglions and neuroplexes around the lumbar and sacral regions of the spine. This reflects in muscular regulation and muscle tonus, and the innervatec femoral and, especially, sciatic nerves. As a result of disruption of the normal innervation, the tonus of the rear thigh muscles increases and they become more subject to traumatic injury, including tears. Analysis of micro- and macro-traumas of the spine and rear thigh muscles shows that these traumas are rarely observed in track athletes with no posture disorders (see Table).

Frequency of Trauma from Posture Disorders
Frequency in Percent

| Type of trauma | Normal spine | Scoliosis | Lordosis |
|---|---|---|---|
| Trauma of the rear thigh muscles | 22 | 35 | 43 |
| Spinal injury | 20 | 42 | 38 |

*Increased lordosis*—also one of the forms of posture disorder, which is expressed by abnormal hyper-extension in the lumbar region of the spine (Drawing 2). The greater the hyperextension of the spine, the greater the change in the position of the pelvis—i.e. the pelvis falls back (anterior tilt). Athletes with such deformations generally have strong back muscles, but the abdominal muscles are relatively weak and are unable to impede the turning of the pelvis.

Curvature of the spine and the altered position of the pelvis lead to disruption of biomechanical integrity and to less effective execution of motor skills for the following reasons. Impaired posture gives rise to faults in running technique (shows up as the characteristic "mold board", which moves the shoulder back), and as a result, execution of the push-off for accelerated forward movement is incomplete (Drawing 3). The more the pelvis is tilted, the greater

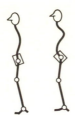

**Drawing 2**
Increased lordosis. Left is the normal position.

is the effort that the athlete must expend in order to lift the thigh, since angle A is less than angle B. The movement becomes constrained and uneconomical. Athletes with similar deficiencies characteristically have less thigh carry and lower leg swing in running.

By altering the biomechanics of the movement, lordosis creates the prerequisites for micro- and macrotraumas. The lumbar region of the spine becomes more sensitive to the various jerks and jolts that an individual continually experiences in life in general, and much more so in athletic activities. Intervertebral discs receive unequal loads. Movement in the intervertebral joints in the region of the greatest hyper-extension begins to exceed physiological capacity and the surrounding tissues become subject to micro-traumatization.

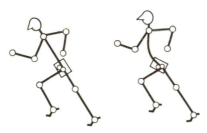

**Drawing 3**
"Mold board" shoulders during running as a result of increased lordosis. Left is the normal position.

As a result of continual microtrauma, various types of aches arise in the lumbar region: lumbosacral radiculitis, ischioradiculitis, trauma of the rear thigh muscle group, etc. Apparently it is no accident that athletes with a tendency toward increased lordosis more frequently traumatize the rear thigh muscles.

Thus, postural disorders dramatically limit the track athlete's capacity for attaining high results. But in spite of the importance of this problem it has been given little attention in sports practice.

Trainers and doctors don't always delve deeply into its nature, but instead separately examine one or another affliction or technique disorder, not examining the real causes. This is why general rules disintegrate into individual, isolated facts and remain unnoticed.

The problem touched upon is subject to deep study by doctors from the one side and scientists of biomechanics from the other. The level of knowledge of the given problem already allows for many effective prophylactic measures for clinical manifestation of postural disorders in athletes.

The basic principle of prophylaxis for the disorders under discussion is elimination of the disproportionate strength development of the individual links of the support-motor apparatus by using localized physical exercises on the non-utilized muscles. For example, for increased lordosis one should strength the rectus abdominus and oblique abdominus muscles so that they can fix the pelvic girdle and impede the excessive extension in the lumbar region of the spine. Considering the great compensatory capacity of the human organism, during the time of exercise, one must take care not only concerning the form of movement but also the correctness of the effort. If not, the exercise will be performed at the expense of well-developed synergistic muscles and will be of less concrete value. The basic criterion for correct selection of the exercises will be agreeably painful sensations in the muscles which need to be strengthened.

Hence, it is clear that, for track athletes, posture disorders in track and field athletes: (1) alter the biomechanics of motor skill, (2) are a predisposing factor for micro- and macrotrauma, and (3) can be corrected through physical improvements.

## COMMENT

The writer disagrees with the Soviet authority on one point only. Anatomically it was proven long ago that the function of the abdominal muscles was to pull the upper trunk forward and downwards. The abdominals do not pull the anterior edge of the pelvis upwards. Lordosis is the result of weakened hip extensor muscles (gluteus maximus and hamstrings) and shortened and contracted hip flexors, which allow the pelvis to tip forward and downwards and thereby create the inward curve of the lower back with short and contracted spinal extensors.

To correct lordosis the gluteus maximus and hamstrings must be strengthened while the hip flexors and lower back spinal extensors are being stretched.

# Glossary

ACCESSORY SCAPHOID or PREHALLUX—Supplementary or extra scaphoid or navicular bone on the inside of the foot.

ACROPARESTHESIA—Attacks of tingling, numbness, and stiffness in the extremities, particularly in the arms, forearms, and fingers.

ADHESIONS—Fibrous bands by which parts abnormally adhere to each other, such as those resulting from an injury to muscle fibers.

ANKLYOSIS—Spontaneous fusion of a body joint leading to extreme stiffness.

ANOMALLY—Marked deviation from the normal standard.

APONEUROSIS—Fascia; white, shining, gristly membrane serving as investment for muscle or connecting muscles with the parts they move.

APOPHYSIS—A bony outgrowth that has never been entirely separated from the bone of which it forms a part.

APOPHYSITIS—Inflammation of an apophysis.

ARCH, INTERIOR TRANSVERSE—Also known as the metatarsal arch.

ARTHRITIS—Inflammation of a body joint.

ARTHRODESIS—A joint fused during an operation.

ARTICULAR—Pertaining to a joint.

ASYMMETRY—Dissimilarity in corresponding parts or organs on opposite sides of the body which are normally alike.

AVULSION—A tearing away of a structure, such as of a tendon from its attachment to a bone.

## -B-

BILATERAL—Pertaining to both sides, such as to both legs.

BILATERAL PEDICLE DEFECTS—A pedicle is a stemlike part by which bone tissue is connected to the basic structure. The two curved spines that project from the central spine are pedicles. When defective, they do not possess the normal thickness.

BURSA—Synovial or saclike cavities filled with a viscid fluid. They are situated at hard parts of the body over which tendons pass, and they serve to prevent friction.

BURSITIS—Inflammation of bursa.

## -C-

CAPSULE—A fibrous sac enclosing a joint and lined with synovial membrane.

CAPSULITIS—Inflammation of a capsule.

CARTILAGE—Gristle; white elastic substance connecting two or more bones at body joints.

CERVICAL PLEXUS—Plexus designates a network of lymphatic blood vessels, veins, and nerves. Cervical pertains to the upper vertebrae of the spine in the neck area.

CERVICO-BRACHIAL—Pertaining to neck and arm.

CHONDRITIS—Inflammation of cartilage.

CHONDROMALACIA PATELLA—Degenerated and softened condition of inner side of kneecap.

COLLAGEN—Main organic constituent of connective tissues.

CONDYLE—Rounded eminence at the articular end of a bone.

CONGENITAL—Existing at or before birth.

CONNECTIVE TISSUE—Tissue which binds together and supports the various structures of the body.

COSTO-CLAVICULAR—Pertaining to the ribs and clavicle.

## -D-

DEFORMITY—Distortion or general disfigurement of any part of body.

DIGITAL NEUROMA—A neuroma is a tumor growing from a nerve. As used here, digital refers to the nerves leading to the toes.

DISTAL—Remote or farthest from the center, origin, or head.

## -E-

EFFUSION—Escape of fluid into a part or tissue.

ENTHESITIS—A group of conditions beginning with inflammatory reactions that are followed by fibrosis and calcification around ligaments, tendons, and muscle insertions.

EPIPHYSIS—A growing portion of bone separated from the main portion in early life by cartilage, but later becoming part of the larger bone.

EPIPHYSITIS—Inflammation of an epiphysis or the cartilage which separates it from the main bone.

EVERSION—Movement of the sole of the foot outward.

EXOSTOSIS—Abnormal bony outgrowth protruding from the surface of a bone.

EXUDATION—Escape of fluid, cells, and cellular debris from blood vessels.

## -F-

FASCIA—A sheet or band of tissue which encloses and connects the muscles.

FASCITIS—Inflammation of fascia.

FIBER—An elongated threadlike structure found in various body tissues.

FIBROMYOSITIS—Inflammation of fibromuscular tissue.

FIBROSIS—Development of excessive fibrous connective tissue.

FIBROSITIS—Inflammation of hyperplasic of white fibrous tissue; generally considered synonomous with intra-muscular rheumatism.

FIBROUS—Composed of fibers.

## -G-

GENU—The knee.

GENU RECURVATUM—Back or hyperextended knees.

GENU VALGUM—Knock-knees.

GENU VARUM—Bowlegs.

## -H-

HALLUX—The big toe.

HALLUX RIGIDUS—A permanent painful flexion of the big toe.

HALLUX VALGUS—Displacement or bending inward of the big toe toward the other toes.

HELBING'S SING—Outward curving of the Achilles tendon as viewed from behind; associated with the pronated or flat foot.

HYPEREXTENSION—Extension of a joint beyond straight alignment.

## -I-

IDIOPATHIC—Due to unknown cause; self-originating.

INFLAMMATION—The condition into which tissues enter as a

reaction to irritation; characterized by pain, heat, redness, swelling.

INSERTION—The place of attachment of a muscle to the bone which it moves.

INTER-ARTICULAR—Situated between articular (joint) surfaces.

INTERIOR TRANSVERSE ARCH—The metatarsal arch.

INTERSTITIAL MYOSITIS—Inflammation of interstices (spaces or gaps in tissues) in connective tissues of body.

INTER-VERTEBRAL—Situated between two adjacent vertebrae.

INTRA—Prefix meaning within.

IRRITABILITY—Ability of a muscle to respond to a stimulus.

-ITIS—Suffix denoting inflammation of the organ or other body part mentioned before it.

### -J-

JOINT—An articulation formed by the meeting of two or more bones of the skeleton, especially one which admits of more or less motion in one or both bones.

### -K-

KINESIOLOGY—Science of human movement.

KOHLER'S DISEASE—A disease or malformation of the scaphoid bone of the foot.

KYPHOSIS—Abnormal curvature and dorsal prominence of the upper vertebral column.

### -L-

LESION—Any pathological or traumatic break-up of tissue or loss of function of a part.

LIGAMENT—A tough fibrous band which connects bones at joints or supports internal organs.

LORDOSIS—An increased forward curve of the spne, usually found in the lower back, but sometimes found in the cervical portion of the upper spine.

LUXATION—Complete dislocation of joint bones.

### -M-

MALLEOLUS—Projection on either side of the ankle joint.

MENISCUS—Crescent-shaped inter-articular cartilage as found in knee joint.

METATARSALGIA—Pain in the metatarsus, usually in the region of the fourth toe.

METATARSUS—Part of foot between tarsus and toes.

METATARSUS VARUS—A condition in which the sole of the foot is turned inward, and the person walks on the outer border of the foot.

MICROTRAUMA—A minute or slight trauma or lesion.

MUSCLE VISCOSITY—Internal resistance factor of muscle.

MYALGIA—Pain in a muscle or muscles.

MYOFASCITIS—Inflammation of a muscle and its fascia, particularly of the fascial insertion of muscle to bone.

MYONEURALGIA—Muscular neuralgia.

MYOSITIS—Inflammation of a voluntary muscle.

MYOSITIS OSSIFICATION—Bony deposits in a muscle associated with inflammation of the muscle.

### -N-

NAVICULAR—A bone in the foot sometimes referred to as the scaphoid bone.

NEURALGIA—Spasmodic pain that extends along a nerve.

NEURITIS—Inflammation of a nerve.

NUCLEUS PULPOSUS—Pulpy mass found in the center of intervertebral disks of spine.

### -O-

OBLIQUITY—Slantedness.

ORTHOPEDICS—Branch of medicine that deals with correction of deformities and treatment of chronic diseases of the spine and body joints.

OS CALCIS—The calcaneus or heel bone.

OSGOOD-SCHLATTER'S DISEASE—Osteo-chondrosis of the tuberosity (upper end) of the tibia.

OSTEO-ARTHRITIS—Degenerative joint disease characterized by softening and thickening of the articular ends of bones.

OSTEO-CHONDRITIS DISSECANS—Softening and partial fragmentation of pieces of inter-articular cartilage into a joint.

OSTEO-CHONDROSIS—Inflammation of bone and its cartilage.

### -P-

PATELLA—The kneecap.

PERIOSTEUM—Tough fibrous membrane covering a bone; possesses bone-forming potentialities.

PERIOSTITIS—Inflammation of the periosteum.

PES—Latin for foot.

PES ADDUCTUS—Forefoot in an adducted (inward) position.

PES CAVUS—Hollow foot; very high arch.

PES PLANUS—Flat foot.

PLANTAR FASCITIS—Inflammation of the fascia of the sole of the foot.

PODIATRY—Branch of medicine which has to do with the care of the human foot in health and disease.

POPLITEAL—Pertaining to the posterior surface of the knee.

PRONATION—Position of feet in which most of the body weight is carried on the inner borders of the feet.

PROXIMAL—Nearer to or on the side toward trunk of body.

PSYCHOGENIC—Originating in the mind.

PSYCHOSOMATIC—Refers to physical disorder caused or influenced by the mind or emotions.

## -R-

RADICULAR—Pertaining to a root.

REFLEX—A reflected action or movement.

## -S-

SCAPHOID—Also known as navicular bone of foot.

SCHEUERMANN'S DISEASE—Osteo-chondrosis of the upper back vertebrae; also called juvenile kyphosis.

SCIATICA—Inflammation of the sciatic nerve of the leg.

SCOLIOSIS—Lateral curvature of the spine.

SESAMOID—Small flat bone developed in a tendon which moves over a hard bony part of the body.

SESAMOIDITIS—Inflammation of sesamoid bones.

SPINA BIFIDA OCCULTA—Incomplete closure of the spinal neural arches.

SPONDYLITIS—Inflammation of a vertebra.

SPONDYLOLISTHESIS—Forward subluxation of the lower lumbar vertebrae.

SPRAIN—Tear of ligament fibers.

STRAIN—Pulled muscle or tendon.

SUBLUXATION—An incomplete or partial dislocation of articulating bones.

SUPINATION—Position of the foot in which weight is borne on outer side; opposite of pronation.

SYNDROME—Set of symptoms that occur together.

SYNOVIAL CAPSULE—Fibrous sac lined with synovial membrane enclosing a joint.

SYNOVIAL FLUID—Transparent fluid secreted by synovial membrane.

SYNOVIAL MEMBRANE—Connective tissue which lines the interior of a joint cavity.

SYNOVITIS—Inflammation of the synovial membrane.

## -T-

TALUS—The astragalus or ankle bone.

TARUS—The instep with its seven bones.

TENDON—Fibrous cord of connective tissue by which a muscle attaches to a bone.

TENDONITIS—Inflammation of tendons and tendon-muscle attachment.

TENOSYNOVITIS—Inflammation of a tendon sheath.

TENOVAGINITIS—Inflammation of a tendon and its sheath.

TONUS—Constant partial or mild contraction of muscle.

TRAUMA—A wound or injury.

TROCHANTERIC—Pertaining to the two processes below neck of femur (upper end of thigh bone).

## -V-

VALGUS—Bent outward.

VARUS—Bent inward.

VASCULAR—Pertaining to blood vessels.

# Acknowledgments

In this world of specialization, no author could write a book containing knowledge drawn from various disciplines without the assistance of many other people. Therefore, I must first extend my deep appreciation to the pioneers to whom this book is dedicated. It was these men who first stimulated my interest in the hidden factors of injury and the subject matter of this volume.

I should like to honor the hundreds of medical specialists and physical education authorities whose effort and knowledge assisted my writing. Credit is given in every instance to all contributors, so far as they can be known. If I have failed to give proper credit, it is an oversight on my part.

Very special thanks are extended to Dr. W. E. Tucker and Dr. J. V. Cerney, whose letters of advice and encouragement enabled me to assemble and read over 1,300 medical and corrective physical education articles, in addition to more than 50 books concerning athletic injuries.

I am deeply indebted to the following publishers, who have granted me permission to quote from medical authorities in their respective books or articles: American Academy of Orthopedic Surgeons; American College of Sports Medicine; American Medical Association; California College of Podiatric Medicine; William Heinemann Medical Books, Ltd.; Houghton Mifflin Co.; J. B. Lippincott Co.; Charles C. Thomas Co.; *Track and Field News*; William and Wilkins Co.; World Publications, Inc.

I also wish to express my deepest appreciation to Drs. Bruce Ogilvie and Charles Tutko, who have regained the copyright to their book *Problem Athletes and How to Handle Them,* for permission to quote liberally from their manuscript.

An expression of gratitude is also extended to the following organizations and publishers, who granted me permission to copy or adapt ideas created by others for illustrations of lower extremity exercise equipment: American Medical Association; Appleton-Century Crofts; Foot King, Inc.; and *The New England Medical Journal* (formerly the *Boston Medical Journal*).

Thanks go as well to Drs. Gene A. Logan, James Dunkleberg, and John H. Arnett, for permission to reproduce the ankle exercise equipment illustrated in my running and wrestling books, and to Reedco, Inc., for permission to reproduce their posture scoring chart, which in my opinion should be used extensively in our elementary and secondary schools.

Any book of this type without descriptive pictures, drawings, and charts would be like a stream without water. I am grateful to Bruce Lee, for the drawings taken from my running book; to Harlan Hiney, for his excellent anatomical drawings taken from my previous books; and to Louis Drake, for his fine drawings of postural faults, foot faults, and foot exercises.

An author is lost without a publisher who believes in the final product, and I wish to thank Donald Duke of the Athletic Press for his patience. Not only did he take many of the photographs in this book, but the idea of an athletic series on strength development, athletic conditioning, and injury prevention for various sports was his to begin with. This volume is the fourth in my series.

Finally, I accept all responsibility for any personal opinions expressed on the subject matter contained in this book. With one exception, they are an analysis of the efforts, and the results of those efforts, of medical and physical education authorities throughout the past 100 years. The exception is expressed in a short conclusion.

# Biographical Index

# Subject Index

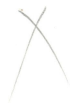